Oxford Medical Publications
Accessing health care

Accessing Health Care: Responding to Diversity

Edited by

Dr Judith Healy

Senior Fellow, Research School of Social Sciences and
Visiting Fellow, National Centre for Epidemiology
and Population Health, The Australian National University,
Canberra, Australia

and

Professor Martin McKee

Professor of European Public Health, London School of
Hygiene and Tropical Medicine, London, UK

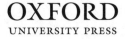

OXFORD
UNIVERSITY PRESS

OXFORD

UNIVERSITY PRESS

Great Clarendon Street, Oxford OX2 6DP

Oxford University Press is a department of the University of Oxford.
It furthers the University's objective of excellence in research, scholarship,
and education by publishing worldwide in

Oxford New York

Auckland Bangkok Buenos Aires Cape Town Chennai
Dar es Salaam Delhi Hong Kong Istanbul Karachi Kolkata
Kuala Lumpur Madrid Melbourne Mexico City Mumbai Nairobi
São Paulo Shanghai Taipei Tokyo Toronto

Oxford is a registered trade mark of Oxford University Press
in the UK and in certain other countries

Published in the United States
by Oxford University Press Inc., New York

A catalogue record for this title is available from the British Library

ISBN 0 19 851618 5

10 9 8 7 6 5 4 3 2 1

Typeset by Newgen Imaging Systems (P) Ltd., Chennai, India
Printed in Great Britain
on acid-free paper by
T. J. International Ltd, Padstow

Foreword

Solomon R. Benatar

University of Cape Town
University of Toronto

This book is about promoting two principles, *equity* in real access to appropriate health services, and *responsiveness* to the needs of the diverse groups of people that increasingly characterize all societies. The extent to which peoples' lives differ and the inequities and lack of responsiveness to health care needs within countries, so well described in this book, are reflected in the now well-known global statistics on life expectancy, burden of disease and annual per capita expenditure on health care.

It is clear that health care services are social constructs – the size, shape and nature of which reflect the social, economic, cultural and political patterns of life in different societies. This is evident from differences in structure, costs and outcomes of health care even within relatively similar industrialized countries. While many believe that medical research is driven by non-value based scientific inquiry, with regret this agenda also reflects power interests – as illustrated by the almost exclusive international focus on diseases that account for 10 per cent of the global burden of disease.

This book's importance lies in the extent to which recommendations for addressing shortcomings in access to and the response of health care services within countries as diverse as Sweden, East Germany and those in which First Nations' people live provide lessons that could be adapted for application at the global level. Globalization has led to movement of people, deterritorialization and less homogeneous populations in almost all countries of the world. The rich, the poor, the elite and the marginalized no longer only live far apart in a north–south distribution but also in closer proximity in different proportions, as small and shrinking 'rich cores' and large and growing 'poor peripheries' in all countries. While physical boundaries have become more porous with erosion of barriers to the movement of people, money, material goods, criminal activity and infectious diseases, the barriers between peoples' hearts and minds have remained distressingly deep. Ongoing and even widening animosity between religious and cultural groups, across different social and economic classes, and between people of different skin pigmentation and gender, perpetuate human suffering on a grand scale.

As the editors point out, 'there is often an enormous gulf between official policies and the everyday reality for those who are meant to implement them as well as those who are subject to them'. As much as this applies within the countries described it applies even more starkly at the global level. Consider for example how many people in the world do not benefit from the Universal Declaration of Human Rights and who lack access to even basic health care. For almost two billion people the progress that has taken place in the past century has been of limited benefit as they have such minimal access to its products. The havoc caused by HIV/AIDS to people's lives and to the economy in Africa exemplifies this.

South Africa offers an additional interesting perspective. While highly visible aspects of its health care system resemble those in much wealthier countries, health care services in that country remain a legacy of those designed and sustained by a powerful minority rather than by a majority that ignores minorities, as in the other countries described in this book. South Africa is a microcosm of the world in its distribution of health and wealth and faces even greater challenges than the countries described in this book in reducing inequities and ensuring greater responsiveness to diversity.

The implications of widening disparities in health should make privileged people deeply introspective. We need to question a value system that fosters and sustains growing disparities. Why do we place so much emphasis on scientific progress as the solution to most of our problems yet neglect to use with wisdom the knowledge we have already acquired? Why did a powerful and wealthy country in conjunction with transnational companies attempt to block the efforts of a middle income country (South Africa) with the heaviest burden of HIV/AIDS in the world to acquire cheap generic anti-retroviral drugs?

Failure of the global economic system to improve the lives of more people, failure of health care systems to deliver more equitable and responsive health care, failure of the medical research endeavour to address the health problems of most of the world's people, the emergence of new infectious diseases and the recrudescence of others in multi-drug resistant forms, the lack of solidarity with fellow humans and neglect of environmental threats, are all signs of instability, entropy and potential collapse of a complex global system. We need to recognize that such a gloomy future is not inevitable and that we can make choices that could favourably alter the prognosis for the future.

Given the universal moral and scientific ideals that potentially bind health care professionals to a common goal, it can be argued that we have an obligation to show moral leadership backed by exemplary action to reshape the future of world health. The agenda will be complex, but it has been the subject of much scholarly thought and the time is ripe to harness the energy of a wider audience. This book reveals inequities at the local level that reflect those at the global level. Similarly the attempts described to narrow these disparities and to increase responsiveness to special and often unique needs are admirable examples of acting locally in the face of powerful global forces that marginalize segments of populations even in wealthy countries. Hopefully, in due course, lessons learned in local contexts may also be applied at the global level.

Preface

Health care systems must take account of increasingly diverse populations: countries contain groups who differ in socio-economic status, culture, ethnicity, and citizenship. This diversity is growing with more population movement in an increasingly globalized world. These diverse groups have particular needs and expectations in regard to health and health care. If a state is to ensure the social and economic well-being of its whole population, it must consider population subgroups in terms of their health status and access to health services.

This book examines this issue in a range of industrialized countries from Europe to North America to Australasia. It explores the nature of claims made by different groups upon health care systems and identifies examples of good (and bad) practice in different settings. A central question underpins this analysis. Should health systems respond to the needs of different people through mainstream care, albeit via services that are sensitive to different needs and expectations, or is it necessary to create alternative services?

We believe that this book is timely for four reasons. First, while much existing analysis considers health systems at the national level, there is now more interest in examining the distribution of health status, service use and outcomes within countries, particularly in relation to social exclusion and poverty. Second, much health systems analysis has concentrated upon economic reform, often with little regard for the impact of such reform on real people. We have taken a more people-centred approach, assessing how reform impacts on different groups, especially the most vulnerable. Third, the discourse on health care reform should be reorientated to take account of the fact that most modern states are composed of diverse cultural groups. Finally, although a large literature addresses the health status of particular groups, defined in various ways, no single volume brings this work together in an international context.

Any project like this can only succeed with the assistance of many different people. We are grateful to the authors of the individual chapters for their (largely) timely delivery of texts and their willingness to keep to the task they were given. We are also extremely grateful to Helen Liepman, Senior Commissioning Editor responsible for medical books at Oxford University

Press, for her encouragement and forbearance, and to Caroline White, who once again proved her ability to make sense of often tangled references, as well as to ensure that the manuscript was delivered in a recognisable format. Finally, we would like to thank our partners, Tony McMichael and Dorothy McKee, for their ongoing support despite the many diverse claims upon their time.

Contents

List of Contributors

Associate Professor Ian Anderson is the Director of the Centre for the Study of Health and Society and the VicHealth Koori Health Research and Community Development Unit at the University of Melbourne. He is also the Research Director for the Cooperative Research Centre for Aboriginal Health. A Koori man, he has worked in Aboriginal health for about 17 years as a clinician, policy maker and academic.

Dr Ian Basnett is Assistant Director of Public Health, North East London Strategic Health Authority, London, United Kingdom. He is disabled and contributes to local and national disability groups. In 1997/1998 he was a Harkness Fellow based at the University of California at San Francisco where his work included how disabled people fared in managed care. He is an Honorary Senior Lecturer at the London School of Hygiene and Tropical Medicine.

Professor Solomon Benatar is Professor of Medicine and Director of the Bioethics Centre, University of Cape Town, Western Cape, South Africa, and Visiting Professor in Medicine and Public Health Sciences at the University of Toronto, Canada. His special interest is in Bioethics with particular emphasis on global health ethics. He is immediate Past President of the International Association of Bioethics.

Dr Dorothy Broom is a Senior Fellow at the National Centre for Epidemiology & Population Health, The Australian National University, Canberra, Australia. For over 30 years, she has studied and taught about issues linking gender and health, and is the author of a number of publications on the subject, including a political history of Australia's unique network of feminist women's health centres.

Professor Reinhard Busse is director of the Department of Health Care Management, Berlin University of Technology and an associate research director of the European Observatory on Health Care Systems. Besides other research interests, he has written extensively about the German health care system, including the Health Care Systems in Transition profile published by the Observatory.

Naaz Coker is Chair of the British Refugee Council and runs her own Executive Coaching Practice. She was previously Director of Race and Diversity at the King's Fund.

Dr Andrew Coyle CMG is Director of the International Centre for

Prison Studies, School of Law, King's College, University of London and Honorary Professor in the Academy of Law and Management, Ryazan, Russia. He is an expert on penal matters for the United Nations and the Council of Europe, including its Committee for the Prevention of Torture.

Peter Crampton is a Senior Lecturer in the Department of Public Health, Wellington School of Medicine & Health Sciences, University of Otago, Wellington, New Zealand. He has a background in general practice and public health medicine. His research is focused on primary care policy, primary care organisation and funding, social indicators and social epidemiology. He teaches undergraduate and postgraduate courses related to public health, health systems and health services management.

Dr Sue Crengle is from the Waitaha, Kati Mamoe and Kai Tahu tribes in Aotearoa/New Zealand. She graduated with her medical and Master of Public Health degrees from the Faculty of Medicine and Health Sciences at Auckland University, and holds specialty qualifications in general practice and public health medicine. She was a recipient of the Harkness Fellowship in Health Policy 1999–2000. She was a Senior Advisor: Mäori in the Ministry of Health, and is currently Head of Discipline, Maori, in the Department of Maori and Pacific

Health, Faculty of Medicine and Health Sciences, University of Auckland and Director of the Tomaiora Mäori Health Research Centre. Her research interests include health services research, quality of care, and the health of the Mäori population.

Dr Jane Dixon is a Fellow, National Centre for Epidemiology & Population Health, Australian National University, Canberra, Australia. Jane is a member of the Scientific Committee of the International Society for Equity in Health and is especially interested in rural health inequalities and the impacts of globalisation on rural societies.

Professor Lesley Doyal is Professor of Health and Social Care, School for Policy Studies, University of Bristol, United Kingdom.

Dr Sandra Eades is a Principal Research Fellow at the Menzies School of Health Research, Darwin, Australia. Dr Eades is a Nyungar and originally from the south west of Australia.

Professor Solvig Ekblad is Adjunct Associate Professor in Transcultural Psychology, Division of Psychiatry, Department of Neurotec, Karolinska Institutet, responsible for research program in Transcultural Psychiatry and Psychology at the R&D at the Department of Psychiatry, Huddinge University Hospital and Head Unit, National Institute for Psychosocial

Factors and Health (IPM), Stockholm, Sweden.

Robert Griew is currently the Chief Executive Officer of the Department of Health and Community Services in the Northern Territory of Australia, a jurisdiction where Aboriginal people approach 30% of the population. He has worked in Aboriginal health since the mid 1990s, when he headed the Commonwealth Office for Aboriginal and Torres Strait Islander Health Services. He wrote his contribution as a doctoral student at the Centre for the Study of Health and Society at the University of Melbourne.

Dr Barbara Hanratty is MRC Research Fellow in Public Health, Department of Public Health, University of Liverpool, Liverpool, United Kingdom.

Dr Virginie Halley des Fontaines is Associate Professor of Preventive and Social Health, Health & Development Institute, Pierre & Marie Curie University, Paris, France. In the early 1980s she ran a humanitarian NGO concerned with immigrants' health. Since then she has supervised several research studies matching intercultural specificities and health services utilisation.

Ms Seeromanie Harding is responsible for the Ethnicity and Health Programme at the MRC Social and Public Health Sciences Unit at the University of Glasgow, Glasgow,

United Kingdom. She is interested in the intergenerational transmission of health risks among ethnic minority groups, particularly about the effects of socio-economic disadvantage and family life. A major focus in the research programme is about the health of UK-born ethnic minorities and whether susceptibility to adverse health outcomes in later life is evident in childhood. It also involves comparative international research about the health of migrants and their children in countries at different stages of social, economic and political development.

Dr Judith Healy was previously with the European Observatory on Health Care Systems, then Visiting Fellow, at the National Centre for Epidemiology & Population Health, Australian National University, Canberra, Australia, and is now a Senior Fellow in the Research School of Social Sciences, Australian National University. Her research interests over the last 20 years have been the comparative analysis of social and health policies and programs.

Professor John S Humphreys is Professor of Rural Health Research, School of Rural Health, Monash University, Bendigo, Victoria, Australia. John is well known for his research on health service provision in rural and remote areas of Australia, rural workforce recruitment and retention, rural health policy and the evaluation of rural health programs. He has undertaken extensive fieldwork on rural health issues throughout rural and remote regions of Australia, and has published widely in books and journals. In addition to his academic career, John has assisted both the Victorian and the Commonwealth Departments of Health in developing National Rural Health Policies.

Dr Martin Kovats is Marie Curie Research Fellow, Budapest University of Economic Sciences and Public Administration, Hungary

Professor Stephen J Kunitz (MD, PhD) is Professor of Community & Preventive Medicine, University of Rochester School of Medicine, Rochester, New York State, USA. He has spent much of his career doing research on the health of American Indians, and of indigenous peoples elsewhere as well. His other areas of research are population and medical history.

Josée G. Lavoie is a Research Associate with the Centre for Aboriginal Health Research, University of Manitoba. She is completing a PhD at the London School of Hygiene and Tropical Medicine, comparing the policies and financing mechanisms in place to support the development of indigenous health organisations in Australia, Canada and New Zealand. Prior to this, Josée spent over a decade working for Indigenous Health Organisations in the Canadian arctic and the sub-arctic.

Professor Martin McKee is Professor of European Public Health, Health Services Research Unit, and a Research Director, European Observatory on Health Care Systems, London School of Hygiene and Tropical Medicine, London, United Kingdom.

Dr Ellen Nolte, is Lecturer in Public Health, European Centre on Health of Societies in Transition (ECOHOST), and a research fellow at the European Observatory on Health Care Systems London School of Hygiene & Tropical Medicine, London, United Kingdom. Her research is looking at the health consequences of the social and political transition in central and eastern Europe and she has completed a PhD at the London School of Hygiene & Tropical Medicine on the health impact of German unification.

Dr Beverly Sibthorpe is Associate Director, National Centre for Epidemiology & Population Health and Deputy Director, Australian Primary Health Care Research Institute, Australian National University, Canberra, Australia. A nurse, anthropologist, then applied epidemiologist and evaluator she has almost 20 years experience in Aboriginal health research and policy.

Baroness Vivien Stern CBE is Senior Research Fellow at the International

Centre for Prison Studies, School of Law, Kings College, University of London. Her publications include *Sentenced to Die? The problem of TB in prisons in Eastern Europe and Central Asia* (1999) and *A sin against the future: imprisonment in the world* (1998). She is the editor of the *Prison Healthcare News*, a bilingual newsletter that promotes better prison and public health in Eastern Europe and Central Asia. She has been awarded Doctorates by Bristol and Oxford Brookes Universities and is an Honorary Fellow of the London School of Economics.

Professor Christina Victor is Professor of Social Gerontology, Department of Public Health Sciences, St George's Hospital Medical School, London, United Kingdom. Her main interests are in health inequalities in later life, the boundaries between health and social care, and social exclusion and older people.

Professor Margaret Whitehead is W.H.Duncan Professor of Public Health and Head of Department of Public Health University of Liverpool, Liverpool, United Kingdom.

Ted Wilkes is an Indigenous Australian, a Nyungar man from the south west of Australia. He has completed a Bachelor of Arts in Social Science and in 1997 was awarded the Alumni Medal of the Curtin University School of Social Science and Asian Language. In 1999 he received a Curtin University Fellow Award. He worked in the West Australian Museum as an Aboriginal Site Recorder for five years and headed up the Aboriginal Studies Unit at Curtin University for six years and worked as the Director of the Derbarl Yerrigan Health Service in Perth WA for 16 years before commencing his current position in May 2002. His work is about creating better quality of life for Indigenous Australians. He is about to commence his Doctorate in Aboriginal Health.

Dr Rory Williams (now retired Head of), Ethnicity and Health Programme, MRC Social and Public Health Sciences Unit, University of Glasgow, Glasgow, United Kingdom.

Professor Alistair Woodward is Professor of Public Health, School of Medicine & Health Sciences, University of Otago, Wellington, New Zealand. With particular interests in environmental health issues, he has worked as a researcher and teacher in Australia, Britain and New Zealand. He was a member of the New Zealand National Health Committee for six years, and currently sits on the Board of the Health Research Council.

Chapter 1

Different People, Different Services?

Judith Healy and Martin McKee

The same but different

We all share a common humanity yet we each have very different health care needs. We include young and old, men and women, rich and poor, and disabled and able-bodied. We come from a wide range of ethnic groups. The societies in which we live may or may not have accepted us as citizens. Our individual uniqueness stems from our position in this multidimensional matrix. Yet our position on each of these dimensions, in other words, our membership of the many groups that exist within our societies, shapes to some extent our particular health needs and our use of health services.

As health care professionals, policy makers and citizens we often seem blind to the diversity that exists around us. Judged by our actions we seem to imply that society consists mostly of middle class citizens of European descent, even when confronted by imagery in advertising and popular culture indicating how widely we differ, a diversity symbolized by one of the most widely recognized advertising campaigns of the 1990s, Oliviero Toscani's provocative photographs for Benetton (Benetton). His most memorable images include those of a white baby feeding at a black breast, and a white and a black arm chained together, challenging our prejudices as to which is the guard and which the prisoner. Yet when we look at our policies it frequently seems that those whose needs and expectations are different to ours are invisible. One reason is that they often *are* invisible to us. They include the migrant workers that clean our offices but who are long gone to their second or third job of the day by the time we arrive for our work each morning. In some countries they include the original indigenous owners of the country whose claims we might prefer to ignore. They include people with disabilities, whose mobility confines them to their homes or whose wheelchair takes them below our line of sight. They include elderly people, our own parents and grandparents, who once would have helped care for our children but who, because of increased labour force mobility, now live far away, out of sight and often out of mind. And they include prisoners, around whom we have erected high walls not just to confine them but also to remove them from our consciousness.

Two basic principles

This book is based on two principles, equity and responsiveness. *Equity* means that everyone should, in practice and not just in theory, be able to access and use appropriate health services. Health services should not only be for the dominant population group. This implies equitable access and use, given that some people will need more health care than others. It also means that we should seek to minimize inequalities in health outcomes. The main elements of a just health care system can be listed as universal access, access to adequate and responsive care, and fairness in financing (Benatar 1996; World Health Organization 2000). Although a just health care system remains an ideal rather than a reality in many countries, we want be clear in this chapter on this goal, while the following chapters go on to discuss some of the strategies required for its achievement.

For example, to ensure equitable access it is simply not good enough to open a health facility, put up a sign saying 'everyone welcome', and think that we have met everyone's needs. Instead we need to ask ourselves a series of questions. Is this facility in the right place? Can everyone get to it? Once they have got there, can they get into and around it? In practical terms, have we ensured that transport links make it accessible to those without a car? Have we ensured access for disabled people? Are our signs legible to the partially sighted or to those who have not mastered the language of their adopted country? Do we, by our attitudes and procedures, make clear that in reality everyone is not welcome, especially if you are poor or from a particular ethnic group? Do we take full account of different cultural requirements, whether related to diet, privacy, or facilities for religious observance, or do we just take the view that it is up to others to conform to our practices?

Second, the principle of *responsiveness* means that we should seek to learn more about the health care needs and experiences of diverse groups in our societies. As different societies have responded to these challenges in different ways there is much that we can learn from each other, both good and bad. Some countries draw reassurance from their failure to look for, and hence find, inequalities in health status and health care among their populations. Others explicitly reject the idea of conducting such research, in some cases because of a reluctance to do anything that will further stigmatize already vulnerable populations. Yet other countries insist that collective care that delivers exactly the same services to everyone is supported by everyone, despite evidence to the contrary.

Even when there is clear evidence of inequalities it is frequently poorly recognized and understood. To take one example, many white Americans are unaware of the much worse life expectancy and infant mortality experienced by their African-American compatriots (Lillie-Blanton *et al.* 2000).

But even when we recognize that there is a problem, do we know what will work and what not if we seek to address it? Do we have the evidence of the effectiveness of policies to reduce inequalities? Are the interests of marginalized populations better served by requiring them to integrate with the dominant culture or by changing society so that it responds to their different beliefs? As all societies are, to some extent, products of their history, does the answer depend on what has gone before in the society concerned?

The problem is accentuated because those advocating quite different policies may each be doing so with the best of intentions. We recognize that these issues are far from simple. There is often an enormous gulf between official policies and the everyday reality for those are meant to implement them (Lipsky 1980) as well as those who are subject to them. Researchers need to understand the experiences of marginalized populations, and not what a national elite thinks is happening. This can be difficult, especially where there is a legacy of distrust by those marginalized populations. For example, such research as has been conducted on the health of the Roma population of central Europe has largely been to serve the interests of the majority population, with its emphasis on the Roma people as a source of contagion, either from the infectious diseases they are alleged to harbour, or from their 'sub-standard' chromosomes diluting the national gene pool (Hajioff and McKee 2000).

Disentangling the causes of disadvantage can be difficult as factors often cluster together. Thus, Navarro has asked whether the much worse health of African-Americans in the United States is 'race or class, or race and class' (Navarro 1991), with more recent work on differential mortality suggesting that both play an important role (Howard *et al.* 2000).

Later in this chapter we look at arguments for and against different ways of addressing these issues. But we also realize that not everyone accepts the importance of adapting health policies to the needs of different population groups and that different values underpin health care systems. We believe that these values should be made explicit so, in the next section, we explore such values and state our position.

Values and beliefs: the nature of social claims

What is the nature of the claims that particular groups within society might make upon the state for special consideration in relation to health care?

Health care is a prime example of an important social good, not just a private commodity, whether delivered by the state or the market. Adjudicating on a 'claim' involves deciding whether a group has a legitimate entitlement to a good or service. To what extent are individuals by virtue of membership of a particular group entitled to any share, an equal share, or a larger share of health resources in a country? Such claims are not absolute but must be mediated by society, and the extent of these claims must be decided relative to those of other people (Mooney *et al.* 1998). We cannot engage in a comprehensive discourse on theories of distributive justice in the space available, but the following paragraphs summarize the main schools of thought.

The theory of entitlement

Writers such as Nozic have developed the theory of entitlement (Nozic 1974), which argues that fairness is simply the right to use one's resources as one chooses. As long as people have acquired their wealth through legitimate means, such as their own labour, a gift or inheritance, or a voluntary exchange, then they should decide what to do with their resources. The result of their decisions will be to create demand for what is wanted, which the 'invisible hand' (Smith 1982) of the market will then supply, at a price that people are willing to pay. The role of the state is limited to enforcing the law in relation to exchanges, in other words, contract law. Thus if people have the money to buy more, better quality or quicker access to health care then they are entitled to do so.

Yet the evidence for market failure in health care is well known (Arrow 1963), even if often ignored by ideologically-driven policy makers. Specifically, the weaknesses of the market impact disproportionately on those already disadvantaged. For example, they are least able to obtain the information to become informed purchasers and their plight is accentuated when that information is in a different language or, increasingly, in electronic form on the Internet, to which they have limited access. Their often greater health needs create an incentive to exclude them. The marginal cost of health services adapted to their cultural needs may exceed those incurred in catering for the dominant groups in society.

Unsurprisingly, no advanced industrialized country has adhered strictly to a model based on a system of entitlement. Even in the highly individualistic United States, about 40 per cent of health care expenditure is by government and this model, which comes closest to the entitlement model, fails on many counts, not least its population health outcomes (in terms of healthy adjusted life expectancy), which are much worse than one might expect given its national wealth and very high per capita expenditure on health care

(World Health Organization 2000). However, the increasing legitimation around the world of health care as a commodity, driven in large part from the United States, is undermining the will of other developed and developing nations to sustain or build a health care system that offers equitable access to affordable health care (Benatar 1998).

Consumer choice is an influential concept within such a market model perspective. Health systems, like other institutions, are subject to postmodernist pressures towards complexity, with a shift away from collective to more pluralist and diverse services (Taylor-Gooby and Lawson 1994; Williams 1992). This more pluralist model emphasizes both consumer choice (a market model perspective) and citizen power (a democratic or a civil society perspective). According to this rationale, everyone is entitled to special consideration from health services, which should be tailored to respond to individuals, rather than being provided in exactly the same way to everyone.

Utilitarianism

A second approach, utilitarianism, based originally on the work of Jeremy Bentham (Hart and Burns 1996), is that decisions on resource allocation should aim to achieve the greatest good for the greatest number. Policies should seek to achieve the greatest improvements in health for a given amount of resources. Furthermore, each action should be judged on what it achieves, rather than how it is done, in other words, the end justifies the means. In a situation of diversity, where the marginal cost of meeting the needs of disadvantaged groups may exceed that of the dominant group, there is a risk that certain actions, while increasing the aggregate well-being of the overall population, do so by further disadvantaging certain already vulnerable groups. Although a basis in utilitarianism may not be stated explicitly, as it is the basis of much contemporary work on cost-effectiveness, it is important to consider the differential impact that policies based on such analyses may have.

Contractarian theory

A third approach is contractarian theory, identified with the work of John Rawls (Rawls 1999). This asks what system of distribution of resources reasonable people would choose if they had to assume they might find themselves in any position in a society to which such rules applied. In other words, if you were the Minister of Health, what system would you design if you thought you might wake up the next morning as a disabled, unemployed black woman?

Rawls argued that most people would seek to maximize everyone's rights to liberties compatible with a similar system of liberties for all, assure equality of opportunity for people with similar abilities, and ensure that those who are worst off benefit. In other words, such a system focuses on ensuring the rights of the worst off in society to obtain necessary care and so would direct priority attention and resources to disadvantaged groups.

A pluralist theory of social justice

These theories offer universal solutions to the question of how to distribute resources within society. However, there are also relativist approaches, such as that of Walzer, who has developed a theory of distributive justice based on a pluralist conception of goods and claims, which argues that different principles operate within different spheres of justice (Walzer 1983). While Walzer advocates a universal basic set of principles, such as the prohibition of slavery and genocide, he argues that different communities should develop a shared understanding of justice, which then applies within different spheres of activity. Each sphere of activity (such as wealth, office, education and health) has its own norms of distributive justice and these norms operate autonomously within different distributive spheres and different societies. Further, no individual should enjoy a significant advantage in one sphere (such as a disproportionate share of health services) just because they are dominant in another sphere (such as wealth or education); while the means of domination may differ between societies, such as money (within a market economy) or public office (within the former Soviet Union). Better health care, in this analysis, could be yet another means by which the powerful dominate (or gain an unfair advantage over) the less powerful. The distributive principles differ for each social good, and in relation to health services, commonly applied distributive principles include need, desert (such as being socially deserving), and citizenship.

The concept of citizenship

Citizenship commonly entitles a person to his or her country's health services, but beliefs about the nature of citizenship, both enshrined in legislation and held as popular beliefs by the public, also shape our health policies (Soysal 1994). The concept of citizenship in the European Union in relation to health care entitlement is changing rapidly, at least in respect of citizens in other European Union member states (Mossialos and McKee 2001). However, for those from other countries, increasingly exclusionary immigration and asylum controls and associated regulations on health and welfare entitlements are widening the gap between countries of emigration and immigration (Lister 2000).

In some countries, such as the United Kingdom, the Netherlands, and Australia (Borowski 2000), there is a widespread acceptance of the concept of multiculturalism, based on mutual respect for other's beliefs. In others, such as France (Jack 2000), those from other cultures largely are expected to conform to the dominant norms. And these beliefs can change. Some countries previously regarded as welcoming to those from other cultures, such as Ireland or Denmark, have experienced a backlash in the face of economic downturn or a perceived excessive level of migration (Fraser 2000), while other countries also have seen an increase in popular support for political parties espousing anti-immigration or anti-refugee agendas, as in Australia and France.

Some countries can be considered to consist of nations within nations. Some population groups may have been incorporated voluntarily or through force, or may be the result of international population movements (Kymlicka 1995). According to Kymlicka, multinational states result from the incorporation of previously self-governing minority cultures through colonialism. Examples of consociational states include Belgium and Switzerland, while examples of polyethnic states include the United States, Canada, Australia and New Zealand. Under the multinational concept, indigenous population groups would have a right to self-government, access to resources to support their cultural practices (polyethnic rights), and the right to special representation within the national parliamentary system. Such a concept therefore would support the goal of self-determination in health care services.

The context is also important since different societies imbue a social good, such as health care, with different social and political meanings; for example, control over health services may have as much to do with political goals as health goals. A pluralist concept of social justice, and hence the relative nature of social claims, makes it important to examine the claims on health care by different groups and within different societies, and hence the distributive principles that may govern health care shares.

Whatever views one holds on these issues, it is important that one has thought them through. In the next section we move from broad principles to specifics, looking at why we believe that health policy makers should be concerned with the needs of different groups in their populations.

Why should we be concerned with diversity?

We argue that the health care system of a country should take account of increasingly diverse populations, particularly since this diversity is growing with greater movements of people between countries in an increasingly globalized world, and where people may have particular needs and expectations with regard to health care. There are several reasons why a country should be concerned about the health care and health outcomes of diverse social groups within its population and we now turn to these.

Legal rights

One reason for health policy makers to be concerned about diversity is simply that governments have committed themselves to doing so. The evolving body of international law in the second half of the twentieth century has established a right to health without regard to individual characteristics. Building on the non-binding, but morally authoritative, *Universal Declaration of Human Rights* (United Nations 1948), governments have agreed numerous multilateral treaties, many of which are legally binding, that support three linked rights: the right to health, the right to enjoy the benefits of scientific progress, and the right to non-discrimination. Thus, the United Nations *International Covenant on Economic, Social and Cultural Rights* (United Nations 1966) recognizes the right of everyone to the highest attainable standard of physical and mental health. Under this covenant, governments are required to report regularly on their progress on a range of measures, including access to health care. They are also asked to identify any groups within their populations whose health situation is significantly worse than that of the majority, to state whether policies have affected them adversely, and to describe measures taken to improve their situation.

There are also binding treaties focusing on the needs of specific groups. These include the *Convention on the Elimination of All Forms of Racial Discrimination* (United Nations 1965), the *Convention on the Elimination of All Forms of Discrimination Against Women* (United Nations 1979), the *Convention on the Rights of the Child* (United Nations 1989), and, with relevance to prisoners, the *Convention against Torture and other Cruel, Inhuman or Degrading Treatment or Punishment* (United Nations 1984).

The principles enunciated in these conventions have subsequently been operationalized in a series of conferences, most notably the 1993 World Conference on Human Rights and the 1994 International Conference on Population and Development, the declarations from which, while not legally binding, have considerable moral authority.

The principle of equity has also been endorsed by the World Health Organization, most recently in its strategy for *Health 21: health for all in the twenty-first century* (World Health Organization Regional Office for Europe 1999). It states that equity underpins the concept of health for all and calls for the removal of unfair and unjustified differences between individuals and groups.

Of course, it is naive to exaggerate the impact of international treaties, even where they have the force of international law or require regular reports by governments, since there is little scope for individuals or groups to press their case or for the supervisory bodies to enforce their views. In addition, many rights conferred under United Nations treaties, especially concerning health, are subject to the principle of 'progressive realization', in which progress towards a goal is contingent on a country's available resources. Yet these treaties do have a value, especially where there are well-organized advocacy groups that can cite the endorsement of these instruments by governments in order to call for policies to meet the needs of disadvantaged groups.

In addition, many countries have incorporated these principles into their constitutions or into other instruments of national law, and have adhered to regional conventions, such as the *European Convention on Human Rights* (Council of Europe 1950), which also outlaw discrimination, and which are often incorporated into national law, as with the United Kingdom Human Rights Act 1998. In a few cases, defined groups may also draw on rights in specific treaties, such as the Mäori in New Zealand under the 1840 Treaty of Waitangi (Brookfield 1999), treaty obligations by the United States government to American Indian tribes (Kunitz 1996), and by the Canadian government to their indigenous peoples (Waldram *et al.* 1995).

Thus for our purposes it is important to recognize that regardless of what they actually do in practice all governments have, to some extent, signed up to the principles of health for all and freedom from discrimination.

Poverty reduction

There is growing support for policies aimed at poverty alleviation, primarily because it is seen as a tool to achieve economic growth. This has been made explicit globally in the International Development Targets (OECD 1996), but it is also a stated goal of many governments. Although membership of a non-dominant group is not automatically linked to poverty, in many cases it does increase one's risk of impoverishment (UK Department for International Development 1997).

Understanding of the relationship between poverty and health is changing. While poverty is an important cause (or risk factor) of disease (Marmot and Wilkinson 1999), it is increasingly recognized that disease is a cause of poverty. The onset of serious disease often causes loss of employment and thus income. In many countries, the financial implications are exacerbated by the cost of obtaining care. Poverty, in turn, can reduce access to effective care, creating a downward spiral affecting not only the affected person but also his or her family (World Health Organization 2000). It is not only those afflicted with catastrophic illness, such as cancer or stroke, who are affected: long-lasting illnesses, such as diabetes, may also lead to impoverishment, especially when coupled with employment practices that make it difficult for those with special health needs to obtain work.

The rationale for health sector reform is increasingly linked to broader social and economic goals. The Commission on Macro-Economics and Health (2002) has begun to quantify the deleterious effect of poor health on economic growth. Other international agencies now see the health care system as a key player in poverty reduction strategies (Asian Development Bank 1999; United Nations Development Programme 1999; World Bank 2000). Studies in the developed world, such as the Wanless Report (Wanless 2002) in the United Kingdom, and work by the Australian Institute of Health and Welfare (Mathers *et al.* 1999), have begun to measure the cost to society of high levels of ill health. Increasingly, for this reason, equitable and affordable health care for all is seen as a key element of an integrated anti-poverty strategy, and health sector reform based on equity and inclusiveness is linked with broader social and economic goals. A healthy population is more likely to become a wealthy population, with advantages for everyone.

Health inequalities

Even where levels of absolute or relative poverty are low, there is an increasing political determination in many countries to confront the health inequalities that have persisted despite the existence of developed welfare states (Whitehead 1992). Inequalities are institutionally embedded in social institutions, including health care systems. A growing literature on poverty and social exclusion focuses, not just on income, but on other tangible and less tangible assets of the poor, such as health care (Askonas and Stewart 2000; MacIntosh 2001). In this view, publicly-funded health services are a potential lever for the state to use in reducing inequalities (Graham 2000). Although health inequalities often have their origins in other sectors, such as economic redistribution, education and housing, it is also clear that many groups do not obtain access to care that is appropriate to their needs.

And the benefits of access to health care are now greater than ever. In the nineteenth century, it mattered little whether one had access to care for most health problems since there was so little that could be done to help, and indeed, the unsanitary conditions prevailing in many hospitals meant that one was often safer at home (Porter 1997).

Writing in the 1960s, McKeown showed how reductions in mortality in the nineteenth and early twentieth century were due mainly to improvements in living conditions (McKeown 1979). However this situation has since been transformed, particularly since the 1960s, by developments in our understanding of the mechanisms of disease, and by advances in pharmaceuticals, in technology, and in effective treatment for many conditions. For example, modern antibiotics mean that many childhood infections are no longer fatal;

chronic diseases such as hypertension, asthma, and epilepsy are now consistent with leading a normal life; common childhood cancers now have cure rates of over 90 per cent.

These advances encompass not only many new means of diagnosis and treatment but, equally important, an explosion of information on what does and does not work, and for whom. Research on effectiveness (Sheldon and Chalmers 1994) has identified many effective treatments that should be used more widely as well as many ineffective treatments that should be dropped, with such knowledge being disseminated through avenues such as the Cochrane collaborations. When linked with active purchasing of health care and programmes of quality assurance the nature of health care has changed immensely.

The impact of modern health care can be illustrated by research on avoidable mortality, that is, conditions from which death should not occur if health care is provided appropriately (Rutstein *et al.* 1976). Mackenbach and colleagues have shown how falls in deaths from conditions amenable to medical treatment accounted for a substantial part of the overall improvement in life expectancy in the Netherlands between 1950 and 1984, (Mackenbach *et al.* 1988) while others came to the same conclusion elsewhere (Albert *et al.* 1996; Bunker *et al.* 1994).

In contrast, in countries such as those in the former Soviet Union, where functioning health care systems have broken down, deaths have increased rapidly from conditions such as diabetes that depend on secure supplies of insulin (Telishevska *et al.* 2001).

Yet this progress does not benefit everyone to the same extent. There is considerable evidence that disadvantaged groups frequently have reduced access to effective health care interventions. Women (Petticrew *et al.* 1993), those living in deprived areas (Ben-Shlomo and Chaturvedi 1995), and people from minority ethnic populations (Shaukat *et al.* 1993), all have lower levels of access to complex cardiovascular interventions. Even when they do obtain care, it may be at a later stage in the disease and treatment may be less intensive. All of these factors combine to explain the consistent finding that cancer survival is worse among the poor (Kogevinas and Porta 1997). It is therefore unsurprising that deaths from conditions amenable to medical care typically exhibit steeper social class gradients than do deaths from other causes (Poikolainen and Eskola 1995).

These findings have led to recognition of 'the inverse care law' (Tudor Hart 1971), which states that those whose health needs are greatest, and who are often to be found among marginalized groups in society, often have the worst access to care. The 'inverse equity hypothesis' suggests that new health programmes initially benefit people of higher socio-economic status and only later reach the poor, so that inequities temporarily increase (Victora *et al.* 2000). In this way, the existing organization of health care systems may actually serve to exacerbate inequalities by benefiting disproportionately those who are already relatively advantaged.

Increasing population diversity

Responding to diversity becomes more important given the increasing population movements between countries and the growth of polyethnic societies. Countries such as the United Kingdom, France and the Netherlands that had overseas colonies have long been multi-ethnic societies, as have countries where European settlers have displaced indigenous populations, such as the United States, Canada, Australia and New Zealand. But the growth of migration is transforming what have until recently been ethnically homogenous populations. The number of migrants worldwide has more than doubled since 1975 with 60 per cent living in developed countries and 40 per cent in less developed countries. In the five years between 1995 and 2000, developed countries received nearly 12 million migrants from the less developed regions, accounting for two-thirds of the population growth in developed regions. About 9 per cent of migrants are refugees with about 3 million currently in developed countries and 13 million in developing countries (United Nations Population Division 2002). The number of refugees each year fluctuates depending upon the waves of civil strife, economic collapse and war around the world, with 12.1 million refuges worldwide in 2001.

Of these refugees, a smaller number ask for permanent asylum in another country. In 2002, there were about 569,000 applications for asylum submitted to the industrialized countries (United Nations High Commission for Refugees 2003). The United Kingdom is the leading country for asylum, accounting for 19 per cent of applications, followed by the United States with 14 per cent, Germany 12 per cent, France 9 per cent, Austria 6 per cent, Canada 6 per cent, and Sweden 6 per cent.

Thus for various reasons, the number of foreigners settling in Europe has almost doubled in the past five years, reaching 1.05 million newcomers in 2001, with Germany now having the highest proportion of foreign-born residents at 9 per cent of the population (Eurostat 2003). Migration has replaced births as the principal source of population growth in industrialized countries. The control of population movements thus is a high priority for migration policies (OECD 2002), and nearly half of developed countries have policies in place to reduce migration levels (United Nations Population Division 2002). Further, many countries are putting up barriers to applications by asylum seekers. Many industrialized countries therefore are ambivalent about the extent to which they are prepared to make their institutions, including their health care systems, more responsive to newcomers.

Stewardship and the role of the state

Given increasing economic and health inequalities and increasing population diversity, there is some reappraisal of the role of the state in ensuring that the needs of all its residents are met. The stewardship concept, advanced in *The World Health Report 2000*, argues that the state has the ultimate responsibility for the performance of a country's health system, and is charged with the careful management of the well being of the whole population (World Health Organization 2000). Since the overall health status of a population may be significantly affected by subgroups within that population, it follows that the health status of particular groups should be considered, and if necessary, addressed. *The World Health Report 2000* set out a system to assess health system performance that includes not just the level of attainment of health and responsiveness, but also their distribution within a country's population. While these measures are still far from perfect, they do at least demonstrate a high level commitment to the achievement of goals based on equity and inclusiveness. A reappraisal of the role of the state, despite or because of increasing health sector privatization, also can be seen in the growing number of national health strategies.

In this section we have argued the case for attention to the needs of diverse groups within a population. The next section explores some issues involved in deciding how this might be done, since services can be delivered in various ways depending in part upon the context.

How might health services be delivered and to whom?

The normative view of a health care system is that the same services should be available to everyone: a mainstream or collectivist position. Historically, however, health systems have responded to diverse groups within populations in different ways, as the following examples show.

In earlier centuries, health services developed separately for the rich and the poor, with the rich treated at home by physicians, while the poor relied on traditional healers and 'nurses'. From the seventeenth century onwards, some western European countries, such as the Netherlands, separated health services on grounds of religion (for example, between Catholics and Protestants), particularly in relation to hospitals, since these were places to prepare for death. The former Soviet health system divided facilities according to age, sex and workplace, with separate polyclinics for children, adults and women's reproductive health, plus many workplace-based services, as well as better quality parallel services for groups such as defence forces and senior party officials (Field 1990).

The rapid advance of medical specialization throughout the twentieth century meant that some physicians and hospitals 'focused on body parts, some on diseases; some on life events, some on age groups' (Porter 1997 p. 381). Some health care reforms in recent years have aimed to organize the delivery of health services more in terms of whole people than bodily parts and conditions: a holistic approach. Finally, many countries now are moving towards structured pluralism in their delivery of health services (Londono and Frenk 1997).

There are thus many organizational models for the delivery of health services, ranging from collectivist services for everyone to setting up a completely parallel system (Healy 1998). Alternative service delivery models tend to concentrate more upon primary health care, but it is theoretically possible (and such systems do exist in practice) to organize a completely parallel health system that includes tertiary care hospitals.

Which service delivery model is the most appropriate in terms of access, use and outcomes for particular population groups? Different groups may prefer different service delivery models. People with disabilities who in the past have been marginalized generally want better access to mainstream services, while in contrast indigenous groups in some countries want to run their own culturally responsive health services. The advantages and disadvantages of different models are not easy to evaluate. For example, advocates of alternative services argue that separate and hence responsive services produce better outcomes, while critics argue that alternative services are often substandard services. We believe that the arguments for and against different models will depend on the groups involved and their circumstances, but we also believe that it is important to understand better what evidence exists to inform these decisions.

We examine three broad categories of people. The first category explores many of the standard sociodemographic descriptors of any population: gender, age, socio-economic status, and urban or rural location. To these we have added disability and imprisonment.

The second category looks at citizenship. Societies everywhere are increasingly exposed to the forces of globalization. International treaties seek to ease the free movement of goods and capital but crucially, not people, or at least not poor people. The criteria for citizenship vary enormously between countries. Citizenship may be acquired through place of birth or by descent, in some cases by virtue of one's ancestral origins many generations previously, and the ease with which it is acquired differs greatly. As a consequence, there are many people now living in advanced industrialized societies who are not part of those societies.

In the third category we look at the challenges of polyethnic societies. In some countries, those in the now dominant group were the migrants, spreading out from Europe in the era of colonialism. In other countries, especially in Europe, the movement has been in the opposite direction, with the colonized coming to the 'mother country'. In others, such as those countries in central Europe with Roma populations, groups have lived together while remaining separate for centuries.

To address the issues identified for this book we have brought together a group of authors that are themselves diverse. They come from different societies (although mostly OECD countries), different disciplinary backgrounds, have experience as policy makers, as academics and as users of services, and focus upon different groups within the society they come from. Their diversity means that they would not normally come together in this way to share perspectives and experiences, which is important since we believe that there is much scope here for mutual learning.

References

Albert, X., Bayo, A., Alfonso, J. L., Cortina, P. and Corella, D. (1996) The effectiveness of health systems in influencing avoidable mortality: a study in Valencia, Spain 1975–90. *Journal of Epidemiology and Communicative Health*, **50**, 320–5.

Arrow, K. J. (1963). Uncertainty and the welfare economics of medical care. *American Economic Review*, **53**, 941–8.

Asian Development Bank (1999) *Health sector reform in Asia and the Pacific: options for developing countries*. Asian Development Bank, Manila.

Askonas, P. and Stewart, S. (2000) *Social inclusion: possibilities and tensions*. Macmillan, Basingstoke.

Benatar, S. (1996) What makes a just healthcare system? *British Medical Journal*, **313**, 1567–8.

Benatar, S. (1998) Global disparities in health and human rights: a critical commentary. *American Journal of Public Health*, **88** (2) 295–300.

Benetton United Colours divided opinions. Available from http://www.benetton.com/wws/aboutyou/ucdo/index.html.

Ben-Shlomo, Y. and Chaturvedi, N. (1995) Assessing equity in access to health care provision in the UK: does where you live affect your chances of getting a coronary artery bypass graft? *Journal of Epidemiology and Communicative Health*, **49**, 200–4.

Borowski, A. (2000) Creating a virtuous society: immigration and Australia's policies of multiculturalism. *Journal of Social Policy*, **29** (3), 459–75.

Brookfield, F. M. (1999) *Waitangi and indigenous rights: revolution, law and legitimation*. Auckland University Press, Auckland.

Bunker, J. P., Frazier, H. S. and Mosteller, F. (1994) Improving health: measuring effects of medical care. *Millbank Memorial Quarterly*, **72**, 225–58.

Commission on Macroeconomics and Health (2002) *Macroeconomics and health: investing in health for economic development*. WHO, Geneva.

Council of Europe (1950) *European convention for the protection of human rights and fundamental freedoms*. Council of Europe, Strasbourg.

Eurostat (2003) europa.eu.int/comm./eurostat accessed 28 February 2003.

Field, M. G. (1990) Noble purpose, grand design, flawed execution, mixed results: Soviet socialized medicine after seventy years. *American Journal of Public Health*, **80**, 144–5.

Fraser, N. (2000) *The voice of modern hatred*. Picador, London.

Graham, H. (2000) From science to policy: options for reducing health inequalities. In D. A. Leon and G. Walt (eds) *Poverty, inequality and health: an international perspective*. Oxford University Press, Oxford.

Hajioff, S. and McKee, M. (2000) The health of the Roma people: a review of the published literature. *Journal of Epidemiology and Community Health*, **54** (11), 864–9.

Hart, H. L. and Burns, A. (1996) *An introduction to the principles of morals and legislation by Jeremy Bentham*. Clarendon Press, London.

Healy, J. (1998) *Welfare options: delivering social services*. Allen & Unwin, Sydney.

Howard, G., Anderson, R. T., Russell, G., Howard, V. J. and Burke, G. (2000) Race, socioeconomic status, and cause-specific mortality. *Annals of Epidemiology*, **10**, 214–23.

Jack, A. (2000) *The French exception*. Profile, London.

Kogevinas, M. and Porta, M. (1997) Socioeconomic differences in cancer survival: a review of the evidence. *IARC Sci Pub*, **138**, 177–206.

Kunitz, S. (1996) The history and politics of US health care policy for American Indians and Alaskan Natives. *American Journal of Public Health*, **86** (10), 1464–73.

Kymlicka, W. (1995) *Multicultural citizenship: a liberal theory of minority rights*. Clarendon Press, Oxford.

Lillie-Blanton, M., Brodie, M., Rowland, D., Altman, D. and McIntosh, M. (2000) Race, ethnicity, and the health care system: public perceptions and experiences. *Care Res Rev*, **57** (1), 218–35.

Lipsky, M. (1980) *Street-level bureaucracy: dilemmas of the individual in public services*. Russell Sage Foundation, New York.

Lister, R. (2000) Strategies for social inclusion: promoting social cohesion or social justice? In P. Askonas and A. Stewart (eds) *Social inclusion: possibilities and tensions*. Macmillan Press Ltd, London and New York.

Londono, J. L. and Frenk, J. (1997) Structured pluralism: toward an innovative model for health system reform in Latin America. *Health Policy*, **41** (1), 1–36.

MacIntosh, M. (2001) Do health systems contribute to inequalities? In D. Leon and G. Walt (eds) *Poverty, inequality and health: an international perspective*. Oxford University Press, Oxford.

Mackenbach, J. P., Looman, C. W. N., Kunst, A. E., Habbema, J. D. F. and van der Maas, P. J. (1988) Post-1950 mortality trends and medical care: gains in life expectancy due to declines in mortality from conditions amenable to medical intervention in the Netherlands. *Social Science Medicine*, **27**, 889–94.

Marmot, M. G. and Wilkinson, R. G. (1999) *Social determinants of health*. Oxford University Press, Oxford.

Mathers, C., Vos, T. and Stevenson, C. (1999) *The burden of disease and injury in Australia*. Australian Institute of Health and Welfare, Canberra.

McKeown, T. (1979) *The role of medicine: dream, mirage or nemesis?* Blackwell, Oxford.

Mooney, G., Jan, S. and Wiseman, J. (1998) 'Communitarian claims' as an ethical basis for allocating health care resources. *Social Science and Medicine*, **47**, 1171–80.

Mossialos, E. and McKee, M. (2001) Is a European health care policy emerging? *British Medical Journal*, **323**, 248.

Navarro, V. (1991) Race or class or race and class: growing mortality differentials in the United States. *International Journal of Health Services*, **21**, 229–35.

Nozic, R. (1974) *Anarchy, state and Utopia.* Basic Books, New York.

OECD (1996) *Shaping the twenty-first century: the contribution of development co-operation.* OECD, Paris.

OECD (2002) *Trends in international migration.* OECD, Paris.

Petticrew, M., McKee, M. and Jones, J. (1993) Coronary artery surgery: are women discriminated against? *British Medical Journal*, **306**, 1164–6.

Poikolainen, K. and Eskola, J. (1995) Regional and social class variation in the relative risk of death from amenable causes in the city of Helsinki, 1980–86. *International Journal of Epidemiology*, **24**, 114–18.

Porter, R. (1997) *The greatest benefit to mankind: a medical history of humanity from antiquity to the present.* HarperCollins Publishers, London.

Rawls, J. (1999) *A theory of justice.* Oxford University Press, Oxford.

Rutstein, D. D., Berenberg, W., Chalmers, T. C., Child, C. G., Fishman, A. P. and Perrin, E. B. (1976) Measuring the quality of medical care: a clinical method. *New England Journal of Medicine*, **294**, 582–8.

Shaukat, N., De Bono, D. P. and Cruickshank, J. K. (1993) Clinical features, risk factors, and referral delay in British patients of Indian and European origin with angina matched for age and extent of coronary atheroma. *British Medical Journal*, **307**, 717–18.

Sheldon, T. and Chalmers, I. (1994) The UK Cochrane Centre and the NHS Centre for Reviews and Dissemination; Respective roles within the information system strategy of the NHS R&D programme, co-ordination and principles underlying collaboration. *Health Economics*, **3**, 201–3.

Smith, A. (1982) *The wealth of nations.* Penguin, Harmondsworth.

Soysal, Y. N. (1994) *Limits of citizenship: migrants and postnational membership in Europe.* University of Chicago Press, Chicago.

Taylor-Gooby, P. and Lawson, R. (eds) (1994) *Markets and managers.* Buckingham, Open University Press.

Telishevska, M., Chenet, L. and McKee, M. (2001) Towards an understanding of the high death rate among young people with diabetes in Ukraine. *Diab Med*, **18**, 3–9.

Tudor Hart, J. (1971) The inverse care law. *Lancet*, **1**, 405–12.

UK Department for International Development (1997) *Eliminating world poverty: a challenge for the twenty-first century.* The Stationery Office, London.

United Nations (1948) *Universal declaration of human rights.* GA Resolution 217A (III), UN GAOR, Resolution, 71, UN Document A/810. United Nations, New York.

United Nations (1965) *Convention on the elimination of all forms of racial discrimination.* UN GA Resolution 2106A (XX). United Nations, New York.

United Nations (1966) *International covenant on economic, social and cultural rights.* GA Resolution 2200 (XXI), UN GAOR, 21st Session, Supplement No 16, at 49, UN Document A/6316. United Nations, Geneva.

United Nations (1979) *Convention on the elimination of all forms of discrimination against women.* GA Resolution 34/180, UN GAOR, 34th Session, Supplement No. 46, at 193, UN Document A/34/46. United Nations, New York.

United Nations (1984) *Convention against torture and other cruel, inhuman or degrading treatment or punishment.* GA Resolution 39/45, UN GAOR, 39th Session, Supplement No. 51, at 197, UN Document A/39/51. United Nations, New York.

United Nations (1989) *Convention on the rights of the child.* GA Resolution 44/25, UN GAOR, 44th Session, Supplement No. 49, at 166, UN Document A/44/25. United Nations, New York.

United Nations Development Programme (1999) *Human development report 1999.* Oxford University Press, New York and Oxford.

United Nations High Commission for Refugees (2003) www.unhcr.ch accessed 28 February 2003.

United Nations Population Division (2002) *International migration report 2002.* United Nations, New York.

Victora, C. G., Vaughan, J. P., Barros, F. C., Silva, A. C. and Tomasi, E. (2000) Explaining trends in inequities: evidence from Brazilian child health studies. *Lancet,* **356,** 1093–8.

Waldram, J. B., Herring, D. A. and Young, T. K. (1995) *Aboriginal health in Canada: historical, cultural and epidemiological perspectives.* University of Toronto Press, Toronto.

Walzer, M. (1983) *Spheres of justice: a defence of pluralism and equality.* Basil Blackwell, Oxford.

Wanless, D. (2002) *Securing our future health: taking a long-term view. Final Report.* HM Treasury, London.

Whitehead, M. (1992) *Inequalities in health.* Penguin, Harmondsworth.

Williams, F. (1992) Somewhere over the rainbow: universality and diversity in social policy. In N. Manning and R. Page (eds) *Social Policy Review 4.* Social Policy Association, University of Kent, Canterbury.

World Bank (2000) *World development report 2000/2001: attacking poverty.* Oxford University Press, Oxford.

World Health Organization (2000) *The world health report 2000. Health systems: improving Performance.* World Health Organization, Geneva.

World Health Organization Regional Office for Europe (1999) *Health 21: health for all in the twenty-first century.* WHO Regional Office for Europe, Copenhagen.

Chapter 2

Sex and Gender in Health Care and Health Policy

Dorothy Broom and Lesley Doyal

In their opening chapter, Healy and McKee call attention to the increasing diversity within national populations, and the challenges such diversity presents to health care policy and planning. Some elements of the diversity canvassed in this volume are especially important because they are always present in every population, cross cutting other dimensions such as culture, ethnicity and citizenship. While the sex ratio may vary between societies or over time, all nations (except the Vatican) contain people of both sexes and all ages. Consequently, the particularities of ethnicity, citizenship, ability and marginalization are always refracted through the lenses of age and gender. Health care policies and services must accommodate the varying needs of different groups such as the poor, asylum seekers or indigenous people. However these groups are themselves not homogeneous, and the needs of individuals within them are influenced by a range of different variables including sex and gender.

In this chapter we concentrate on the way gender shapes health and health care. We begin with a broad overview of how sex and gender relate to health status, experiences of illness, and health care needs. We go on to consider women's health activism in the United Kingdom and Australia, comparing their very different histories and exploring the ways in which feminist activism has influenced national health policy and services.

Becoming aware of gender and health

Until the 1970s, the term 'gender' was not much in use, and the field that might now be labelled 'gender and health' was limited to women's sexual and reproductive health. In poor societies (and among the poor in wealthy societies), low levels of maternal and infant health signalled the need for improved primary health care services (including birth control), and improved access to existing services. By contrast, in rich societies, specialist obstetrics and gynaecology services were becoming increasingly dominant forces in women's health care.

The advent of 'second wave' feminism in the late 1960s brought with it claims that women were not being well served by mainstream medicine, and that medical care often failed to meet women's health needs and sometimes contributed to their oppression (Dreifus 1977). In the USA, the United Kingdom, Australia, and other developed countries, feminists launched women's health movements that sought to enhance the appropriateness and quality of health services, striving for a revolution in the ways service providers interacted with women, and to make services more accessible to women in need.

Partly as a result of these campaigns and of recent advocacy for men, health services planners and providers are now becoming more aware of the importance of taking gender into consideration. Although considerable research has amplified and complicated the picture during the last three decades, the underlying analysis that originally motivated second wave feminists still informs thinking about how gender and health are related.

Beginning with women

Biological differences between the sexes have generally been accepted as relevant to health, or at least to women's health. The implications of those differences, however, have been more controversial, with some people believing that 'biology is destiny'. The women's movement argued strongly that although access to birth control and high-quality maternity care are essential, women's health care needs cannot be met only within the arena of obstetrics and gynaecology. Feminists showed conclusively that everyday existence, life chances and health are shaped not only by biological differences, but also by the social distinctions between females and males – their roles, responsibilities, and social expectations (Annandale and Hunt 2000).

Some advocates have claimed that women suffer worse health than men because of their social roles, low incomes, powerlessness, and the inadequacy of health services in meeting their needs. Although the family home is often represented as a refuge from health hazards, responsibility for domestic work and the care of children and other family members may contribute to a range of physical and mental health problems such as fatigue, anxiety and depression which are more prevalent among women (Astbury and Cabral 2000; Lee and Porteus 2001). Household work and childcare also constrain women's ability to compete on equal terms with men in the paid workforce and in the public sphere more generally, thus diminishing their mobility, income and political power.

Violence against women – including family violence – was also placed squarely on the agenda as a women's health issue. A feminist analysis construes violence as a health problem in itself because of the morbidity and mortality it causes, and also as a symptom of women's comparative powerlessness. Thus, shelters for women and their children escaping domestic violence are, from the feminist perspective, understood as essential elements of adequate women's health services.

Second wave feminists were also concerned about women's access to conventional medical goods and services (especially but not only birth control, including abortion) and the quality of women's relationships with service providers. Sex based assumptions, prejudice and discrimination led some doctors to deny reproductive health services to unmarried women, to impose birth control on disabled and other disadvantaged women, and to ignore the particular needs of migrants, lesbians, adolescents and older women. Gender stereotyping has also complicated women's relationships with service providers, prompting some doctors to treat women in condescending, insulting or even sexually exploitative ways.

In addition to gender bias in the relationship between female patients and service providers, there is now evidence that doctors do not always deliver the same treatments to male and female patients presenting the same medical condition. For example, there is now abundant proof of what might be called gender bias in medical care for several important conditions, including cardiovascular disease (Foster and Mallik 1998; McKinlay 1996; Sonke *et al.* 1996; Steingart *et al.* 1991).

The women's health movements in Australia and Britain were both motivated by similar patterns of discrimination and bias. But while feminist starting points were similar, the strategies have taken very different trajectories in the two nations.

Taking action: Australian community activism

Beginning in the 1970s, innovation in Australian women's health care was driven by vigorous political advocacy and practical action by a feminist women's health movement. Feminist pressure was sustained despite constraints and political reversals over two decades.

Along with the feminist movement and other generally progressive social initiatives (Broom 1991; Ruzek 1978), a number of developments were occurring in the health field. The 'new public health', community health movement and health consumerism all contributed to the articulation of a critical orientation to biomedicine (Milio 1988; Nettleton 1996; Petersen and Lupton 1996). Lay people were being encouraged to ask questions and inform themselves, and to take more responsibility for their own bodies and health. The women's health movement worked in concert with these activities, often exercising a strong leadership role.

Drawing on the broad agendas of political action at the time, themes of oppression and liberation permeated women's health activism. The term 'sexism' appeared, and analogies were drawn to racism. Academic women's studies supplied conceptual and analytical tools that helped activists formulate perspectives on problems and strategies for response. The women's health movement was a focus for a range of activities, from private discussions about dissatisfaction with doctors to feminist consciousness-raising to public meetings, lobbying, advocacy and community-based service provision. Beginning with amateur pamphlets and extending to highly professional publications such as *Our Bodies Ourselves* (Boston Women's Health Book Collective 1971), women seized the initiative of defining their own health priorities and generating their own sources of information. Producing and distributing health advice may seem uncontroversial from the vantage point of the twenty-first century, but when a booklet called *What Every Woman Should Know* was distributed to Sydney high school girls in the early 1970s, it provoked vigorous efforts to have it banned.

Action and information on women's health were framed initially in terms of a vocabulary of resistance to patterns labelled as *patriarchal* and a conception of biomedicine as male-dominated (Broom 1995; Broom 1984). The language of the women's health movement referred to discrimination and injustice, notions around which it was easy to mobilize a vigorous and diverse constituency in the activist 1970s. The election of the Whitlam Labor government in 1972 created a national political environment of innovation and responsiveness particularly in the health field, with such significant initiatives as the national public health insurance scheme and the Community Health Program.

A major focus of the Australian women's health movement was the creation of community-based feminist women's health centres (the first of which were funded by the Community Health Program). Between 1974 and the 1990s, approximately 50 such centres were opened around the country. It has been said that Australia has more such centres per head of population than any other country. They are not the only activity relating to women's health (and the majority of women in Australia never attend one). Nevertheless, the centres have played an important role in shaping the changing face of women's health services and policies. They have applied a dual strategy of supplying services to women while also working with mainstream services in order to advance the diverse agenda of the movement.

The culmination of these developments occurred in 1989. Following a long and democratic process of consultation in which more than one million women throughout Australia participated (Broom 1991; Gray 1998), a comprehensive National Women's Health Policy (NWHP) was endorsed by all health ministers (Commonwealth Department of Community Services and

Health 1989). This innovative policy was internationally recognized as the first of its kind in the world and was especially valued for its recognition of diversity among women themselves.

Indigenous women and those from non-English speaking backgrounds emphasized somewhat different priorities from those advanced by Anglo-Australian women. For example, Aboriginal women were more concerned about the coercive imposition of fertility control than access to abortions (Goodall and Huggins 1992). And migrant women gave urgent priority to improvements in occupational health and safety and mental health services. Women of all racial and ethnic backgrounds were united, however, in their call for a voice in personal health care decisions and in the formulation of health policy. The NWHP sought to reflect this diversity by formulating both broad principles, and targeting women disadvantaged by age, ethnicity or disability.

The policy was a highly visible government response to women's health advocacy. Getting women's health squarely on the political agenda for the Commonwealth and all States was a major accomplishment for the women's health movement. The NWHP was a watershed because it signified that the Commonwealth was encouraging governments to innovate, promote and expand women's health initiatives. It also gave women's health an ongoing national significance.

The policy affirms a social view of health, and highlights (among other things) violence against women, occupational health and safety, mental and emotional health, provision of health information, and women's involvement in health decision-making. At the time it was adopted, many people still assumed that 'women's health' was equivalent to reproductive and sexual health, so the priorities set by the policy legitimized a very different understanding, one that was more in tune with what women themselves have identified (Redman *et al.* 1988).

From dual strategy to mainstreaming

In the late 1990s the emphasis began to shift towards a policy of mainstreaming (Rees 1999). The climate that had produced the NWHP was transformed by the election of more politically conservative governments with a strong emphasis on containing public spending. The move toward mainstreaming women's health was justified by a number of gradual changes such as the recruitment of more women into medicine (Pringle 1998), numerous family planning clinics opening, and four national women's health conferences, as well as the activities for the implementation of the NWHP. Nevertheless research conducted in the 1990s showed that most of the concerns that had motivated the foundation of the original women's health centres and later prompted the NWHP were still very much alive (Broom 1998; Brown and Doran 1996), and women are still seeking an approach that is difficult or impossible to obtain from other sources (Broom 1997).

From 1985 until 1998, Australian women's health initiatives (including the NWHP and programs for its implementation) were guided nationally by the Australian Health Ministers' Advisory Council Subcommittee on Women and Health which consisted of the women's health advisers (from the Commonwealth and all States and Territories), plus representatives of several NGOs and professional bodies (Broom *et al.* 1993). However, special purpose funding for implementing the NWHP ended in the late 1990s, the Subcommittee was dissolved and, except for continuing national oversight of breast and cervix screening programs, women's health activities effectively became the responsibility of the States and Territories.

What happens to women's health policies and programs in such an environment? Because of the dual strategy in women's health, collaboration with mainstream agencies has been occurring for some time on certain issues. For example, many feminist organizations supplying services to women experiencing domestic violence and sexual assault had instigated successful cooperative programs with police, the criminal justice system and hospitals.

Furthermore, within State health departments, there is considerable strategic development designed to support mainstreaming of women's health. For example, in 2000 and 2001, the health departments in both New South Wales and South Australia published women's health frameworks to guide planning and practice for their departments (Gay and Dwyer 2000; NSW Health Department 2000a; NSW Health Department 2000b), and the government of Victoria released a *Women's Health and Well-Being Strategy* in 2002.

In addition, Australia has several national health priority areas (for example injury, heart disease, diabetes) and numerous national public health strategies such as HIV/AIDS and nutrition as well as other national programs, all of which could be shaped by an appreciation of the relevance of gender to health, health promotion and protection, and health service needs. To date, however, there have been no systematic or sustained efforts to ensure that a women's health – let alone gendered – perspective informs any of these activities.

Worlds apart? The British women's health movement

Like their counterparts in Australia, women in the United Kingdom have participated in the development of broad-ranging critiques of contemporary health care systems. They have identified gender bias in the provision of health care at a number of different levels and have highlighted the links with gender inequalities in the wider society. However they have been much less successful in translating these insights into practical changes in the delivery of services. This reflects the different health care systems of the two countries as well as the different trajectories of wider feminist politics in the two settings.

Health activism by women in the United Kingdom was founded on very similar principles to those in Australia (Doyal 1993) including the early focus on sexism and patriarchy, and the use of small groups for consciousness raising and knowledge building. During the 1970s, British activists worked hard to validate their understanding of their own bodies, challenging the superior status accorded to the clinical knowledge of doctors (O'Sullivan 1987). However these new ideas did not lead to the development of separate feminist services as happened in Australia and in the USA, mainly because of the existence of the British National Health Service (NHS).

The NHS is a system of socialized medicine set up in 1948 and based on the principle of health care free at source to all those in need. Throughout its history it has symbolized the values of a society based on collective solidarity. This made it very difficult for many women to criticize the health care they were being offered. The creation of alternative services outside this framework was also seen as politically problematic since it appeared to condone the privatization of health care (Doyal 1983). Such services would be likely to attract a mainly middle class clientele, leaving those in greatest need to cope with the (patriarchal) rigours of the NHS. As a result, only a few explicitly feminist services were set up, mostly offering limited reproductive care such as pregnancy testing. Some psychotherapy services for women were also initiated, reflecting the near total absence of such facilities within the NHS itself.

The early stages of women's health activism in the United Kingdom therefore focused mainly on women taking care of themselves and each other. There was a commitment to ensuring that women had access to information about their own bodies, non-discriminatory health care and fertility control. However radical change in the way services were delivered was difficult to achieve while the NHS itself retained almost iconic status.

These ideological constraints on women's willingness to challenge the status quo in health care were exacerbated after 1979 by the policies of the new conservative government led by Margaret Thatcher. With the introduction of monetarist policies and efforts to reduce public spending, some feared that the existence of the NHS in its original form could no longer be taken for granted. The creation of what was called an internal market and pressures towards the privatization of service delivery all appeared to put the NHS under threat. Under these circumstances the defence of the NHS itself (and other public services) became the major priority for those who might otherwise have been campaigning more directly on women's issues.

In the United Kingdom, as in other developed countries, it is women who are the major users of health care. This reflects their specific needs associated with biological reproduction but also their greater longevity. They have more to lose than men if the quantity and/or quality of services decline. This is especially true in the context of community services which are used most frequently by women (and those for whom they are responsible) but often receive the lowest priority in situations of fiscal restraint. During the Thatcher era for example, there were marked reductions in family planning and abortion services (Doyal 1983; Kennir 1990). Given this gender discrimination, many women chose to resist NHS cuts in ways that highlighted their particular needs.

The form of these campaigns reflected women's importance not only as consumers of health care but also as health workers. Throughout its history, female workers have made up more than 70 per cent of the NHS workforce but they have had little power or influence. As a result they have often been most at risk from deteriorating conditions and intensification of work. In response to these developments, women health workers joined trade unions in increasing numbers during the 1980s. They also initiated new campaigning groups based on their occupational status. These organizations of nurses, midwives, health visitors, medical students and doctors were committed to broadly-based feminist ideas, which they tried to combine with defence of the NHS. A long (and ultimately unsuccessful) campaign was waged for example, to keep open the only women's hospital left in London (Doyal 1983).

Thus, women from a number of different constituencies fought during the Thatcher years to keep the health service they had, but also to reshape it in ways that met their needs more effectively. However this was not a hospitable climate for progressive change, and successes were few and far between (Robinson and LeGrand 1993). In 1997 a Labour government was returned with a manifesto to maintain and improve the NHS. This has meant more funds for some parts of the service and an ambitious 'modernization' agenda (UK Department of Health 1997). However there has been little evidence of an increased commitment to reflect the particular needs of women in this process.

Small groups of women have struggled under both Conservative and Labour governments to achieve greater influence over the running of the NHS and to ensure that services are delivered in more effective and appropriate ways. However this has been a very ad hoc process. Unlike the experience in Australia, there has been no systematic debate about the value of specialist women's services versus gender mainstreaming. The United Kingdom has never had a women's health policy and gender has had low priority in the context of the broader inequalities agenda. Under these circumstances women's efforts can most accurately be described as 'seizing the moment'. Lacking the political power for a sustained push to achieve major reforms, they have pursued a more limited strategy. This strategy has involved seeking out the fault lines created by the modernization of the NHS and using them to push for improvements in care for women.

One of the most visible pressures on health care providers has been the imperative to increase the number of patients treated while resources in some areas are contracting. Many old models of care have become unsustainable and new ways have been sought for organizing services and deploying staff. For example, nurses are replacing junior (sometimes senior) doctors in carrying out a wide range of patient care responsibilities (Doyal *et al.* 1998). These strategies have offered new opportunities for (mostly female) nurses to develop their capacity for autonomous work. At the same time female service users appear to have been the major beneficiaries of these initiatives, which often offer greater continuity of care and higher quality interpersonal communication (Bell 1998).

Over the same period, the development of what has come to be called 'evidence-based medicine' has meant a rapid growth in the monitoring and evaluation of clinical practice as well as more critical consideration of the way medical knowledge is produced. Women in the United Kingdom have tried to ensure that sex and gender issues are highlighted in this process. Drawing on experiences in the US, they have called for regulation to ensure the inclusion of both women and men in clinical trials in appropriate numbers. They have also highlighted the growing evidence of gender bias in diagnosis, treatment and rehabilitation in heart disease and other health problems affecting both sexes (Sharp 1998).

As part of the reshaping or modernization of the NHS, for the first time in the history of the service, the purchasers or commissioners of health care have been required to meet the needs of the population they serve in ways that are open to public scrutiny. For example, the planning process must include consultation with the various groups served, and women have used this opportunity to express their particular needs (Griffiths and Bradlow 1998). In some areas, coalitions of primary care workers, women's groups and community health councils have used this opportunity to obtain an increase in NHS funding for abortion services (Abortion Law Reform Association 1997). Similarly, the question of whether to fund infertility treatment is now being openly discussed in many parts of the country in ways that would previously have been done behind closed doors. (Australia had a prolonged and vigorous debate on this issue during the 1980s.)

There have also been major policy initiatives to bring health and social care closer together in an effort to make service delivery more effective. At the same time there has been a shift towards more care in the community. In some areas, women have been able use the spaces created by these developments to set up small-scale projects which could serve as models for larger initiatives (Amos *et al.* 1998; Wilton 1998). These include new approaches to caring for women with AIDS and new models of support for those with mental health problems. Many have involved collaboration between the NHS and the voluntary sector but too often they have remained as one-offs, cited as examples of good practice but not mainstreamed into the wider NHS (Mills 1996).

As the physical and economic shape of the NHS has been changed there has also been a gradual shift in its basic underlying philosophy, moving away from narrowly focused biomedicine towards a social model of health. Though the response to these developments has been more muted in the United Kingdom than it was in Australia, there has been a growing acceptance of the links between health, illness and daily life. Again this has offered women a new arena for action. Drawing on a wide literature on gender and well-being they have campaigned for greater gender sensitivity in the development of health promotion strategies concerning issues such as smoking, exercise and nutrition (Daykin and Naidoo 1995; Graham 1998). However their influence in these areas continues to be limited.

British women have played an important part in developing the theoretical and conceptual analysis of gender, health and health care. They have also been active in non-governmental organizations (NGOs) and international organizations concerned with the pursuit of gender equity in health on global scale. However they have made relatively little impact on the delivery of health care in their own country.

Global analysis, local strategy: Australian and British initiatives in gendered health

As we have seen, Australian and British feminists were motivated by a common analysis, but they were operating in different political environments, and responding to distinctive national health services regimes. Consequently, they devised very different strategies to advance women's health, and to move forward the broader feminist project. The Australian women's movement has worked within as well as against the state (London Edinburgh Weekend Return Group 1980), manifesting a deep ambivalence towards this institution as simultaneously a protector of dominant (male) interests, and a vehicle for the pursuit of feminist reform (Dowse 1984). Australia has been noted for the numbers of feminists employed in the public service, leading to the neologism 'femocrat' (Sawer 1990). Consequently the Australian women's health movement had friends inside the public sector bureaucracy who contributed to their effectiveness in advocating for funding and policy.

By contrast, a review of feminist politics in the United Kingdom reveals that second-wave women's movements have been characterized by their separation from the activities of state institutions at both local and regional level. Unlike the situation in Australia or the US, British women have not been seen (and have not acted) as a key political constituency. Hence their influence in all areas of policy development has been more limited. Though equal opportunities legislation has been passed, the mechanisms for its implementation remain relatively weak and there are few opportunities for women's voices to be heard in the corridors of power. Thus, the contrast between the achievements of the British and Australian women's health movements can be attributed in part to the nature of their respective health systems; but it also reflects the relative lack of political power of British women and their limited engagement with the state.

Despite these differences, in more recent years, there have been parallels in the direction of political and academic developments surrounding gender and health. For example, in both nations, increasing attention is now being paid to men's health. High quality research is being conducted in the field of men's health, often with direct reference to women's health research (Cameron and Bernardes 1998; Lyons and Willott 1999; Sabo and Gordon 1995; Watson 2000).

There are also developments in policies and services for men. In Australia, in addition to commercial establishments that focus on men's sexual insecurities, and a national research centre in male sexual and reproductive health announced in 1999, several men's health inquiries, projects and programs have been instigated by governments and NGOs. A draft national men's health policy did not become government policy, but there have been four national conferences (1995, 1997, 1999 and 2001) and a report on research priorities in men's health (Connell et al. 1999). New South Wales has a men's health strategy (NSW Health Department 1998, 1999), and some links are being formed between women's health activists and the pro-feminist men's movement (Pugh and Caleidin 2001). Similarly, in the United Kingdom, the Department of Health has also been developing a men's health policy, although in this case, there is no women's health policy to complete the picture.

It remains to be seen how such nationally distinctive histories of gendered health action will affect the array or quality of services available. In the context of growing international emphasis on gender equity (Doyal 2000) and mainstreaming (Rees 1999), Australia and the United Kingdom may become more similar in the next three decades than they have been in the last, at least as far as gendered health services are concerned. On the other hand, the foundations laid during the latter part of the twentieth-century may continue to shape the directions for services and policy, even in the changed political environment.

References

Abortion Law Reform Association (1997) *A report on NHS abortion services.* ALRA, London.

Amos, A., Crossan, E. and Gaunt-Richardson, P. (1998) Women, low income and smoking: developing a 'bottom-up' approach. In L. Doyal (ed.) *Women and health services: an agenda for change*, pp. 178–88. Open University Press, Buckingham.

Annandale, E. and Hunt, K. (2000) *Gender inequalities in health.* Open University Press, Buckingham.

Astbury, J. and Cabral, M. (2000) *Women's mental health: an evidence based review.* World Health Organization, Geneva.

Bell, K. (1998) The establishment of a women-centred gynaecology assessment unit. In L. Doyal (ed.) *Women and health services: an agenda for change*, pp. 141–6. Open University Press, Buckingham.

Boston Women's Health Book Collective (1971) *Our bodies, ourselves: a book by and for women.* Simon and Schuster, New York.

Broom, D. H. (1984) Natural resources: health, reproduction and the gender order. In D. H. Broom (ed.) *Unfinished business: social justice for women in Australia*, pp. 46–62. George Allen & Unwin, North Sydney, Australia.

Broom, D. H. (1991) *Damned if we do: contradictions in women's health care.* Allen & Unwin, Sydney.

Broom, D. H. (1995) Masculine medicine, feminine illness: gender and health. In G. M. Lupton and J. M. Najman (eds) *Sociology of health and illness: Australian readings*, second edn, pp. 99–112. MacMillan, Melbourne.

Broom, D. H. (1997) The best medicine: women using community health centres. *Australian and New Zealand Journal of Public Health*, 21 (3), 275–80.

Broom, D. H. (1998) By women, for women: the continuing appeal of women's health centres. *Women & Health*, 28 (1), 5–22.

Broom, D. H., Dewar, R., Otorepec, M., Ramsay, J. and Renwick, M. (1993) *Health goals and targets for Australian women.* AGPS, Canberra.

Brown, W. J. and Doran, F. M. (1996) Women's health: consumer views for planning local health promotion and health care priorities. *Australian and New Zealand Journal of Public Health*, 20 (2), 149–54.

Cameron, E. and Bernardes, J. (1998) Gender and disadvantage in health: men's health for a change. In M. Bartley, D. Blane and G. Davey Smith (eds) *Sociology of health inequalities*, pp. 115–34. Blackwells, Oxford.

Commonwealth Department of Community Services and Health (1989) *National women's health policy: advancing women's health in Australia.* Australian Government Publishing Service, Canberra.

Connell, R. W., Schofield, T., Walker, L., Wood, J., Butland, D., Fisher, J., *et al.* (1999) *Men's health: a research agenda and background report.* Commonwealth Department Of Health and Aged Care, Canberra.

Daykin, N. and Naidoo, J. (1995) Feminist critiques of health promotion. In R. Bunton, S. Nettleton and R. Burrows (eds) *The sociology of health promotion: critical analyses of consumption, life style and risk,* pp. 59–69. Routledge, London.

Dowse, S. (1984) The bureaucrat as usurer. In D. H. Broom (ed.) *Unfinished business: social justice for women in Australia,* pp. 139–60. George Allen & Unwin, Sydney.

Doyal, L. (1983) Women, health and the sexual division of labour: a case study of the women's health movement in Britain. *Critical Social Policy,* 7, 21–33.

Doyal, L. (1993) Changing medicine? Gender and the politics of health care. In J. Gabe, D. Kellahar and G. Williams (eds) *Challenging medicine.* Tavistock, London.

Doyal, L. (2000) Gender equity in health: debates and dilemmas. *Social Science & Medicine,* 51 (6), 931–39.

Doyal, L., Dowling, S. and Cameron, A. (1998) *Challenging practice: an evaluation of four innovatory nursing posts in the South West.* Policy Press, Bristol.

Dreifus, C. (ed.) (1977) *Seizing our bodies: the politics of women's health.* Vintage, New York.

Foster, S. and Mallik, M. (1998) A comparative study of differences in the referral behaviour patterns of men and women who have experienced cardiac related chest pain. *Intensive and Critical Care Nursing,* 14 (4), 192–202.

Gay, J. and Dwyer, S. (2000) Plan for change: integrating women's health and well being services in rural communities in South Australia, pp. 205–15. Paper presented at International Conference: Primary Health Care 2000 – Creating Healthy Communities. Melbourne.

Goodall, H. and Huggins, J. (1992) Aboriginal women are everywhere: contemporary struggles. In K. Saunders and R. Evans (eds) *Gender relations in Australia: domination and negotiation,* pp. 398–424. Harcourt Brace Jovanovich, Sydney.

Graham, H. (1998) Health at risk: poverty and national health strategies. In L. Doyal (ed.) *Women and health services: an agenda for change,* pp. 22–38. Open University Press, Buckingham.

Gray, G. (1998) How Australia came to have a national women's health policy. *International Journal of Health Services,* 28 (1), 107–25.

Griffiths, S. and Bradlow, J. (1998) Involving women as consumers: the Oxfordshire health strategy. In L. Doyal (ed.) *Women and health services: an agenda for change,* pp. 213–20. Open University Press, Buckingham.

Kennir, B. (1990) *Family planning clinic cuts: a survey of NHS family planning clinics in Greater London.* Family Planning Association, London.

Lee, C. and Porteus, J. (2001) Experiences of family care-giving among middle aged Australian women. *Feminism and Psychology,* 12 (1), 79–96.

London Edinburgh Weekend Return Group (1980) *In and against the state,* revised and expanded edn. Pluto Press, London.

Lyons, A. C. and Willott, S. (1999) From suet pudding to superhero: representations of men's health for women. *Health: An Interdisciplinary Journal for the Social Study of Health, Illness and Medicine,* 3, 283–302.

McKinlay, J. B. (1996) Some contributions from the social system to gender inequalities in heart disease. *Journal of Health and Social Behavior,* 37 (1), 1–26.

Milio, N. (1988) *Making policy: a mozaic [sic] of Australian Community Health Policy development.* Department of Community Services and Health, Canberra.

Mills, M. (1996) Shanti: An intercultural psychotherapy centre for women in the community. In K. Abel, S. Johnson, E. Staples, M. Buscewicz and S. Davison (ed.)

Planning community mental health services for women a multiprofessional handbook. Routledge, London.

Nettleton, S. (1996) Women and the new paradigm of health and medicine. *Critical Social Policy*, **48**, 33–53.

NSW Health Department (1998) *Strategic directions in men's health: a discussion paper.* NSW Health Department, Sydney.

NSW Health Department (1999) *Moving forward in men's health.* NSW Health Department, Sydney.

NSW Health Department (2000a) *Gender equity in health.* NSW Health Department, Sydney.

NSW Health Department (2000b) *Strategic framework to advance the health of women.* NSW Health Department, Sydney.

O'Sullivan, S. (1987) *Women's health: a* Spare Rib *reader.* Pandora Press, London.

Petersen, A. and Lupton, D. (1996) *The new public health: health and self in the age of risk.* Allen & Unwin, St Leonards.

Pringle, R. (1998) *Sex and medicine: gender, power and authority in the medical profession.* Cambridge University Press, Cambridge.

Pugh, L. and Caleidin, C. (2001) In the interests of whom? Gender equity in public health practice. Paper presented at Fourth Australian Women's Health Conference, Adelaide.

Redman, S., Hennrikus, D. J., Bowman, J. A. and Sanson-Fisher, R. W. (1988) Assessing women's health needs. *Medical Journal of Australia*, **148**, 123–7.

Rees, T. (1999) Mainstreaming equality. In S. Watson and L. Doyal (eds), *Engendering social policy*, pp. 165–83. Open University Press, Buckingham.

Robinson, R. and LeGrand, J. (1993) *Evaluating the NHS reforms.* Kings Fund Institute, London.

Ruzek, S. (1978) *Women's health movement: feminist alternatives to medical control.* Praeger, New York.

Sabo, D. and Gordon, D. F. (1995) *Men's health and illness: gender, power and the body.* Sage Publications, Thousand Oaks, CA.

Sawer, M. (1990) *Sisters in suits: women and public policy in Australia.* Allen & Unwin, Sydney.

Sharp, I. (1998) Gender issues in the prevention and treatment of coronary heart disease. In L. Doyal (ed.) *Women and health services: an agenda for change*, pp. 113–26, Open University Press, Buckingham.

Sonke, G. S., Beaglehole, R., Stewart, A. W., Jackson, R. and Stewart, F. M. (1996) Sex differences in case fatality before and after admission to hospital after acute cardiac events: analysis of community based coronary heart disease register. *British Medical Journal*, **313** (October), 853–5.

Steingart, R. M., Packer, M., Hamm, P., Colianese, M. E., Gersh, B., Geltman, E. M. *et al.* (1991) Sex differences in the management of coronary artery disease. *New England Journal of Medicine*, **325** (4), 226–30.

UK Department of Health (1997) *The NHS: modern and dependable.* Stationery Office, London.

Watson, J. (2000) *Male bodies: health, culture and identity.* Open University Press, Buckingham.

Wilton, T. (1998) Gender, sexuality and health care: improving services. In L. Doyal (ed.) *Women and health services: an agenda for change*, pp. 147–62. Open University Press, Buckingham.

Chapter 3

Services for Older People

Christina R. Victor

Introduction

As a society, the United Kingdom has developed a variety of services in response to the perceived needs of older people and 'old age' more generally. In this chapter we consider health sector responses to the issues of ageing in terms of the services designed for or used by older people. Policy makers in the United Kingdom, as in many other countries, are concerned about the anticip- ated 'burden' upon health services as a result of population ageing trends, described by Jefferys (1983) as a 'moral panic'. At the level of individual service provision, a strong humanitarian tradition within British policy development and within gerontology has led to a move away from the stereotyped emphasis upon ageing as a problem both for the individual and the wider society. However, as we are examining issues concerned with service needs, delivery and use, the problem-orientated approach to the issues facing individuals and populations will figure more prominently in this chapter. At both the individual and societal level, policy makers see old age as a tragedy or crisis, which requires a response. This chapter focuses upon the delivery of health services and their responses to the problems presented by older individuals. However, all elements of service provision and development are located within the broader macrocontext of how governments understand and respond to the issue of population ageing. We start by offering a brief history of the development of health and social welfare services for older people in the UK. This historical context forms the backdrop against which to examine the patterns of health care need presented by older people and their utilization of these services, and to present some of the key policy debates. Although this chapter draws mainly upon the experience in the UK, the issues raised have a wider resonance.

The development of health services for older people

Within the British social welfare context it is only fairly recently that 'the elderly' were identified as a specific social problem group set apart from the general mass of the indolent, the poor and the destitute. In the Victorian period, the problems of 'aged paupers' were distinguished and, with the establishment of a system of pensions, the state made separate provision to respond to these problems. Older people were considered a 'deserving' group and arrangements were put in place to respond to their basic needs. Old age was, for the pauper at least, conceptualized by the Victorians as a personal tragedy to which measured responses were required. The introduction of the first pensions in the nineteenth century marked a change in thinking. Before this, older people were predominantly the responsibility of the family and were not identified as a separate social group or one with distinct problems. Since the development of the post-war welfare state, which began in 1948, older people have had access to a wide range of health and social welfare services. However, in undertaking a review of patterns of need, utilization and key policy debates, it is important to remember that comparatively few such services were designed specifically for older people per se. Rather, older people use the generic provisions encompassed within the broad structure of the welfare state, which was designed to cater for all 'from cradle to grave'.

The chronological definition used by governments and policy makers to define older people has remained remarkably constant over the last eight decades and is linked to the age of eligibility for the state retirement pension, currently 65 for men and 60 for women (although this is being equalized upwards for women). These threshold ages were established in the 1920s when longevity in the UK was considerably less than the current 76 years for men and 80 years for women, while the 'average' 60-year-old can expect to live for another twenty years. As a result of this demographic change, 75 per cent of the population can expect to reach their late seventies. The welfare state generally, and health services specifically, has been slow to respond to the universalization of the experience of old age.

The increase in the numbers of older people has led scholars and researchers to recognize the greater heterogeneity of this population and, consequently, considerable variation in their needs for health care (Phillipson 1998). However, the diverse nature of the older population is rarely recognized in policy terms. Rather, government policy for older people articulates two main stereotypes of old age. The most enduring stereotype conceptualizes older people as being both 'needy' and 'deserving' (similar to the earlier distinction between the deserving and undeserving poor). They are presented as being lonely, isolated, neglected by their family, in poor mental and physical health, badly housed and poor. This presumption as to the experience of old age has been highly influential and has generated considerable research in the humanitarian 'old age as a social problem' type of approach, for example, the work of Tunstall (1963).

It has also influenced the development of services with older people being seen as having a single set of needs, a common set of social circumstances that have merited a universalist type of response. More recently, a new stereotype has emerged with the discovery of the WOOPIE (the well off older person) and the development of consumption-based definitions of old age, such as the distinction between the 'third' and 'fourth' ages (Gilleard and Higgs 2000). Recognition of the greater diversity of the older population, the varying needs presented, and the variety of possible service responses, has resulted in a greater emphasis upon assessment before the delivery of care packages. Whilst we can see evidence of a more sophisticated evaluation of service needs, it is not yet clear that service responses, especially for those with intensive care needs, have matched the articulated demands.

Unlike the United States, there are no specific acts in the UK concerned with older people. With no equivalent to the Older Americans Act, services have developed in different ways, although it is still possible to identify the 'ageing enterprise' proposed by Estes (1979). The ageing enterprise consists of the myriad of professional and voluntary organizations, professionals and special programmes and projects involved in the care of older people. Estes argues that all of these enterprises have a vested interest in the maintenance of the 'separateness' of older people, and in perpetuating stereotypes of a universal set of needs that can be met by a uniform set of policy responses. Despite the development of selected specialist services for older people, such as geriatric medicine, the general development of health services for older people in Britain has been within the universalist model. However, we can still see evidence of the ageing enterprise in the often spatial separation of older peoples' services from the mainstream, and by the outposting of specialist services for older people away from the main hospital sites.

The provision of health services in Britain

The National Health Service (NHS), created in 1948, provides health services in the UK. The mission statement of the NHS includes a commitment (or aspiration) to an ideology of social and spatial equity by providing users with equal access to care of equal quality. Clinical need is the criterion for the provision of services, which are largely provided free of charge at the point of consumption and funded largely out of general taxation. Unlike, for example, the US, where entry to programmes such as Medicare is based upon chronological age, it is clinical need that determines entitlement to health services in the UK. Hence claims to the services provided by the health service tend to be articulated in terms of clinical categories, such as mental health services or HIV services, rather than in terms of population groups such as older people (although there are some exceptions). Debates concerning entitlement are, therefore, often articulated in very different terms from those conducted in insurance/private health care systems. An example of the population claims approach is illustrated by the recent debate about pension provision and entitlement, although this remains an underdeveloped line of debate within a UK health care context. Entitlement to health and social welfare is based more upon need than age, although chronological age may frame how those needs are defined and met. However, age is clearly an important factor both in designing services and as an organizational principle. For example, the remit of screening services, such as breast and cervical screening, is based upon age, which is used as an indicator of increasing risk, although for both these cancers those at highest risk of death are excluded. Similarly, some services, such as paediatrics, are developed around the chronological age of the client group; others, such as cardiology, are organized around the treatment requirements of specific conditions or body systems: the major organizing principle for hospital/secondary care.

The British health care system makes a major distinction between primary care and secondary care. Primary health care is provided via a system of general practitioners who act as gatekeepers to secondary care and other specialist services, such as various forms of therapy, specialist disease-based management clinics and a range of health promoting initiatives. Every member of the population is registered with a practice, which may range from a single doctor to a large health centre operated by a group of practitioners from different health care professions. The members of the primary health care team, involving doctors, nurses, and health visitors, work together to provide a comprehensive service to patients. The importance of the role of primary care should not be underestimated, as it is both a direct care provider and the entry point to specialist care. Thus primary care has a key role both in treating older people and in referring them on to secondary services. In both these facets of operation there is obviously scope for variation in the way older people are treated.

The NHS from its creation in 1948 incorporated the three existing non-profit hospital sectors (public, voluntary and public assistance) into one system. Hence we nationalized existing inequities in both access to care and quality of care for older people and the population more generally. Each sector had catered for a different type of patient and could exert varying degrees of power over who they would (and would not) admit. For example, voluntary hospitals were run on a charitable basis and, as such, could choose the type of patients they wished to treat, often developing an admissions policy focusing upon the acutely ill and the exclusion of the chronic sick. This pattern was adopted by the main public hospitals, so that it was left to public assistance hospitals to look after the chronically sick, most of whom were elderly. These latter hospitals were largely detached from developments in mainstream medicine and health care. This professional and spatial separation of the chronic and acute sick is a feature that still pervades the modern organization of hospital-based medicine in the UK. It took the establishment of the Emergency Medical Service during the Second World War to 'rediscover' the plight of the chronically sick by drawing attention to the large number of beds, required to treat war casualties, that were occupied by this group of patients (Means and Smith 1998).

Whilst there is little evidence of macro-scale debates about the claims of older people to health care in the UK, there are vigorous debates as to the legitimacy of older peoples' claims to certain components of the health care system. Almost from the start of the NHS, the entitlement of older frail patients to treatment in an acute hospital setting has been contested. The issue of the 'appropriate' use of hospital beds by older people is a constant theme running through the history of health care provision for older people and has been a fruitful topic for researchers and policy makers alike (Means and Smith 1998). The National Beds Enquiry (Department of Health 2000; Goddard 2000), for example, report that up to 20 per cent of bed-days for older people are used 'un-necessarily' and that such individuals are best treated outside the acute sector.

The development of geriatric medicine

The stimulus for the creation of specialist medical services for the old came from a variety of sources, reflecting both general trends within medicine and concerns specific to older people. As the twentieth century progressed the range of treatments available, combined with the changing nature of disease, resulted in the increasing specialization of medicine and the emergence of new specialities, such as paediatrics and cardiology. We can see the emergence of geriatric medicine as part of a general trend within the medical profession towards increasing specialization. Within the hospital sector there were both positive and negative factors involved in the creation of the new speciality. The negative factors focus upon the perceived problem of bed blocking and delayed discharge by older patients. It was widely felt that large numbers of hospital beds were occupied by older people who, although medically fit for discharge, could not be sent home because of inappropriate social circumstances, thereby blocking beds. Concerns about the costs of treating older people were also raised because of their long length of stay and its consequent economic implications. However, the impetus to develop specialist hospital-based medical services for older people was not entirely negative. In the 1950s, pioneers of effective rehabilitation (Dr Marjorie Warren at the West Middlesex Hospital) and early post-operative mobilization and rehabilitation (Mr Cosin at Orsett Hospital in Essex) demonstrated that older patients could be treated and managed effectively within the context of a modern health service. It was argued that the creation of a specialist geriatric medicine department within a general hospital, concentrating upon the clinical, preventive, remedial and social aspects of health and disease in old age, would improve the quality of care received by older patients and optimize the use of hospital resources by reducing the blocking of beds and length of hospital stay. Hence, although there were concerns with quality of care, geriatric medicine has also used arguments concerned with effective resource use to justify its existence.

The defining features of geriatric medicine are concerned with the assessment, diagnosis, rehabilitation and continuing care of older adults. However, a continuing debate is whether geriatric medicine is a true medical speciality and whether it is the most effective way of responding to the health care needs of older adults. Are there principles of care that are unique to the clinical management of the older adult? Can a speciality be based upon age as a key defining criterion? Although the age focus of geriatrics is questioned, paediatrics does not have similar problems in justifying its existence, except perhaps at the adolescent end of the age spectrum. Whilst the founding principles of geriatric medicine remain fairly constant, there have been profound changes in the nature of the older population and the treatment potential available to them. Initially the age focus of geriatric medicine was all those aged 65 years and over. This group now represents about 35 per cent of all hospital episodes and 60 per cent of bed days. The age-focus of geriatric medicine thus has moved ever upwards with an emphasis now upon those in their late seventies and older. In addition, the scope and effectiveness of interventions for older people available in other branches of medicine, such as cardiology, renal medicine and orthopaedics, has expanded considerably. Hence older people who once were the client of the geriatrician are now treated in other medical specialities.

Hospitals are organized according to two main models of care. In the specialist model, departments of geriatric medicine treat all patients, acutely or chronically ill, above a defined age; in the generic model, geriatric and general (internal) medical services are integrated, with certain consultants having a special interest in the care of older people. A recent survey by the British Geriatrics Society reported that there has been a move away from an age related model towards a more integrated model of service delivery. At the inception of the NHS, Amulree recommended the evaluation of the effectiveness of both the NHS and its newly created departments of geriatric medicine (Amulree 1955).

Despite this forward-looking statement that anticipates the recent development of evidence-based health care, there has been little research on the effectiveness of hospital treatment of the old or on the effectiveness of different models of care. The absence of conclusive evaluation data makes it difficult to be definitive as to the best (i.e. most effective) model of care. To some degree, the preferred model of care reflects current fashion and thinking as to the relative merits of generic/specialist services within the NHS more broadly. It also reflects the changing nature of the older population, in terms of health care needs, the potential interventions available in other branches of medicine and the availability of other types of services. For example, older people being cared for in long-term care show much higher levels of frailty and disability than in the early days of the NHS. This 'dependency creep' is evident in other parts of the health care system, since increasingly frail elders are maintained at home rather than in institutions. As 'care in the community' is the main focus of government policy for older people, the increasing frailty of the acute hospital population may be taken as an indicator of the success of this policy.

Need for health services

Older people account for the major concentration of health problems within modern western societies. In England and Wales, of the 532,498 deaths in 2000, 80 per cent were aged 65 years and over (Office for National Statistics 2002). Rates of both mortality and morbidity, as measured by long-standing health problems, increase with age. For example, death rates increase from 14 per 1000 for those aged 65–74 years to 158 per 1000 for those aged 85 years and over, whilst rates of long-standing illness double for the same age groups (from 37 per cent to 60 per cent) (National Centre for Survey Research 2002). Similar patterns are evident for other measures of morbidity, such as disability or mental health.

Within this broad pattern of increasing mortality and morbidity with age, there are important variations in the health status of older people. Although men are less likely to reach old age, those that do demonstrate lower levels of chronic illness than their female counterparts. Similarly, those from more privileged social backgrounds demonstrate consistently lower levels of health problems than the less privileged. Hence old age is characterized by profound inequalities in health status and these largely represent a continuity of earlier phases in the life cycle. Since until recently, the presumption was that older people represented a homogeneous group in terms of health status because all old people were ill, little attention has been given to enumerating and combating inequalities in health in later life. For example, Victor (1991) demonstrates that a male aged 85 and over from the highest social classes 1 and 2 has a lower rate of long-standing limiting illness than his 65–69 year old counterpart from the unskilled/semi-skilled manual classes. Even less attention has been paid to inequities in access to treatment and the quality of care offered to older people. There is some evidence of gender variations within the older age groups in terms of both access to care and the quality of care offered to older people (Bowling 1999). However, the situation for class and ethnicity is unclear.

Levels of provision and utilization of services

What services should we provide and in what quantities? Health services for older people have developed in a piecemeal and pragmatic fashion with central government reluctant to formulate any detailed norms of provision or prescribe models of care. Although the NHS aspired to the vision of equal access to services of equal quality for all subjects, the reality is wide variations in access to care, quality of care and care outcomes. In the late 1990s the English Department (Ministry) of Health initiated a series of initiatives to improve and standardize the quality of care provided in the NHS. These included the creation of a new body, the National Institute for Clinical Excellence (NICE), which was given the task of developing a response to 'post-code prescribing', whereby patients with the same needs had differential access to treatment depending upon where they lived. NICE issues guidance upon the availability of drugs, such as Viagra and other medical interventions. It also has developed National Service Frameworks (NSF), that draw upon evidence assessed rigorously by expert panels, contain guidelines for prevention and treatment of disease, and are focused either on broad disease areas, such as cardiovascular disease, or upon the needs of designated groups, such as older people. The long-term aim of these developments is to reduce inequalities in health in terms of access, quality of care and outcomes.

The National Service Framework for Older People

The Older People's National Service Framework, published in 2001, is a ten-year programme designed to promote the development of 'fair, high quality, integrated health and social care services for older people'. It is intended to support independence in later life, promote health, develop specialized services for key conditions and ensure that older people and their carers are treated with respect, dignity and fairness. The four main principles of the NSF are:

+ To root out age discrimination;
+ Provide person-centred care;
+ Promote health and independence; and
+ Match services to needs.

These aims are to be achieved via the implementation of eight standards , each of which has milestones and performance monitoring elements. The response has been mixed. The Framework is certainly a positive development in that it recognizes age discrimination and the importance of older people to the health service (and vice versa). However, some commentators are more critical. For example, Grimley Evans and Tallis (2001) interpret the move towards 'intermediate care' as a not very subtle way of excluding older people from the acute hospital and recreating a warehousing solution to the (perceived) problems of providing care to older people. By extension, such policy solutions raise the spectre of poor quality care provided to a low status patient group in poor quality accommodation away from the main hospital campus. Hence the popularity of the intermediate care solution may be seen as another manifestation of the debate concerning the entitlement of older people to acute hospital beds.

Apart from these general guidelines, the British Geriatrics Society has a very old consensus statement as to staffing and minimum levels of provision, such as 10 beds per 1000 population aged 65 years and over (Vetter *et al.* 1981). These are rather outdated, and do not sit easily with the new rhetoric of needs rather than service-led arrangements, as they are formulated entirely in terms of resources. The comparison with the National Service Framework standards illustrates how far we have travelled in the last few decades in terms of our thinking about the health service provision for older people. It remains, however, a matter of speculation as to how much difference changes in rhetoric make to the care received by older people. The old guidelines had an aspirational quality as to the numbers of staff and resources required for running a comprehensive geriatric service, recognizing that it is difficult to provide good quality care without adequate physical or staffing resources. In comparison, the National Service Framework for older people is rather more coy about the resources required to provide adequate care, although it is much stronger on the processes required and has a more multidisciplinary focus and a clear implementation timetable.

Utilization of services

What use do older people make of the three main components of welfare state health services: the institutional sector, acute hospital services; and community health and medical services? Expenditure on health services for older people is considerable in both absolute and relative terms (Seshamani and Gray 2002). In England and Wales, total health expenditure in 1998–99 was £32.7 billion, of which 35.6 per cent was accounted for by those aged 65 and over. Per capita expenditure increased over the age range from £1088 for those aged 65–74 years to £2517 for those aged 85 and over (approximately five times that for a person aged 16–44). However, these authors demonstrate that the percentage of expenditure on those aged 65 and over decreased from 40.2 per cent in 1985–87 to 35.6 per cent in 1998–99 (despite both and absolute and relative increase in this age group). This is in sharp contrast to Japan, Australia and Canada where expenditure increased. The decrease in health expenditure in England and Wales thus may well reflect the shift of the costs of long-term care to the social care and income support budgets as well as to private individuals.

Apart from calculating expenditure, we can examine the use made by older people of health services in two distinct but complementary ways. The first approach investigates older people as a part of all users of health care. The second approach examines what percentage of all older people use health services. Both perspectives are adopted here as each is informative as to the resources provided in response to the 'problems' of old age. The first approach examines routine hospital data in terms of finished consultant episodes. This NHS measure of hospital activity describes a defined period of care under a specific consultant (specialist), although it does not neatly equate to a stay in hospital, which may include several individual consultant episodes. Older people are consistently the major 'user' group for most branches of hospital medicine. In 2000/01, there were over 12 million finished consultant episodes in England of which 33.8 per cent were accounted for by those aged 65 and over, even though this age group is only 15 per cent of the population (14.2 per cent were aged 65–74: 13.4 per cent were aged 75–84 and 6.2 per cent were aged 85 and over) (Department of Health 2002b).

The other way to look at service use is to consider what percentage of the target population, in this case older people, use different types of services. The percentage of people reporting an inpatient stay in the previous year increases with age, as does the length of stay. For example 18 per cent of those aged 75 and over had been admitted in the previous year and had an average of 16 nights in hospital per annum. In addition, 10 per cent of those aged 75 and over had been treated as day case patients. About 20 per cent of older people report a GP consultation in the 14 days and those aged 75 and over have, on average, six consultations a year. Given the predominance of older people as clients of both hospital and community-based services, perhaps such services should regard older patients as the norm and design services with their needs in mind, rather than treating older users as a deviant minority group. Clearly, in terms of both expenditure and utilization older people receive more health services than do the young. However, given the concentration of morbidity in older age groups, this high use reflects clinical need: therefore, services are being allocated in line with the main criterion of clinical need.

Key issues in organizing health services for older people

Within the broad British social policy context health service responses to the perceived problems of old age and older people may be categorized in several different ways, reflecting wider debates about how best to organize effective service delivery to those in need. Four major themes may be identified:

- The type of care needs presented;

- Who provides care;

- The location of care provision; and

- Access to care.

Within each of these areas, major policy issues operate at different levels ranging from macro (societal) to micro (individuals and families).

Classifying care needs

There is an important policy and provision demarcation between the types of needs (or problems) presented by the older person – or indeed any other age group. Policy makers draw a distinction between those services concerned with meeting health needs from those concerned with meeting social care needs. This reflects the two arms of the post-1945 welfare state, which differentiated health services, designed to cater for those with health problems, and social care services, designed for those with non-health problems such as personal or house care needs. The presumption that health care needs can be clearly and distinctly separated from social care needs is at the heart of the British system of social welfare (Means and Smith 1998). Hence health care provision for older people involves a series of potentially frustrating boundary disputes (between acute and chronic care and between health and social care). Emblematic of the notion of the contested boundary is the requirement by older people for help with bathing. Approximately 7 per cent of those aged 65 and over in Britain (680,000 people) are unable to bath/shower. The need to maintain personal hygiene is central to maintaining the dignity and independence of the older person, and the requirement for a service response, where there are no other sources of help, is clear and incontrovertible. However help with bathing is defined variously as a social or a health need and has become the subject of demarcation disputes between the caring agencies (Twigg 2000). The consequences of such organizational disputes can, however, be very profound for the older person who simply wants to maintain his or her personal hygiene!

Similarly, boundary disputes can characterize the entry of older people into long-stay care. Although the providers of long-stay care have changed dramatically over the past two decades, the basic duality of the system has not. The residential care sector cares for those who, though frail, only need care and attention, whilst the nursing home sector (which has replaced long-stay wards in hospitals) cares for those with health needs. With the development of nursing homes the NHS has virtually withdrawn from direct long-stay provision (although it remains responsible for funding where people need continuing medical care). Long-stay hospital beds were a relic of the chronic sick wards of public and poor law institutions inherited with the creation of the NHS. Further, the UK was virtually unique in being the only country that had hospital beds for which the length of stay was, in principle at least, indefinite. The withdrawal of the hospital sector from direct long-stay provision reflects the NHS redefinition of hospital care in terms of acute care, and the consequent shift of the cost of long-term care from the hospital sector to social services and individuals. Hence the claim of older people to state-funded, health service-provided long-term care has been undermined. This represents another example of the debate about claims to care being conducted in terms of what types of care different groups can access rather than whether they can legitimately access care at all.

Clearly, given older peoples' often complex needs it is problematic to draw this distinction between health care needs and social care needs. This point was made almost from the inception of the British system (Means and Smith 1998), when concerns were expressed about those who would fall between the remits of the different services, or whose complex needs would mean that they would become the contested responsibility of both parties. This requirement for services to categorize needs into social or health is not simply an issue of interest to academics and policy makers. Rather, as the example of bathing illustrates, it is important for individual service users, as the different arms of the welfare state have differing philosophies, structures and eligibility criteria that can have important consequences for older people and their families. If an older person has health needs then these are provided free to the user, whilst needs that are defined as falling within the remit of social care may require users to pay. This meant that those who entered long-stay care because of health problems received free care whereas those who had social care needs had to contribute to the costs (if they had sufficient means). This anomaly resulted in a report (Royal Commission on Long-Term Care 1999), which concluded that whilst the nursing element of long-term care should be free, other components such as personal care should be charged. This remains the position in England, but as a result of devolution the Scottish assembly has determined that all long-stay care for older people in Scotland should be free. Claims for care are, therefore, being articulated and defined in terms of nationality and residence.

What is the best model of care?

This debate incorporates several differing dimensions relating to whether generic or specialist staff and agencies should provide services for older people. Again, this debate is not confined to issues concerning older people. Rather, there are echoes as to how we respond to the needs of children, to special groups within the population such as homeless people or refugees, or to complex and emerging diseases such as HIV/AIDS. This debate centres upon the most effective and appropriate ways to provide care. Those in favour of the specialist approach argue that, given the difficulties the health/welfare system has dealing with those with complex needs or difficult circumstances, such groups are best served by specialist, expert services. The generic argument holds that, however complex or difficult the needs presented by a specific client group, the general system should be of such good quality in terms of administration and quality that it can care for all groups. The generic argument implies, if not specifically articulates, that to deal with groups outside of the mainstream both marginalizes, stigmatizes and ghettoizes such groups and those who work with them. Hence the care of older people becomes someone else's problem. A recent British Geriatrics Society survey (2002) suggests that the integrationist model is in the ascendancy.

This debate is illustrated within the health service where there has been persistent concern as to the most appropriate model of care for older people. Should services be specialist and age based, with care to people above a threshold age provided by specialist services (variously called medicine for old age, health care for older people, geriatric medicine etc.), or are older people best served by the generic services? This specialist versus generic debate is not exclusive to older people and can be seen in other areas such as the treatment of stroke or HIV/AIDS. Perhaps it is within the realm of the specialist services for older people that we can see elements of the ageing enterprise thesis advanced by Estes (1979). Are older peoples' needs best met by services where age is the criterion for entry, or do such services serve to detach older people from the mainstream and thereby isolate and stigmatize them and provide an implicit justification for the delivery of sub-standard care? There is some limited evidence, based upon observation data, that older people have a better outcome after treatment in geriatric medicine rather than general medicine (Victor and Vetter 1989) and that length of stay is shorter (Rai et al. 1985). However, the absence of rigorous evaluation data comparing outcomes makes it is difficult to come to a firm conclusion as to the best model of care. It is clear, however, that older people in an acute hospital setting often experience poor quality care and show evidence of neglect such as malnourishment (Hospital Advisory Services 2000). Such failings may reflect the level of resources rather than limitations of the model of care.

Coordinating care

Within the current configuration of the welfare state, different agencies are involved in the provision of health care to older people, even more if we include social care. Within the health service, both primary and secondary care sectors are heavily involved (including independent contractors). Even considering only the most basic aspects of the health service response to older people, it is obvious that this variety of agencies all have varying professional objectives and differing modes of working. Such dislocations in care pathways are most evident at specific transition points, such as admission and discharge from hospital or arranging assessment and admission to long-term care. The issue of discharging older people from hospital back into the community exemplifies the organizational problems that beset the care of those groups within the population whose needs cross the boundaries of the caring services. There is a significant body of research dating back to the early days of the NHS documenting the numerous dislocations in the delivery of care when older people are discharged from hospital back to the community (Means and Smith 1998), such as the blocking of hospital beds by older people awaiting discharge (Victor *et al.* 2000). Both delayed discharge and problematic discharges reflect the interplay of differing factors. Healy and Victor developed a model with four sets of factors associated with delayed discharge: predisposing factors such as age, enabling factors such as presence of a family carer, health/functional factors such as level of dependency, and organizational factors such as type of multidisciplinary team and supply of resources (Healy *et al.* 1999). They also note that discharge problems reflect the much deeper structural tensions across the health/social care and primary/secondary care interfaces. Where caring agencies have differing eligibility criteria, assessment methods and underlying philosophies then dislocations in care are to be expected.

Where is care provided?

We can also distinguish between the locations where services for older people are provided, and again there are vigorous debates as to the most appropriate locations for the provision of care. One debate concerns the boundaries between primary and secondary care. Hospital services have been extended beyond the hospital buildings with the development of 'hospital at home' schemes. Perhaps the most important debate within the post-war British welfare state surrounds the respective merits of institutional- versus community-based responses to groups such as older people. The idea of caring for older people in group or institutional settings is neither novel nor recent. Rather, it has been an enduring component of the development of services for older people in Britain (Means and Smith 1998). Thus Townsend (1964), in his book *The last refuge*, attacked the quality of residential care provided for older people in post-war Britain. He drew attention to inappropriate buildings (usually old workhouses), inadequate facilities and the regimented quality of life for the residents. These empirical data meshed in a rare synergy with the theoretically informed writings of Goffman (Goffman 1963, 1968), who noted the inhuman, depersonalizing and all pervasive timetabled nature of life within an institutional setting. The notion of the 'total institution' resonated with the empirically based critique proffered by Townsend. Academic research and sociological theory, combined with the revelation of systematic and sustained abuse in various British long-stay hospitals, merged to create a powerful perception that institutional care was inherently a bad thing. Irrespective of the resources and funds involved, institutional care solutions were seen as being inherently ineffective and inhumane. Hence the concept of community care is imbued with both positive attributes (the cosy and comforting image of the caring community as personified by some radio and television soap operas) and important negative ones (i.e. it is not institutional care!). This is another example of policies being defined in terms of negative outcomes (what they are not or are seeking to avoid) rather than being based upon a more positive goal.

Community care remains the favoured policy goal for the care of the older people, although it is now a very different conceptualization – care being largely provided *by* the community rather than *in* the community – (Victor 1997) from that conceived by the original proponents of community care. In our acceptance of the posited expense of institutional care, its inherent inhumanity and presumed therapeutic ineffectiveness, we have not always examined community care with the critical, in the sense of reflective and questioning, gaze that such major policy goals deserve. The presumed implicit financial advantage of community care, at least for people with intensive needs, is highly questionable. Furthermore, the term 'community care' has been subject to an Orwellian redefinition. Less attention has been paid to questioning the inherent advantages of community-based solution in terms of therapeutic effectiveness and humanity. There are comparatively few studies that have compared community versus institutional forms of provision for those with long-term care needs. Clearly, there are schemes that are effective in terms of preventing or delaying entry to long-term care and others where, for example, community-based physiotherapy compares well with group provision such as in day hospitals. There are also effective 'hospital at home' schemes. However, the recipients of these services are not entirely comparable with the types of people and services found in the institutional sector. Overall, the research evidence suggests that community-based solutions may be as effective as those provided in institutional settings, such as hospitals, day hospitals or nursing/residential homes, but the debate about cost-effectiveness is more problematic. Less interest has been expressed in looking at the presumed humanitarian advantage of people staying on in their own home in the community. However, in theory at least, the care of very dependent people within their own home can reproduce many of the undesirable features associated with institutions such as a constrained lifestyle, lack of choice and routines established for the benefit or providers rather users.

Providing services or assessing needs?

As originally organized, the British welfare state established a series of health and social care services, which were service rather than needs led. Within the health service context, a framework of acute district general hospitals was established, underpinned by a primary care family doctor service and domiciliary nursing services. The initial social care framework of the welfare state was largely service rather than needs based and came to be typified by three specific services: home help, meals on wheels and community nursing. Why were these services identified and how appropriate are they for meeting older peoples needs and achieving the wider policy objective of maintaining older people in the community? Similar points are made about health care services, where they are often provided in terms of medical specialities such as ophthalmology and cardiology, rather than dealing with a particular condition, such as diabetes, in an integrated fashion. To some degree the development of service frameworks may be seen as an attempt to develop treatment in terms of diseases rather than subdivisions of the medical profession.

More recent policy developments have attempted to overcome these fundamental limitations by developing a needs-led service, based upon comprehensive single assessment process and the design of an appropriate care package. This perspective is exemplified in standard two of the National Service Framework for Older People and the development of the single assessment process. Although the philosophy has changed, it is not yet clear whether service delivery has become more innovative, and whether this has resulted in real improvements in the quality of care provided or the lives of older people. Certainly, the Framework offers guidance as to what to include in the single assessment and offers a timetable for the implementation of the process. It is, however, silent upon the issue of resources required to respond to identified needs. To date, the emphasis is more concerned with the process than the outcome of assessment. In terms of data collection, routine statistics still collate information about home care services and routine surveys, such as the General Household Survey, continue to ask questions about the receipt of traditional services such as home help, mobile meals, district nursing and health visiting, medical specialities or operations undertaken. Such service-led data preclude a vigorous debate as to the effectiveness of services in meeting needs.

Who provides care?

The recent history of the NHS is of a creeping trend towards the privatization of care, especially in the field of long-stay care provision and domiciliary based caring services. In addition, the health service, especially the secondary care sector, has sought both to draw its boundaries to exclude chronic health problems and to shift the costs of caring for such groups upon to the social care sector and individual users. In the UK about 5 per cent of those aged 65 years and over are in long-term care. The privatization of long-term care has developed rapidly such that 92 per cent of homes and 85 per cent of all places are now provided by the private sector (this includes the voluntary bodies). The expansion of private sector care, in both institutional and community environments, has been encouraged by an ideological debate about the provision of welfare that has preoccupied Britain for the past two decades. The philosophy underpinning the development of private sector involvement within a state welfare system is rooted in the primacy of individual responsibility, a belief in the efficiency of the market as a method of organizing the distribution of goods and services, and a repudiation of state-provided welfare services as inefficient, unresponsive, mediocre in standards and unresponsiveness to the needs and wants of users (or consumers). The development of private care solutions has been justified by reference to the following themes:

(1) Meeting the existing, but unsatisfied, demand for care;

(2) Expanding the choices and autonomy of older people (and their relatives);

(3) Decreasing the power of professionals and 'experts';

(4) Reducing inequality in old age by extending the available choice;

(5) Improving quality for with private care providers the older person has the freedom to move if (s)he is dissatisfied with the standard of care provided; and

(6) The comparative failure of the public sector to respond to the changing nature of the older population and their needs and wants.

However, there remains scant evidence to support the view that private care has driven up standards in either long-term care or domiciliary settings.

Access to care

The final issue relates to the access to care by older people. The National Service Framework for Older People has taken up the battle against ageism and age discrimination as its first challenge. This a complex issue with several different elements, including entitlement to care (should we use age to ration care?), simple access to services (can older people get the care they need?), and the quality of care (are older people treated to the same quality of care as other groups?) The debate is further complicated by differences in how the varying subgroups of the older population are treated. Are older men more likely to receive care than older women? Do issues of class and race matter? Clearly, the whole debate around ageism and age-discrimination is highly complex, especially when the primary/secondary care distinction is included.

There are essentially two positions in terms of the attitudes towards age-based rationing of health care and the relative entitlement or claims of different groups within the population to care. Williams (1997) argues for the 'fair innings' thesis, in that once a certain age has been achieved then priority for treatment should be given to other age groups. Consequently, above a certain age there should be no entitlement or claim to care and societal debate would determine where this boundary should be drawn. In this scenario, the older person's previous contribution to society does not bring with it an open-ended claim to (limited) health care resources. For example, we could determine that no acute interventions such as dialysis or pacemakers should be prescribed to people aged 80 and over, or that those above a certain age should not be resuscitated in the event of a collapse. Overt ageism with specific age bars to services such as cardiology are less evident but covert ageism is more difficult to identify (Bowling 1999). The Department of Health (2002b) reports that 41 health service areas have age-related policies (some of which positively discriminate in favour of older people). There is clear evidence that older people experience discrimination in accessing care and in the quality of care provided, and that differing groups within the older age groups are differentially treated. The Department of Health report acknowledges the lack of clarity concerning terms such as age discrimination and the widespread nature of implicit age discrimination.

Grimley Evans (1997) supports the view that age is a very imprecise mechanism by which to allocate care and that we should treat older people individually according to their needs. This view suggests that, irrespective of chronological age, older people have a legitimate claim to care rooted in past contributions to society and the intergenerational contract. Clearly this is the view accepted by the NHS, and the first standard is concerned with eradicating age discrimination and negative attitudes towards older people.

Conclusion

The history of health service development for older people in the UK is characterized by responses to a variety of factors, including disenchantment with institutionalized care, the expense of providing such care, fears about the numbers of older people requiring care, and a perception that community care is a cheap option compared with other forms of provision. Perhaps the most interesting feature of the development of policy for older people is the way that it has evolved in a highly pragmatic fashion, with little reference to the needs and wants of the consumers of care, perhaps because the UK lacks an effective political age-based lobby group or because of a stereotype of the universal nature of the health care needs of older people. Policy developments for older people are driven more by the needs of professional groups than the expressed wishes of older people themselves. The power of professional vested interests continues to strongly influence policy development. In particular, there is still a tendency to deny the autonomy of older people and to provide them with the sorts of services we think are good for them, rather than responding to their expressed wishes. Furthermore, services have tended to promote a universalist set of responses to the needs of the older person. Remarkably little attention is paid to the variations within older age groups, in terms of gender, class and ethnicity, and how these might influence service needs. There has been little explicit recognition of the importance of health inequalities within the older age groups in terms of health status, access to care and health outcomes. The predominantly negative perception of the health of older people means that little emphasis has been given to promoting and enhancing the health of older people, despite the potential of such interventions for improving the quality of life of older people (Ginn *et al.* 1997; Killoran *et al.* 1997; Victor and Howse 2000).

Many of the recent policy developments related to older people are designed to prevent specific adverse outcomes predominantly (inappropriate) hospital admission, delayed discharge (often pejoratively termed bed blocking), hospital readmission or admission to nursing/residential homes. It is policy-makers who define the adverse outcomes to be avoided, rather than older people or society more widely. These adverse outcomes appear to be predicated upon the implicit assumptions that older people are using such services excessively or inappropriately and that the legitimacy of older people's claims upon the health care system are tenuous. These assumptions have rarely been tested to determine their veracity. Furthermore, it is presumed that these resonate with the wishes of older people (or other groups), although it seems likely that some outcomes (such as preventing admission to long-term care) may be more acceptable than others (would older people rather be treated in hospital rather than at home?). These broad policy objectives are not very inspirational or aspirational in terms of the quality of life of older people. Most policies attempt to prevent the negative rather than promote the positive. Hence the emphasis is upon preventing admission to care (either hospital or long-stay nursing/residential homes) rather than focusing upon providing high quality, appropriate and effective care within these settings. This does not offer a very positive image of policy development: it is usually reactive in trying to contain costs rather than promote more positive outcomes (either for older people themselves or society more generally). The entitlement of older people to health care services is secure within the broad remit of a national health service. However, the arguments concerning care of older people are largely conducted in terms of claims to different sorts of care. The legitimacy of the claims of older people to access the acute hospital and to occupy a hospital bed remains contested. Grimley Evans and Tallis (2001) argue that this approach is inherent within the recent National Service Framework for Older People (Department of Health 2001) and that such policies amount to 'institutional ageism'. Clearly, there is still much work to be done in systematically involving older people in the design and delivery of services, in evaluating models of care, in challenging 'institutional ageism', and in securing for older people access to high quality services that meet their needs.

References

Amulree, L. (1955) Modern hospital treatment and the pensioner. *Lancet*, **17** September, 571–5.

Bowling, A. (1999) Ageism in cardiology. *British Medical Journal*, **319**, 1353–5.

British Geriatrics Society (2002) *Service models; results of a BGS survey*, BGS Online Newsletter, September. Available from http://www.bgsnet.org.uk/Sept02%2ONL/15service.htm. British Geriatrics Society, London.

Department of Health (2000) *National beds enquiry – shaping the future NHS*. The Stationery Office, London.

Department of Health (2001) *National service framework for older people*. Available from http://www.doh.gov.uk/nsf/olderpeople.htm. The Stationery Office, London.

Department of Health (2002a) *National service framework for older people: interim report on age discrimination*. Available from http://www.doh.gov.uk/nsf/olderpeople.htm, accessed 13 August 2002.

Department of Health (2002b) *Health and Personal Social service Statistics – England.* Available from http://www.doh.gov.uk/HPSSS/INDEX.HTM. Department of Health, London.

Estes, C. (1979) *The aging enterprise.* Jossey Bass, San Fransisco, CA.

Gilleard, C. and Higgs, P. (2000) *Cultures of ageing.* Prentice Hall, London.

Ginn, J., Arber, S. and Cooper, H. (1997) *Researching older people's health needs and health promotion issues.* Health Education Authority, London.

Goddard, M. (2000) Measuring appropriate use of acute beds: a systematic review of methods and results. *Health Policy,* **53,** 157–84.

Goffman, E. (1963) *Stigma – notes on the management of a spoiled identity.* Penguin, Harmondsworth.

Goffman, E. (1968) *Asylums – essays on the social situation of mental patients and other inmates.* Penguin, Harmondsworth.

Grimley Evans, J. (1997) Rationing health care by age: the case against. *British Medical Journal,* **314,** 822.

Grimley Evans, J. and Tallis, R. (2001) A new beginning for care for elderly people? *British Medical Journal,* **322,** 807–8.

Healy, J., Thomas, A., Seargeant, J. and Victor, C. (1999) *Coming up for care: assessing the post-hospital needs of older patients.* Policy Studies Institute, London.

Hospital Advisory Services (2000) *Not because they are old: an independent enquiry into the care of older people on acute wards in general hospitals.* Hospital Advisory Services, London.

Jefferys, M. (1983) The over eighties in Britain; the social construction of a moral panic. *Journal of Public Health policy,* **4,** 367–72.

Killoran, A., Howse, K. and Dalley, G. (1997) *Promoting the health of older people: a compendium.* Health Education Authority, London.

Means, R. and Smith, R. (1998) *From poor law to community care,* second edition. Policy Press, Bristol.

National Centre for Survey Research (2002) *Health survey for England 2000: the health of older people.* Available from http://www.doh.gov.uk/healtholderpeople2000.htm. The Stationery Office, London.

Office for National Statistics (2002) *Health statistics quarterly,* 14. Available from http://www.statistics.gov.uk/products/p6725.asp. The Stationery Office, London.

Phillipson, C. (1998) *Reconstructing old age.* Sage, London.

Rai, G. S., Murphy, P. and Pluck, R. A. (1985) Who should provide hospital care for elderly people. *Lancet,* **I,** 683–5.

Royal Commission on Long Term Care (1999) *With respect to old age: long term care: rights and responsibilities,* Cm 4192-I, Sutherland Report. The Stationery Office, London.

Seshamani, M. and Gray, A. (2002) The impact of ageing on expenditures in the National Health Service. *Age and Ageing,* **31** (4), 287–94.

Townsend, P. (1964) *The last refuge.* Routledge and Kegan Paul, London.

Tunstall, J. (1963) *Old and alone.* Routledge and Kegan Paul, London.

Twigg, J. (2000) *Bathing – the body and community care.* Routledge, London.

Vetter, N. J., Jones, D. A. and Victor, C. R. (1981) Variations in the care for the elderly in Wales. *Journal of Epidemiology and Community Health,* **35,** 128–32.

Victor, C. R. (1991) Continuity or change; inequalities in health in later life. *Ageing and Society*, **11**, 23–39.

Victor, C. R. (1997) *Community care and older people*. Stanley Thornes, Cheltenham.

Victor, C. R., Healy, J., Thomas, A. and Seargeant, J. (2000) Older patients and delayed discharge from hospital. *Health and Community Care*, **8** (6), 443–52.

Victor, C. R. and Howse, K. (2000) *Promoting the health of older people*. Health Education Authority, London.

Victor, C. R. and Vetter, N. J. (1989) Measuring outcome after discharge from hospital: a conceptual empirical investigation. *Archives of Gerontology and Geriatrics*, **16**, 87–94.

Williams, A. (1997) Rationing health care: the case for. *British Medical Journal*, **314**, 820.

Chapter 4

Meeting the needs of people with disabilities

Ian Basnett

Introduction

Disabled people have begun to fight back against many of the inequities in health care provision that they have experienced, inequities that are becoming increasingly explicit as a consequence of policies such as managed competition and rationing.

The aim of this chapter is to increase understanding of the implications of health care organization and provision for disabled people, and so provide evidence that can help to make services more appropriate to their needs. The challenges faced by disabled people in obtaining appropriate health care can only be understood by looking at the societal context within which disability exists. Thus, I begin by reviewing the historic evolution of approaches to the provision of health services as it has affected disabled people. This chapter will highlight the greater stake that disabled people have in the provision of health services, and show how different approaches to the funding and organization of healthcare and the attitudes of healthcare providers affect minority groups such as disabled people. It will then show how the pressure to create a more inclusive model of health care has mirrored the wider fight by disabled people to achieve inclusion in mainstream society. However, inclusion must also reflect diversity, so while the move towards a more inclusive, generic health service chimes with the aims of the disability movement, there are also models of specialist services that are strongly supported by their users and clinicians.

In writing about disability and health, many textbooks discuss disability in very medical terms, describing different causes of impairments, such as multiple sclerosis, cerebrovascular accidents, muscular dystrophy or schizophrenia. Yet this contrasts dramatically with much of disabled people's experience with disability, where the impairment they experience is not necessarily equivalent to ill health; indeed, many disabled people lead healthy lives. The experience of many disabled people is that their disability results more from barriers and

Table 4.1 An overview of the International Classification of Functioning, Disability and Health

	Part 1 Functioning and disability		Part 2 Contextual factors	
Components	Body functions and structures	Activities and participation	Environmental factors	Personal factors
Domains	Body functions Body structures	Life areas (tasks, actions)	External influences on functioning and disability	Internal influences on functioning and disability
Constructs	Change in body functions (physiological) Changes in body structures (anatomical)	Capacity: Executing tasks in a standard environment Performance: Executing tasks in the current environment	Facilitating or hindering impact of features of the physical, social and attitudinal world	Impact of attributes of the person
Positive aspect	Functional and structural integrity Functioning	Activities Participation	Facilitators	Not applicable
Negative aspect	Impairment Disability	Activity limitation	Barriers/hindrances	Not applicable

Source: World Health Organization. Permission sought.

attitudes within society. This understanding that disability is in large part a function of the society we live in, most obviously in terms of physical barriers but more subtly in terms of things like attitudes, employment policies, isolation and the availability of personal care, is known as the Social Model of Disability (DeJong 1979; Oliver 1985; Zola 1979). This model has informed much of the thinking among disabled people and researchers for the last 30 years and has influenced the International Classification of Functioning, Disability and Health (ICF), developed by the World Health Organization (WHO) to complement the International Classification of Disease (World Health Organization 1999). The ICF considers both functioning and disability and contextual factors, with each having positive and negative features (Table 4.1).

Meeting the health needs of disabled people

Even the WHO ICF model is rejected by some disabled people, who view disability principally as a political issue originating from oppression, disability is complicated, multidimensional and a product of the cultures and societies in which people live and work, so a global definition that fits all circumstances is very difficult (Altman and Barnartt 2000; Slater *et al.* 1974). However, there are common categories of health problems that many disabled people face. First, some disabled people may be more prone to common illnesses, such as respiratory disease or urinary infections, and may be more seriously affected. Second, disabled people may not be able to undertake exercise and other health promoting activities as easily as others. Third, chronic health conditions may have an earlier onset amongst disabled people, for example, cardio-vascular disease or renal disease because of a neurogenic bladder; there may be related functional losses, such as arthritis due to self propulsion in a wheel-chair. Fourth, illnesses may have a more profound effect on disabled people and recovery may be more complicated and take longer. Fifth, there may be a need for sustained pharmacological support, which may be specific to an impairment such as mental illness or spasms. Sixth, there may be a need for assistive technologies and medical equipment, such as wheelchairs or adapted computers, and for long-term personal support services. Finally, there are specific health care needs for individual impairments, such as sickle cell anaemia, bipolar depression or muscular dystrophy (American Congress of Rehabilitation Medicine 1993; Bockeneck *et al.* 1998; DeJong 1997; DeJong and Basnett 2001).

For all of these reasons, disabled people are more frequent and more inten-sive users of health care than are the general population and so have a greater stake in the organization and delivery of health services. In the UK in 1994, persons of working age with a long-standing illness, disability or infirmity comprised around 17 per cent of the working age population, but they accounted for 35 per cent of visits to primary care and 45 per cent of hospital-izations (Bockeneck *et al.* 1998). Similarly, in the USA, disabled people com-prised 16 per cent of the population, but in 1996 accounted for 34 per cent of visits to a physician, nearly half of all hospital discharges and 46 per cent of all adult health care expenditure (DeJong and Basnett 2001; Tepper *et al.* 1997).

This does not, of course, mean that disability is, nor should it be, defined by health needs. Indeed, the disability movement has long struggled to move away from a medical definition of disability and the paternalism that is often associated with it, as will be illustrated in the next section.

Despite greater need for and use of health services, disabled people face greater barriers to access. In the USA DeJong and colleagues have defined these as falling into physical, social and communication barriers, and financial and health plan coverage barriers (DeJong *et al.* 2002). The physical, social and com-munication barriers will be familiar to disabled people worldwide, whether inaccessible buildings or unusable equipment, a lack of understanding of the health care needs of disabled people, or more subtle social or communication barriers. The financial and organizational issues impact in different ways in different health systems. For example, American disabled people face barriers in authorization and health insurance coverage, spend more on prescriptions, and those with the most severe mobility impairments receive less preventive care: the evidence is that disabled people who have the greatest need for services have the most difficulty obtaining them (Beatty and Dhont 2001; Beatty *et al.* 2003).

The evolving paradigm of care for disabled people

The approach to providing health care for disabled people has varied enormously over time, with changing practice partly explained by two broad themes; the quest for rights for disabled people, and the recognition that disability is not simply a health issue but has wider socio-political dimensions. At the same time, health and welfare systems evolved to be more inclusive and 'patient-centred', as paternalism declined. (It takes time though: this week a nurse in outpatients looked over my shoulder and asked someone with me 'What does he weigh?'.)

Drake has identified four phases over the twentieth century in societal attitudes to people with disabilities (Drake 2001). The first was a period of containment. Before the First World War, health care for disabled people, as with welfare in general, centred on institutionalization, initially in workhouses and then hospitals and residential homes. In some degree this reflected the inability of society to offer more complex alternatives in the community; this was in part due to a fear of disability and disabled people. Disability has at times been categorized in some societies as being a threat; something to be feared, perhaps bringing bad luck (Drake 2001).

The experiences of the First and Second World Wars brought about a major change in the approach towards providing welfare and health care to disabled people. Disabled people were seen as the victims of a struggle waged on behalf of the rest of society and so deserving of recompense. Drake characterizes this as a period of compensation. Yet their health care continued to be kept largely separate from much of mainstream society.

Drake terms the third phase the period of care, during which society recognized that various groups, including disabled people, were deserving of care and that this should be provided collectively. However, the disability was still seen as the focus of the problem, which called for an essentially medical approach. The fourth period is the emergence of an approach based on rights as the basis for the provision of welfare and health care.

The change to this more rights-based approach to health care has emerged in parallel with a realization that disability is in part a socio-political issue, which is as much about changing the environment and attitudes as it is about changing an individual's impairment. Disabled people have fought to be included within mainstream society and have led this shift in societal attitudes, with support from law makers who have enacted anti-discrimination legislation. At last, legislation has codified the place of disabled people in society, placing them on an equal footing with others.

These changes have in part been due to the understanding that disabled people have rights that demand their inclusion, not only within society as a whole, but also in how health care services should be provided. However, the actual models of provision vary hugely between countries, with differing results. For example, in the UK, where the health system is underpinned by the strongly held value of universal health care, a more paternalist approach has predominated until recently. In contrast, in the USA, a more rights-based culture exists and access can be greater where those rights are clearly defined, as with renal dialysis. However, despite the existence of Medicare and Medicaid, and a legislative framework in the Americans with Disabilities Act (ADA 1990), many disabled Americans struggle to obtain decent healthcare. Further, ADAPT (American Disabled for Attendant Programs Today) is still fighting to enable more disabled Americans to live in the community rather than in nursing homes.

The extent to which good quality health care is provided for disabled people depends on the overall societal commitment to the provision of health care for all, the extent to which societies have moved through the stages listed above, and their values with regard to equity of access. These factors overlay the questions of health system organization examined in the next section.

Contemporary approaches to health care for disabled people

While the organization of a health care system ought not necessarily to impact on the care received by disabled people, there is evidence that it does. Two broad models can be distinguished. The first, a third-party model, involves bodies responsible for purchasing care on behalf of a population, exemplified by the purchaser–provider split in the UK. An agency is responsible for assessing the health needs of a population and purchasing health care to meet those needs. This model stresses flexibility and adaptability with few enshrined legal rights for the health care user. Thus, the United Kingdom Disability Discrimination Act (DDA) applies to access to buildings, employment and the provision of goods and services, but excludes decisions on the allocation of resources or whether to treat an individual. Much depends on societal values and on the particular interests of the individuals involved; there are examples of good practice, but in many places health care provision is oblivious to the needs of those with disabilities.

The second, a rights-based model, gives a greater role to the individual, whose position is strengthened by explicit legal rights. This can been seen in the USA, where health care is largely market based, albeit with a safety net for disabled, older and poor people. This rights-based approach is exemplified by the Americans with Disabilities Act, which requires long-term care to be provided in the most inclusive setting. It could be argued that a rights-based approach to health care is more likely to benefit disabled people, if it can guarantee equal access to treatment based on a principle of equal worth for all members of society. However, the picture is mixed, especially as a consequence of pressures to contain costs in American managed care organizations. As described earlier, the evidence is that disabled people who have the greatest need for services have the most difficulty obtaining them (Beatty and Dhont 2001; Beatty et al. 2002). In managed care, people with disabilities are more likely to have a regular primary care provider (Beatty and Dhont 2001), although less likely than others to obtain the physician of their choice (Neri et al. 2001) or to access specialty care (Beatty et al. 2002; Wholey et al. 1998). There are some innovative examples of managed care carve-outs for disabled people, allowing fuller integration of health and social care. They include the Community Medical Alliance in Boston, the Shepard Care Network in Atlanta and the Community Living Alliance in Wisconsin (Bockeneck et al. 1998 p. 628). However, these examples remain remarkable partly because they are exceptional and have received project funding.

As this brief analysis shows, very different funding and delivery systems can achieve good or bad results, with much depending on the underlying attitudes to disability.

Integrated versus specialist care

The balance between completely integrated health care systems and some specialist elements, such as for HIV/AIDs, mental health and spinal injuries is discussed here as part of the push by the disability movement towards greater integration. However, some people with some specific impairments are strong supporters of specialist services for medical reasons. As I described above, the health care problems that disabled people suffer can include the generic, presenting in the usual ways and requiring standard treatment, although these may be exacerbated by disability, or may present differently, or there may be specialist health problems. These latter health problems may not be obvious, making management difficult for physicians not specializing in that disability. Conversely, specialists may have only limited knowledge outside their own area and be unable to offer comprehensive care. Hence the balance between provision by specialists and generalists is much debated.

For example, I have a spinal injury. Spinal injury units revolutionized the care for people with spinal injuries, dramatically improving their survival. Although not perfect, they are good models of highly specialist units for a specific impairment, dealing with the immediate spinal injury, follow-up and any complications. Such units are often highly valued by people with spinal injuries who feel confident that their generic care and their specific needs, such as skin care and personal hygiene, will be dealt with competently. Many would prefer that all of their acute healthcare problems were dealt with in such units. However, if I have an acute general medical problem I will be admitted to my local hospital, and if an uncomplicated problem, such as a urinary tract infection, then the clinical management of that condition may be fine. However, whilst in hospital I still need general personal care and a non-specialized hospital (at least in the UK) often struggles with, for example, my bowel care. Many common interventions, such as general anaesthesia for otherwise generic surgical problems, may be more complex in a high quadriplegic and require a clinician who is familiar with the potential problems. Yet the alternative, with disabled people obtaining all their health care in specialist units, would pose logistical problems. It would be difficult to have sufficient units to ensure local access and the relatively small numbers of skilled staff in spinal units, already under pressure, would be swamped.

Which elements of care are provided in which settings for those with particular impairments involves balancing factors, such as the prevalence of the impairment, the power of patient and clinician lobby groups, and the role of external factors: for example, war led to the development of spinal injury units.

Where the current balance lies differs in different countries, depending on the division between primary and secondary care. Thus, in the UK, the dichotomy between generic and specialist health care is particularly marked, and the vast majority of health care is provided in primary care. Primary care professionals will diagnose and treat many problems, and act as gatekeepers referring on to more specialist services if necessary. In the USA and in many European countries patients are more likely to have direct access to specialists.

Which model best meets the needs of disabled people is highly dependent upon the impairment and the problem. For many impairments with potentially complex health problems it is impossible for a generalist to be sufficiently well informed. However, all of us face common general health problems, such as viruses and skin rashes, which a specialist in an impairment is less well placed to manage. There are benefits from having easy access to both generalists and specialists: what matters is the pathway between the two to ensure an appropriate division of care. Health care providers need better training in disability issues, both in general terms as well as in specific medical issues. The problems that disabled people face are often not acute medical ones and stretch beyond the domain of medicine, but doctors are trained to medicalize problems. Knowledge about the health and other problems that many disabled people face is often thin, especially in primary care, constituting what DeJong and colleagues describe as a lack of 'disability literacy' (DeJong *et al.* 2002).

Attitudes and rationing

The organization of care is, of course, a secondary issue to the more important one of whether care is provided at all. Beliefs about the quality of life experienced by disabled people can have profound implications for the decisions made on their behalf by professionals. Whether due to discrimination or simply a lack of knowledge, health professionals often make entirely unjustified assumptions about what is in the best interest of the patient. Health professionals reflect the attitudes of the society of which they are part, but they do bear a greater responsibility to be better informed about their patients.

My own experience as a physician who became disabled after qualifying illustrated this for me personally (Basnett 2001). When I suddenly became severely disabled I found myself only too aware of how inaccurate were my own perceptions of life as a disabled person. It is not a bed of roses, especially as society has some way to go in terms of its attitudes and responses, but it is not the life worse than death that I had imagined. The corollary is that any judgements I might have previously made about the importance of health interventions to save disabled people's lives would have been grossly misinformed.

These misplaced attitudes are not unusual amongst health professionals (Basnett 2001; Gardner *et al.* 1985; Rothwell *et al.* 1997 pp. 452–5). For example, when asked to place themselves in a hypothetical situation, providers of emergency care imagined a strikingly more negative quality of life and outcome than that reported by people with quadriplegia. Ninety two per cent of people with quadriplegia reported being glad to be alive, whilst only 18 per cent of emergency care providers imagined they would be glad to be alive if they were quadriplegic. The researchers describe the attitude they unearthed as 'better off dead' (Gerhart *et al.* 1994).

Whilst these attitudes clearly have their origins in our society, it is possible that the training undergone by health professionals, and especially doctors, exacerbates these prejudices. So might the system of selecting students, since students in medical schools where the student body is more diverse are more likely to value an emphasis on diversity in the curriculum (Kahtan *et al.* 1994).

As health professionals, we most often come into contact with disabled people when they are unwell and most dependent on others, and we very rarely have contact with them as equals. Medical training emphasizes biomedical factors and prioritizes cure over care, even though the prospect of a cure is impossible for many disabled people. There is limited consideration of the social origins of disability (Wagner and Stewart 2001), although this is at last changing, albeit slowly. Some medical schools make particular efforts to address this issue, however, with evidence that it is possible to promote more positive attitudes to disability (Crotty *et al.* 2000), and some medical schools are involving disabled people in curriculum design (Wells *et al.* 2002).

The attitudes of health professionals matter for a number of important reasons. On an individual level, some health professionals that we encounter are tremendous, but attitudes can vary between the benign paternalistic, simply clumsy and inappropriate and even the aggressive (often originating in uncertainty or fear). Attitudes also impact on decisions about things like whether to resuscitate a potentially disabled baby and how actively to treat someone with quadriplegia.

A particular example of the impact of attitudes to disabled people is the debate on assisted suicide. An assumption underlying much of the debate is that the quality of life for severely disabled persons is poor and helping them to take their lives is appropriate and humane. I would argue that actually helping someone to kill themselves is the wrong intervention. It is more appropriate to look at society's attitudes towards disability, personal care support systems, education and employment. Some reported cases of assisted suicide in the USA are especially disturbing, since these individuals had been subjected to the withdrawal of education and employment opportunities or the refusal of personal care before their suicide (Basnett 2001 p. 455).

The current debate on the human genome also illustrates an area where judgements about the quality of life of a disabled person matters a great deal. Based on those, and other issues such as cost, it is debated whether impairments could be substantially avoided. Clearly, this already happens with Down's syndrome and spina bifida via *in utero* diagnosis.

Attitudes also matter because they affect higher level investment and rationing decisions (Peters 1995). These decisions are influenced profoundly by views on the pre-existing or potential quality of individual's lives, views that are informed by the adaptations made by people with disabilities (Menzel *et al.* 2002). This is of growing importance as technological advances make the potential scope of health care ever greater, while health system developments, such as managed competition and other efforts to contain costs, lead to explicit resource allocation decisions. It is important to recognize that disability has been used for many years as a reason for not providing health care.

Increasing emphasis on 'rational' approaches to the allocation of resources has given rise to a number of initiatives based on a utilitarian approach to resources; for a given investment how can maximum benefit be obtained in terms of overall quality of life for a population? This can lead to disabled people faring much worse if their underlying quality of life is assumed to be poorer than able-bodied people and having less potential marginal gain. Decisions about presumed quality of life may further disadvantage disabled people because of stereotypical views about how disability lowers quality of life (Asch 2001 p. 317). However, Wasserman argues that there may also be circumstances in which disabled people can benefit from a utilitarian approach, where their relative disadvantage offers scope for an intervention to yield a high marginal utility (Wasserman 2001 p. 235). In practice, however, it is increasingly recognized that explicit rationing methods are essentially a means of deflecting criticism from politicians who are unwilling to provide adequate health care resources, as exemplified by the highly criticized New Zealand system of allocating scores to patients on surgical waiting lists (Gauld and Derrett 2000).

A contrasting rights-based approach, where each individual is considered of equal worth, assuming that the benefits of an intervention outweigh the disbenefits for that individual, means that he or she should have access to care, irrespective of the potential that these benefits are reduced relative to others by the presence of a coexisting disability (Asch 2001; Orentlicher 1986 p. 317). Indeed, society could additionally decide that disabled people who are worse off should benefit most (Asch 2001; Orentlicher 1986 p. 317).

Even in countries with explicit rationing strategies, there are often contradictions, either between rhetoric and reality, or between different elements of policies. Thus, in England and Wales, the National Institute for Clinical Effectiveness has adopted an informal cut-off of £30,000 (€45,500) per Quality Adjusted Life Year that should be sought when recommending interventions for use in the National Health Service. In contrast, the recent Fair Access to Care Guidance requires social services departments to focus on those with most needs (Department of Health 2002).

Notwithstanding the arguments of Wasserman, in my view a strongly utilitarian approach to allocating resources is most likely to impact adversely on disabled people, particularly if judgements about the quality of life of disabled people are ill informed, as the evidence shows that they are. This then gives rise to what Asch has described as a substitution of social decisions with their prejudices about the utility of life, for what should be medical decisions (Asch 1998).

Health care reform

Health care systems are continually changing as they struggle to address ever more rapidly changing circumstances. The challenge is to ensure that this process of reform benefits rather than disadvantages people with disabilities. A report of an American Study Group on Health Care Reform, People with Disabilities, and Independent Living (1992) made a series of recommendations in 1992 that remain applicable today, and while many of their recommendations related to the unique circumstances of the USA, such as the need to ensure equitable access to health care financing, others have more general relevance. In the USA, wholesale health care reform aside, one is left with trying to 'manage the market', but the absence of good risk adjustment methods and the data to support them means health plans have incentives to avoid disabled people. In general terms, however, there is a need for a paradigm shift, away from the current episodic sickness model of health care and toward a long-term partnership between patients, health care providers, and those responsible for paying for care, with the goal of achieving the optimum well-being for all individuals. In reality, much of the rhetoric of health care reform is driven by the objective of delivering ever more discrete packages of care, exemplified by the drive to introduce payment systems such as Diagnosis-Related Groups. This creates perverse incentives not to provide optimal services that meet the needs of those with chronic disorders and with disabilities.

There is a need to emphasize cost-effectiveness over cost containment, with decision-making informed by a knowledge of the meaning of disability for those affected. Most health care providers still have little understanding of disability and many people with disabilities continue to have to educate their health care providers about their health status, the impact of their disabilities on their general health, and the types of interventions that are most effective in addressing their chronic and acute health problems.

Any health care reform initiative should include mechanisms to promote professional responsiveness to consumer needs. Even in the most advanced health care systems, the ability of many health care providers to listen and respond to the needs of disabled users is questionable.

Other measures

Measuring quality in health services is an evolving science. Even in the USA where a great deal of work has been done, few measures are appropriate to disabled people. There are important research tasks to investigate the extent to which the current measures provide useful information about disabled people, to develop new, easily applied indicators of quality which are accessible, and to understand how these can be used to improve quality (DeJong *et al.* 2002).

The Internet and telemedicine are both expanding areas in health care provision. Whilst only a small proportion of disabled people use the Internet, 10 per cent in an American study (Kaye 2000), well validated information could help disabled people navigate themselves through the health care maze.

Telemedicine is expanding in many countries and offers the potential to expand access, particularly for people with mobility impairments, although this remains to be evaluated in many settings.

A great deal of valuable research has been undertaken into health service provision and disability, but relative to research into other marginalized groups it is less well supported (DeJong *et al.* 2002). Research into better ways of training and educating health care providers about the needs of disabled people, better models of service delivery, risk adjustment in market systems, how to measure quality and improving its quality are amongst the priorities.

Moving forward

So what should be done to enable health care systems better to meet the needs of disabled people? In this chapter I have identified several issues that should be considered by policy makers:

- The funding mechanism and the organizational model, for example a single national provider, such as the NHS in the UK, or a mixed economy of unstructured providers, many operating for profit, such as the USA;

- The balance between provision by generalists, especially primary care, or specialists;

- Attitudes towards disabled people and the ethos of the healthcare system;

- The legal frameworks to protect people with disabilities, which differ radically between countries.

- Measuring quality and developing a research agenda.

There is conflicting evidence as to how disabled people fare in market driven systems. It is certainly true that unless adequate safeguards are in place, disabled people, whose care can often be expensive, will lose out. Putting such safeguards in place can be difficult.

With regard to integration versus specialist care, the debate is one of balance as much as one model or another. The evidence to guide us is somewhat thin and many decisions have to be pragmatic, in the context of a particular health care system and an individual's particular impairments. Some models of primary care, whether social care or disability-specific services, have been positively evaluated, but these exist in a health care system where the alternative is much less structured and were developed and supported by enthusiasts. Thus their generalizability remains to be demonstrated.

Specialist services for particular impairments are often highly valued by their users. This is partly because people are confident that they will see professionals who understand their problems and will be seen in a supportive environment. Hence there will always be a need for disabled people to navigate their way through generic health care systems, especially if they have a rare impairment. This means all health care providers must effectively address the basic issues of access, attitudes, knowledge, acceptance of the expert patient and a willingness to seek specialist help.

In the USA, the principal legal source of protection for disabled people, the Americans with Disabilities Act, is under attack while in the UK the government has been slow to strengthen the Disability Discrimination Act. It is important that the principle of equality of access for disabled people is supported in law but the direction of change is not all positive.

More fundamental, however, is improving knowledge and changing attitudes within society and the health professions. We may have come a long way, but there is still some way to go. Attitudes towards disabled people matter hugely in determining the care that they receive. These attitudes affect decisions and interactions at an individual level, for example, how we are treated as individuals, decisions about whether to intervene to support individuals at the beginning of life or in life threatening situations. At a programme level, these attitudes affect investment and rationing decisions; for example, is the amount spent on disabled people's care services, such as wheelchairs, personal assistance and mental health, on making all primary care physically accessible, or offering renal dialysis to disabled people.

At a societal level, there needs to be broad acceptance that disabled people have an entitlement based on rights supported in law, rather than at the mercy of paternalism. Most importantly, the health professions need to change. Whilst they are in part a reflection of broader society, they have a particular responsibility for being knowledgeable about disabled people's quality of life and making decisions informed by that knowledge and not by broader prejudices. Training health professions in disability awareness is making some progress, but it is patchy and not always well received when at variance with the expectation of cure.

Almost all of these issues raise important health service research questions that are difficult to answer without more support for disability related research. It is time that health care for disabled people receives the same attention as other disenfranchised groups and that equal access becomes the norm.

Acknowledgements

I am grateful to Professor Gerben DeJong for his comments and suggestions, although the final responsibility for the chapter is mine.

References

American Disabled for Attendant Programs Today. Available at http://www.adapt.org.

Americans with Disabilities Act (1990) Available at http://www.usdoj.gov/ada/adahom1.htm.

Altman, B. and Barnartt, S. N. (2000) *Expanding the scope of social science research on disability*. JAI Press, Greenwich, CT.

American Congress of Rehabilitation Medicine (1993) Addressing the post-rehabilitation health care needs of persons with disabilities. *Archives of Physical Medicine and Rehabilitation*, **74**, S8–12.

American Study Group on Health Care Reform, People with Disabilities, and Independent Living (1992) Available at http://www.ilru.org/mgdcare/greenbook.html.

Asch, A. (1998) Distracted by disability. *Cambridge Quarterly of Healthcare Ethics*, **7**, 77–87.

Asch, A. (2001) Intellectual disabilities – Quo Vadis? In G. Albrecht, K. D. Seelman and M. Bury (eds) *A handbook of disability studies*. Sage, Thousand Oaks, CA.

Basnett, I. (2001) Advocacy and political action. In G. Albrecht, K. D. Seelman and M. Bury (eds) *A handbook of disability studies*. Sage, Thousand Oaks, CA.

Beatty, P. and Dhont, K. (2001) Medicare health maintenance organisations and traditional coverage: perceptions of health care amongst beneficiaries with disabilities. *Archives of Physical Medicine and Rehabilitation*, **82**, 1009–17.

Beatty, P., Hagglund, K., Neri, M., Dhont, K., Clark, M. and S, H. (2003) Access to health amongst people with physical disabilities and/or chronic illness: patterns and predictors. Archives of Physical Medicine and Rehabilitation (in press)

Bockeneck, W., Mann, N., Lanig, S. I., DeJong, G. and Beatty Lee, A. (1998) Primary care for people with disabilities. In J. DeLisa and B. Gans (eds) *Rehabilitation medicine: principles & practice*, 3rd edition, pp. 905–28. Lippincott-Raven, Philadelphia, PA.

Crotty, M., Finucane, P. and Ahern, M. (2000) Teaching medical students about disability and rehabilitation: methods and student feedback. *Medical Education*, **34**, 659–64.

DeJong, G. (1979) Independent living: from social movement to analytical paradigm. *Archives of Physical Medicine and Rehabilitation*, **60**, October, 435–46.

DeJong, G. (1997) Primary care for people with disabilities: an overview of the problem and opportunities. *American Journal of Physical Medicine and Rehabilitation*, **76**(3), Suppl. 1–7.

DeJong, G. and Basnett, I. (2001) The political economy of the disability marketplace. In G. Albrecht, K. D. Seelman and M. Bury (eds) *A handbook of disability studies*. Sage, Thousand Oaks, CA.

DeJong, G., Palsbo, S. E., Beatty, P. W., Jones, G. C., Kroll, T. and Neri, M. T. (2002) The organisation and financing of health services for persons with disabilities. *Milbank Quarterly*, **80** (2), 261–301.

Department of Health (2002) *Fair access to care services: guidance on eligibility criteria for adult social care*. London, Department of Health.

Drake, R. F. (2001) A sociological approach. In G. Albrecht, K. D. Seelman and M. Bury (eds) *A handbook of disability studies*. Sage, Thousand Oaks, CA.

Gardner, G. P. R., Theocleous, J. W., Watt, J. W. and Krishnan, K. R. (1985) Ventilation or dignified death for patients with high level tetraplegia. *British Medical Journal*, **291**, 160–222.

Gauld, R. and Derrett, S. (2000) Solving the surgical waiting list problem? New Zealand's 'booking system'. *International Journal of Health Planning Management*, **15**, 259–72.

Gerhart, K. A., Koziol-McLain, J., Lowenstein, S. R. and Whiteneck, G. G. (1994) Quality of life following spinal cord injury: knowledge and attitudes of emergency care providers. *Annals of Emergency Medicine*, **23**, 807–12.

Kahtan, S., Inman, C., Haines, A. and Holland, P. (1994) Teaching disability and rehabilitation to medical students. Steering Group on Medical Education and Disability. *Medical Education*, **28**, 386–93.

Kaye, H. S. (2000) *Disability and the digital divide*, Disability Statistics Abstract 22. U.S. Department of Education, National Institute on Disability and Rehabilitation Research, Washington, DC.

Menzel, P., Dolan, P., Richardson, J. and Olsen, J. A. (2002) The role of adaptation to disability and disease in health state valuation: a preliminary normative analysis. *Social Science & Medicine*, **55**, 2149–58.

Neri, M., Beatty, P. and Dhont, K. (2001) *Individuals with disabilities are less likely to have the primary care doctor of their choice – especially in managed care*. Health and Disability Data Brief. NRH Center for Health and Disability Research, Washington, DC.

Oliver, M. (1985) *Understanding disability: from theory to practice*. Macmillan, Basingstoke.

Orentlicher, D. (1986) Destructuring disability rationing: rationing of health care and unfair discrimination against the sick. Harvard Civil Rights. *Civil Liberties Law Review*, **31**, 48–88.

Peters, P. G. (1995) Health care rationing and disability rights. *Indiana Law Journal*, **70**, 491–547.

Rothwell, P. M., McDowell, Z., Wong, C. K. and Dorman, P. J. (1997) Doctors and patients don't agree: cross-sectional study of patients' and doctors' assessment of disability in multiple sclerosis. *British Medical Journal*, **314**, 1580–3.

Slater, S. B. P., Vukmanovic, T., Macukanic, T., Prvulovic, T. and Cutler, J. I. (1974) The definition and measurement of disability. *Social Science and Medicine*, **8**, 305–8.

Tepper, S., Sutton, J. P., Beatty, P. and DeJong, G. (1997) Alternative definitions of disability: relationship to health care expenditures. *Disability and Rehabilitation*, **19**(12), 556–8.

Wagner, A. K. and Stewart, P. J. (2001) An internship for college students in physical medicine and rehabilitation: effects on awareness, career choice, and disability perceptions. *American Journal of Physical Medicine and Rehabilitation*, **80**, 459–65.

Wasserman, D. (2001) The uneasy home of disability in literature and film. In G. Albrecht, K. D. Seelman and M. Bury (eds) *A handbook of disability studies*. Sage, Thousand Oaks, CA.

Wells, T. P., Byron, M. A., McMullen, S. H. and Birchall, M. A. (2002) Disability teaching for medical students: disabled people contribute to curriculum development. *Medical Education*, **36**, 788–90.

Wholey, D., Burns, L. and Lavizzo-Mourey, R. (1998) Managed care and the delivery of primary Care to the elderly and chronically ill. *Health Services Research*, **33** (2), 322–53.

World Health Organization (1999) *International classification of functioning, disability and health*. Geneva, World Health Organization.

Zola, I. (1979) Healthism and disabling medicalization. In I. Illich, I. Zola, J. McKnight, J. Caplan and H. Shaiken (eds) *Disabling professions*. Calder & Boyars, London.

Chapter 5

Health Care for Rich and Poor Alike

Margaret Whitehead and Barbara Hanratty

People living in poverty have resources so seriously
below those commanded by the average individual or
family that they are, in effect, excluded from ordinary
living patterns, customs and activities.
Townsend 1979 p. 31

Poverty and social exclusion

Across Europe as a whole, east and west, many millions of people are experiencing poverty and social exclusion. The exact figure depends on how poverty
is defined, but there is no dispute that the magnitude of the problem is both
serious and unacceptable.

Absolute poverty is equated with insufficient income to survive in a physically
fit condition, but human needs go beyond mere physical survival, and income
is not the only resource that is important. Increasingly poverty is seen as an
inadequacy of a range of resources needed to reach and maintain well-being –
including health and education, environmental well-being and income. The
recently defined concepts of relative poverty and social exclusion can be found
in Peter Townsend's original definition of poverty quoted above (Townsend
1979). This lack of opportunity to participate in activities that are considered
normal in a particular country is echoed in notions of social exclusion gaining
ground in Europe, for example, in the definition proposed by the Centre of the
Analysis of Social Exclusion (CASE) at the London School of Economics:

> An individual is socially excluded if a) he or she is geographically resident in a society,
> b) he or she cannot participate in the normal activities of citizens in that society, and
> c) he or she would like to participate, but is prevented from doing so by factors
> beyond his or her control.

Burchardt *et al.* 1999 p. 229

This chapter outlines the evidence on the link between relative poverty and health, exploring the key mechanisms in this relationship, before going on to consider the role of the health system. A central premise of this chapter, in common with the rest of the book, is that universal entitlement means that everyone, in practice not just in theory, should be able to access and use appropriate health care. This is a particular challenge for poorer groups in society, and the final section of the chapter deals with the barriers that the poor face and successful strategies to overcome them.

Better health status for those with more money and power

Looking at the mountain of evidence across Europe, we see a clear pattern of better health status for those with more money and power and, conversely, worse health for those who are poor and excluded (Whitehead and Diderichsen 1997). Compared with their more affluent counterparts, people in poverty tend to have shorter lives – up to five years shorter in terms of life expectancy; they also suffer more years of disability before they die, and experience greater severity of illness (Blank and Diderichsen 1996).

The cycle of disadvantage, poverty and ill-health starts from conception and runs throughout life. For example, low birth weight is more common in lower social classes: on average the babies of less skilled manual workers are 130 gm lighter than offspring of managers and professionals (Office for National Statistics 1997). These low birth weight babies then grow into children and adults at increased risk of a range of diseases, including non-insulin dependent diabetes and ischaemic heart disease (Barker 1998).

This common social patterning of ill-health applies to all parts of Europe: north, south, east and west. In the North, for example, Finnish women from the lowest educational group have eight fewer years of disability-free life expectancy after the age of 25 than women in the top group. For Finnish men the situation is even worse, with a 13-year gap between the lowest and the highest educational groups (Valkonen et al. 1993). In Spain, large differentials have been found between the wealthiest and poorest districts for standardized mortality ratio, life expectancy and years of potential life lost in the 1990s, and these differentials have widened since the 1980s (Borrel and Arias 1995; Navarro and Benach 1997).

Eastern Europe has faced impoverishment on a large scale since 1990, and massive psychosocial stress as societal structures broke down (Cornia and Paniccia 1995). This turmoil was accompanied by an overall decline in life expectancy for the populations of some of the countries, and a more severe effect for the poorer sections of society in each country.

In Britain, many studies have looked at health by deprivation of the area of residence, and found premature mortality increases with increasing levels of area deprivation (Shaw *et al.* 1999). A recent British report on the impact of poverty on children concluded that the highest number of 'excess' deaths occur in the poorest areas and that more children die in areas where child poverty is highest (Mitchell *et al.* 2000). Further afield, studies reporting a widening gap in mortality between educational and income groups are raising concern. In the USA, the richest country in the world, for example, the proportion of mortality attributable to poverty in American adults has increased in recent decades, and by the mid-1990s was comparable to that attributable to cigarette smoking (Hahn *et al.* 1995).

What causes poorer people to have poorer health?

A large body of evidence demonstrates that these inequalities in health are, to a large extent, generated by differential exposure and differential vulnerability to social, environmental and behavioural causes of disease (Acheson *et al.* 1998). Poorer groups and poorer areas are exposed to a greater number and extent of health-damaging factors, whether in terms of poorer living conditions, more dangerous, stressful jobs or having to live in more polluted neighbourhoods. Furthermore, exposures are cumulative over the life course: children who suffer deprivation in childhood are more likely to suffer further disadvantages at critical stages throughout their adult life and so are more vulnerable to adverse influences.

The exact mechanisms through which poverty leads to poorer health are complex, but at least three main pathways can be distinguished. First, and perhaps the most obvious, is through lack of financial resources to obtain the basic prerequisites for health. Poor people have insufficient money for decent food, shelter, heating, schooling, health care and so on. Inadequate access to these prerequisites is linked with malnutrition, inadequate housing and perhaps exposure to unhealthy working environments. In turn, this leaves poorer people vulnerable to injuries, illnesses such as bronchitis and heart disease, and poor obstetric outcomes. Suboptimal nutritional and immunological status, and disadvantaged living conditions may also leave the poor ill equipped to recover rapidly from illness.

The second pathway is through psychosocial stress caused by the stigma, humiliation and loss of control associated with living day-to-day in poverty. Some of the higher rates of anxiety, depression, and suicide observed in low-income groups and people without jobs have been attributed to the soul-destroying effect of being denied self-respect and dignity (Wilkinson 1996). This is exacerbated by the loss of social contacts that comes from having little money. The evidence is mounting for an additional effect of psychosocial stress on physical heath problems, particularly an increased risk of coronary heart disease (Hemmingway and Marmot 1999).

The third pathway is through behavioural change, triggered by social isolation and loss of hope. Tobacco and alcohol use may offer a welcome distraction from a life in poverty (Graham 1993); and the pressures of struggling to survive on a low income may leave little time or money for recreational exercise. Such behaviours are likely to have significant physical and psychological impacts on health, as well as having financial consequences for the household. Low income also restricts dietary choices – often to the cheaper, fatty foods that may be detrimental to health. Indeed, higher levels of overweight and obesity are found amongst poorer people, a major and increasing health risk (Joint Health Surveys Unit 1999). None of these pathways are mutually exclusive, and elements of all three are likely to affect poor families. They illustrate the potential complexity of the relationship between poverty and ill-health and have important implications for the nature of interventions needed to break this link, which will be discussed at the second half of this chapter.

In all this, inequalities in access, quality and outcome of curative health care services play a minor role compared with the wider social determinants in generating the observed differences in health status between rich and poor. Access to essential health services can, however, play a vital part in dealing with or ameliorating the health damage caused by wider societal influences, since the health care system can intervene at strategic points in some of the above pathways.

Health care for rich and poor – a basic human right?

As Healy and McKee point out in Chapter 1, health care is not just a private commodity, but is widely considered an important social good. That is why no government anywhere leaves access to health services entirely to the market. People are not left on the streets to die because they cannot afford emergency care after an accident, nor are elderly people denied curative care because they are not as productive as working age people, or because it would be 'less efficient' to treat them. Across Europe, and even in the strongly market-oriented USA, public provision is made for vulnerable sections of society, including the poor, the very young and older people. At the very least, a basic safety net is provided where poor people can use specially provided public facilities without charge, or they can have their medical fees waived for private services by a means-tested procedure.

Practical questions arise in such basic systems about quality and comprehensiveness – how limited is the package of services to which vulnerable groups have access and are they of an acceptable quality? This leads into more fundamental questions of an ethical nature concerning access of the whole population to good quality health care. In the human rights approach, health is seen as a very basic human need in itself and, crucially, it also influences access to other human rights. People need their health to enjoy any of their democratic rights as citizens (Sen 2000). The benefits of medical interventions are not only seen in terms of improved physical health, but within a wider perspective of improved quality of life, including, for example, good quality palliative care and freedom from pain (Dahlgren and Whitehead 1992).

Access to good health care services according to need, not ability to pay, is the fundamental base for the human rights approach, recently restated in the British ten-year plan for the NHS:

> NHS core principles: Principle One: Healthcare is a basic human right. Unlike private systems the NHS will not exclude people because of their health status or ability to pay.
>
> Department of Health 2000

The human rights approach puts the onus on governments to ensure access to essential health care. Allocation cannot be on the basis of payment. In practical terms, the unequal distribution of sickness within societies poses a challenge for the fair organization of a health care system, and for resource allocation in particular. It means, for example, that poorer people, due to their greater morbidity and risk of mortality, have greater need for health care services. They may need more help in gaining access to services and, even when they do receive health care, they may not respond to treatment as well, or as rapidly, as their more affluent peers. Thus, the health care system is obliged to deal with the health damage caused by other processes and determinants in society.

What is known about access to and use of health services by poorer people?

While the human rights approach outlined above suggests that need should be the overarching principle guiding the provision of health care, it is not always the case in practice.

In this section, we review the current state of knowledge of inequities in health care for socio-economically disadvantaged groups. For pragmatic reasons, such studies tend to approach the measurement of poverty or disadvantage in one of two ways. The first approach attempts to measure the poverty of individuals (using indicators such as the type of work a person does and the social status of that job, family income or educational level of the family member). Alternatively, deprivation of the area in which patients live is assessed, using indicators such as the rate of unemployment in the area, the proportion of overcrowded houses in the neighbourhood, and so on, with several indicators sometimes combined into a composite index of area deprivation. It needs to be borne in mind when interpreting area-based (ecological) studies that not all people who live in deprived areas will be poor, and not all poor people live in deprived areas.

The inverse care law

'The availability of good medical care tends to vary inversely with the need for it in the population served' (Tudor Hart 1971 p. 405). Although the seriousness of the situation varies in different systems, there seems to be an almost universal phenomenon in all countries – dubbed the 'inverse care law' by Tudor Hart (1971) – that the availability and quality of health services is inversely related to the need for those services. Thus poorer groups and disadvantaged areas suffering the worst health often have access to fewer and poorer quality services. This 'law' can be seen to operate right through the different levels of service, from preventive to primary, secondary and tertiary care. Most of the empirical studies quoted below measure utilization of services as a proxy indicator for access to health care. Whilst this mirrors policy makers' emphasis on the measurable, it needs to be remembered that utilization may not capture all the important differences in the way in which health services are delivered to different groups. Crucially, studies need to control for level of morbidity when comparing the health care utilization of different social groups. If this is not done, then higher utilization by lower social groups may mistakenly be taken to indicate that their needs are well catered for and there are no barriers to access. We emphasize here those studies that have adjusted for the differences in morbidity across the social groups.

Primary care

Disturbing trends have been noted for the Swedish national health service in relation to primary care. Studies in the 1970s and 1980s showed that, after controlling for health status, no socio-economic differences were found in the proportion that had visited a primary care doctor (Dahlgren *et al.* 1984; Haglund 1984). By the mid-1990s, however, inequalities in access had appeared, with lower use of GP and outpatient services by manual workers compared with professionals and other non-manual groups, after controlling for morbidity (Whitehead *et al.* 1997). A reverse trend has been found for the British health service, with early evidence from the 1970s indicating a 'pro-rich' bias in GP services (Blaxter 1984; Le Grand 1978), transforming in the 1980s (O'Donnell and Propper 1991) and the mid-1990s to a 'pro-poor' bias in NHS consultations with GPs. This pro-poor bias did not extend to outpatient clinics at hospitals (Whitehead *et al.* 1997).

In many health systems, the primary care doctor provides the bulk of basic health care, is the gatekeeper to more specialist services, and is a central figure in facilitating access to care. This is most clearly seen in countries such as the Netherlands, which operate parallel private and public insurance systems, with a prominent role for the GP in the latter. The strong gatekeeping role of the GP is evident in the reduced use of secondary care amongst the publicly insured (Bongers *et al.* 1997). Thus, access to primary care has great potential to both reduce and create inequities in health care. However, the decision to consult a primary care physician will be influenced by many factors, ranging from the patient's own health beliefs and expectations to the availability of alternative forms of care.

Referral to secondary care is an important outcome of consultation with primary care practitioners. It is cause for concern, therefore, that people living in socio-economically deprived areas or working in manual occupations are less likely to be referred to secondary care by their general practitioners in the UK (Hippisley-Cox *et al.* 1997; Hippisley-Cox and Pringle 2000; Majeed *et al.* 2000; O'Donnell 2000). A similar picture is apparent in other health systems, such as Canada (Dunlop *et al.* 2000).

Hospital services

The availability of hospital services in relation to need has received less attention from researchers. Keskimaki and colleagues have looked at socio-economic differences in hospital care across the whole of Finland (1995), controlling for patterns of mortality and prevalence of self-perceived illness. The trend to high hospital use in lower socio-economic groups was mirrored by social gradients in mortality and morbidity, suggesting equity in treatment, although this may also reflect the substitution of hospital care for appropriate primary care by poorer people. Accounting for differences in the severity of illness is also important, as otherwise aggregate data may conceal important differences in the process and outcomes of care. For example, less affluent patients may be seen later in their illness, with consequent reduced chance of curative care. This was illustrated by a study of patients with glaucoma at three London hospitals, where people who presented late for care, and were therefore at greater risk of blindness, tended to live in more deprived areas and to be of lower occupational social class than other patients (Fraser *et al.* 2001).

Ischaemic heart disease, responsible for one in four deaths in developed countries, is now recognized as a disease of poverty rather than affluence. Socio-economic inequalities in cardiovascular disease are apparent in most industrialized countries, with commonly the lower social classes and less well educated being more severely affected (Mackenbach *et al.* 2000). Similar social patterning should therefore be expected in the use of services. Re-vascularization procedures for ischaemic heart disease have been the subject of a large number of research studies, and the results are remarkably consistent. It does not appear to matter which country is being studied, or the method used to determine socio-economic disadvantage, the more deprived people in societies are less likely to gain access to investigation (angiography) and re-vascularization procedures (percutaneous transluminal angioplasty or coronary artery bypass grafting) (Ancona *et al.* 2000; Black *et al.* 1995; Hippisley-Cox and Pringle 2000; Keskimaki *et al.* 1997; MacLeod *et al.* 1999; Payne and Saul 1997). Adjustment for need, using either mortality rates (Black *et al.* 1995; Keskimaki *et al.* 1997) or community surveys of symptom prevalence (Payne and Saul 1997), support the idea that patients were not being prioritized for admission on the basis of their clinical condition. The more deprived also waited longer for admission to hospital (Pell *et al.* 2000).

In contrast to the low rates of routine referral to specialist care, poorer people have high rates of emergency hospitalizations and admissions. This is neatly illustrated by a study of hospital admissions within one English health authority area. Deprivation at the level of general practice was positively correlated with emergency, but not routine admissions (Reid *et al.* 1999). Similar patterns of hospital use have been described in Canada (Roos and Mustard 1997), the USA (McMahon *et al.* 1993) and Finland (Keskimaki *et al.* 1995).

Preventive services

Infectious diseases are closely associated with poverty, and immunization programmes have the potential to have an impact on inequalities in health (Jimenez 2001). Yet, in countries where universal programmes are available, vaccine coverage is still lower for children from lower social groups or deprived areas (Essex *et al.* 1993; Hull *et al.* 2001; Simonetti *et al.* 2002). There is also evidence from the United Kingdom of a lower provision of health promotion clinics for poorer social and economic groups (Gillam 1992).

How could health services take poverty into account?

The previous section has described a complex association between health service use and socio-economic disadvantage, with examples of the inverse care law in operation, especially in relation to secondary care. Although poorer people are less likely to be referred routinely to hospital, they are more likely to be admitted as emergencies and, in universal systems, to stay for longer. Before ways can be devised to address such differentials in access and use of services, searching questions need to be asked about what stops poorer groups gaining appropriate access to the services they need. In this respect, it is useful to distinguish between different kinds of access, because they each imply distinct actions. The next sections will focus on financial, geographical and cultural barriers to health care access, and successful strategies to overcome them.

Improving financial access and reducing the medical poverty trap

There may be numerous financial barriers placed in the way of poor people who need access to health care. In the most extreme situation, people on low incomes may be inhibited from seeking care altogether because they cannot afford it. Untreated, their health may deteriorate until their condition becomes chronic, or they require emergency care – both scenarios incur high health care costs. A related situation arises when people obtain some form of care when they fall sick, but the expenses involved force them to take out loans or sell assets that may be needed for their long-term livelihood. As a consequence, they may fall into a medical poverty trap in which medical expenses push people into poverty, or deepen already existing poverty. When this happens the health system itself becomes one of the causes of poverty (Whitehead *et al.* 2001).

The situation may be exacerbated by the behaviour of the providers of health services. Patients from disadvantaged groups are often more costly to treat than the average, because they are more likely to suffer from more expensive and long-standing conditions and may take longer to recover from treatment due to their generally poorer health. Against this background, providers of medical care may try to avoid those patients who are likely to be costly, and instead cream off the healthier, 'profitable' patients. Alternatively, the services provided for a set price may be of lower quality in a deprived area, to cope with the extra demand and keep within the budget. Invisible barriers, such as unofficial under-the-table payments for services, are becoming increasingly important for patients in many central and eastern European countries and clearly constitute a serious problem for the poor.

Even with universal services, free at the point of use, financial barriers may arise. Dental services offer a very clear example of the role played by fees in preventing access to health care, as dental fees are charged in many European countries, even when other aspects of health care are free. Official statistics show that annual courses of treatment fell by almost one quarter in the UK when free check-ups were abolished and charges increased in the late 1980s (Yuen 1999). This is sure to have had a particularly profound effect on the disadvantaged in society, and may contribute to the marked socio-economic variation in edentulouness seen in the UK (Watt and Sheiham 1999).

France has recently revised the way in which it funds health care, to remove financial barriers faced by the poorest section of the population. Before 2000, health insurance was provided via social security contributions from employed people. The basic cover offered partial reimbursement of health care costs for employees and their families, then workers were expected to purchase supplementary insurance to cover part or all of their remaining costs. However, reclaiming expenses involved a complex and stigmatising procedure for low-income patients. This system left the poorest 2 per cent of the population without basic cover, and a further 16 per cent without supplementary cover. A study in 1997 found that many of those excluded from cover had not sought the treatment they needed because of the costs (Aligon *et al.* 2001). Two years after the introduction of universal health insurance for low-income people, Cuverture Maladie Universelle (CMU), 1.2 million people are receiving the basic CMU, and 4.7 million, or 7.8 per cent of the population, the supplementary CMU. In a study of CMU recipients after 12 months of the new scheme, 65 per cent said that they had used at least one of the services that they had previously not taken up because they could not afford to pay (Van-Ingen 2002).

From such experiences, strategies for improving financial access to essential care for the poor can be gleaned, including:

◆ Breaking the link between sickness and payment by sharing the risks out across the whole population and by including medicines in the cover.

◆ Devising less stigmatizing processes for claiming the cover that a person is entitled to under the law.

◆ Reforming the way the system is structured and services are delivered, in order to minimize interference with people's jobs and livelihoods.

◆ Auditing services for equity in order to identify who is getting what services and at what cost, and most importantly, who is effectively denied the services they need because they cannot afford them.

More sensitive cultural access and tackling discrimination

Cultural access is mainly concerned with the contacts between health workers and patients since a good relationship is a prerequisite for high quality care. Poorer groups in society often face significant barriers. Differences in educational and cultural backgrounds of academically qualified professionals and unskilled workers, for example, may make establishing a dialogue more difficult and lead to all kinds of communication problems. This may result from both differences in health beliefs and knowledge, as well as social distance. A lack of appreciation of the difficulties of living on a low income may mean that professionals give unrealistic advice or fail to provide the extra support needed to ensure a speedy recovery.

Even in the face of apparently equitable access, disadvantaged patients may not receive the same services as the rest. Much of the research evidence suggests that poorer people have a different experience of primary care. For example, their consultations are shorter (Stirling *et al.* 2001; Wiggers and Sanson-Fisher 1997), they are more likely to be passive recipients of instructions (Bochner 1983), and may be less able to actively seek information (Boulton *et al.* 1986). In other community services, such as pharmacy, differences have been noted in the advice given, according to the socio-economic status of the area in which the service is located (Rogers *et al.* 1998).

Some disadvantaged patients may be unhappy with their primary care options since a high proportion of attendees at accident and emergency departments with 'primary care' problems are poorer people. Whilst this earns the label 'inappropriate' hospital use from health professionals (Murphy 1998), it may reflect people's views on the alternatives available, or a desire to exercise more control over their use of health care. For example, a study in Glasgow found that dissatisfaction with daytime provision in general practice was a factor in the heavy use of out-of-hours care by disadvantaged people (Drummond *et al.* 2000).

Strategies for improving cultural access for the poor include:

- Ensuring that professional training for health care staff includes considering the needs of poorer patients and the ethical principles that should guide their interaction with all patients, including the disadvantaged.

- Adapting service times to fit the family and work patterns of patients working in unskilled and blue collar jobs.

- Adapting the timing and staffing of services to fit in with religious or cultural practices, and training or employing staff with additional language and cultural–anthropological skills to overcome communication barriers.

Provision of additional preventive and supportive services to minimize the health damage caused by living in poverty. Services are needed to help people to cope better with the risks they face, so that they are less likely to fall ill when they experience hardship. These include counselling services to help prevent a decline in mental health following unemployment and misfortunes, and social support for all families living in disadvantaged circumstances.

Improving geographic access for poorer groups

Health services, even when officially free, may be few and far between in disadvantaged areas, making them geographically inaccessible to poor or marginalized groups. In most European cities, for example, it is common to find that health care providers have gravitated towards the more affluent parts of town, which are over-provided for, while at the same time there are severe shortages of primary care facilities and staff in the run-down inner city or in social housing estates on the outskirts of town. This pattern has been noted for Stockholm following an increase in private practitioners (Dahlgren 1999) and greater provision of primary care facilities has been found in more affluent districts within Scottish cities (Sooman and Macintyre 1995). The recruitment of doctors to work in deprived urban areas in England is now said to be in crisis (Hastings and Rao 2001). It is not just quantity, but quality that is affected. General practices in poor areas demonstrate fewer of the characteristics associated with high quality care. They are more likely to be run by single-handed practitioners, they tend to be less responsive to recommended changes in policy and slower to develop new services (Leese and Bosanquet 1995).

This apparent lower quality of care may be for a mixture of reasons, ranging from the fact that it is easier to make a living by serving affluent fee-paying patients, rather than poor ones, to the understandable preference of many practitioners to live and work in pleasant surroundings. A similar differential may exist between urban and rural localities. For poor people who live in the under-served areas, however, poorer geographic spread of services may mean that they have to spend more time and more money in transport costs and loss of earnings to gain access to the available services.

In a study in four low-income areas of Liverpool, for example, one-third of families had neither car nor telephone. Respondents were asked to describe what was involved for them in attending a 9.30am clinic appointment at the nearest hospital. The trip there and back for a short clinic appointment often took half a day and involved complicated arrangements for transport and care of children or vulnerable dependants left at home (Pearson *et al.* 1992). It is little wonder that there are high rates of non-attendance for pre-booked medical appointments in some parts of the NHS, especially among patients from disadvantaged areas. Health professionals may not fully appreciate the problems posed by barriers to geographic access. However, the increased tendency for UK general practitioners to visit disadvantaged patients at home and out-of-hours does suggest that some services are becoming responsive to needs.

Strategies for addressing barriers to geographic access for the poor include:

♦ Ensuring that the volume and quality of health services match the pattern of ill health found in communities and groups. Social inequities and poverty create an increased need for medical care. Thus, the Netherlands, Sweden and the United Kingdom have all endeavoured to devise more equitable resource allocation formulae, for example, allocating extra funds for services to deprived populations with greater health care needs (Diderichsen *et al.* 1997; Rice and Smith 2002).

♦ Providing long-term financial and other incentives for health professionals to work in poorer areas.

♦ Devising outreach services by taking clinics to marginalized groups or hard-to-reach rural populations, rather than waiting for them to come to the services.

More direct attacks on poverty

Increasingly questions are being asked about the scope of direct action by the health sector to reduce or prevent poverty and unemployment. How, if at all, can the health system influence the amount of money that low-income people have to spend on the prerequisites for health? How can it help people find jobs and enhance their skills to increase their chances of employment?

These are questions that the 26 Health Action Zones (HAZs) in England have been addressing under government initiatives to break the link between poverty and ill health. HAZs are designated administrative localities selected because they contain the most disadvantaged, socially excluded populations in the country. Set up in the late 1990s, HAZs cover around 13 million people, or one quarter of the English population. Within each zone, the local statutory agencies are charged with working with the voluntary sector and with the people suffering deprivation to deliver the public services more sensitively and effectively. They are also required to explore new ways of using their resources to tackle the wider determinants of health beyond the health sector. To do this, ring fenced funding of £330 million (Euro 525 million) has been provided, over the first four years (*www.haznet.org.uk*). It is still too early to tell whether HAZs are having any impact on the health of the public. Attributing changes in population health to such interventions is always difficult, and new methods of evaluation are being developed, appropriate to complex, community initiatives (Judge 2000).

As well as working on different aspects of access to health care, some NHS agencies in particular have gone further and considered how they could use their considerable influence in the local economy. Examples include:

♦ Deliberate attempts by local NHS providers to stimulate employment and provide job opportunities within the deprived communities that they serve, for example, by setting up 'back-to-work' training schemes and by encouraging local recruitment to job vacancies in the health services.

- ◆ Auditing their own performance as a fair employer, such as looking after the rights and needs of its workforce for a healthy work environment and a fair wage.
- ◆ An explicit policy on the part of local health services to use their considerable purchasing power to buy goods and services from suppliers in surrounding disadvantaged areas, thus helping to stimulate the local economy.
- ◆ Primary care providers offering welfare rights advice in their premises to help patients claim the social security benefits to which they are entitled. These schemes have helped low-income patients claim large amounts of extra income (Paris and Player 1993).

Conclusion

It is possible to devise separately financed and provided services for the poor but there is a great danger, as Titmuss famously remarked, that a service for the poor will become a poor service (Titmuss 1968). To meet both ethical and practical concerns, it is preferable to aim for a universal service, but one that makes special efforts to reach the worst off in society. The special efforts need to include attention to the barriers faced by poorer people, including the financial, geographic and cultural issues outlined above. Too many systems are blind to the barriers they erect and the first step to improvement is to monitor more sensitively what happens to low-income people when they attempt to gain access to care. It is not just an issue of quantity but most especially of quality of care.

It is clear from the evidence reviewed in this chapter that we know far more about the nature of the problems of access to care than how to resolve them. This area of research has been neglected right across Europe. In some countries, such as the UK, the challenges are well documented, and attention should turn now to developing successful intervention strategies, including implementation research. In other countries, inequities in access to health care for poorer people have yet to be acknowledged, and there is much work to be done in monitoring and raising awareness of the problems faced by these groups. If, as we suggested at the beginning of the chapter, appropriate health care is to be universally available for rich and poor alike, this huge agenda for research and evaluation cannot be ignored. Action should not stop there, however. Not only do health systems need to put their own houses in order, they could, and should, look beyond their own boundaries and join with others to tackle poverty head on.

References

Acheson, D., Barker, D., Chambers, J., Graham, H., Marmot, M. and Whitehead, M. (1998) *Report of the independent inquiry into inequalities in health.* The Stationery Office, London.

Aligon, A., Com-Ruelle, L., Dourgnon, P., Dumesnil, S., Grignon, M. and Retailleau, A. (2001) *La consommation medicale en 1997 selon les caracteristiques individuelles. CREDES n°1345*. Centre de Recherche d' Etude et de Documentation en Economie de la Santé, Paris.

Ancona, C., Agabiti, N., Forastiere, F., Arca, M., Fusco, D. and Ferro, S. (2000) Coronary artery bypass graft surgery: socioeconomic inequalities in access and in 30-day mortality. A population-based study in Rome, Italy. *Journal of Epidemiology and Community Health*, **54**, 930–5.

Barker, D. (1998) *Mothers, babies and health in later life*. Churchill Livingstone, Edinburgh.

Black, N., Langham, S. and Petticrew, M. (1995) Coronary revascularisation: Why do rates vary geographically in the UK? *Journal of Epidemiology and Community Health*, **49**, 408–12.

Blank, N. and Diderichsen, F. (1996) Social inequalities in the experience of illness in Sweden: a 'double suffering'. *Scandinavian Journal of Social Medicine*, **24**, 81–95.

Blaxter, M. (1984) Equity and consultation rates in general practice. *British Medical Journal*, **288**, 1963–7.

Bochner, S. (1983) Doctor, patients and their cultures. In D. Pendelton and J. Hasler (eds) *Doctor-patient communication*. Academic Press, London.

Bongers, I. M., Van der Meer, J. B., Van den Bos, B. J. and Mackenbach, J. P. (1997) Socio-economic differences in general practitioner and outpatient specialist care in the Netherlands: A matter of health insurance? *Social Science and Medicine*, **44**, 1161–8.

Borrel, C. and Arias, A. (1995) Socio-economic factors and mortality in urban settings the case of Barcelona. *Journal of Epidemiology and Community Health*, **49**, 460–5.

Boulton, M., Tuckett, D., Olson, C. and Williams, A. (1986) Social class and the general practice consultation. *Sociology of Health and Illness*, **8**, 325.

Burchardt, T., Le Grand, J. and Piachaud, D. (1999) Social exclusion in Britain 1991–1995. *Social Policy and Administration*, **33**, 227–44.

Cornia, G. and Paniccia, R. (1995) *The demographic impact of sudden impoverishment: Eastern Europe during the 1989–1994 transition*. UNICEF Innocenti Occasional Papers, Economic Policy Studies, No. 49. UNICEF, Paris.

Dahlgren, G. (1999) Strategies for reducing social inequities in health – visions and reality. In E. Ollila, M. Koivusalo and T. Partonen (eds) *Equity in health through public policy. Report on the expert meeting in Kellokoski Finland 1996*. Stakes, Helsinki, Finland.

Dahlgren, G., Diderichsen, F. and Spetz, C.-L. (1984) Health policy targets and need based planning. *SOU 1984: 40 Allmänna Förlaget, Stockholm* (in Swedish).

Dahlgren, G. and Whitehead, M. (1992) *Policies and strategies to promote equity in health*. World Health Organization, Copenhagen.

Department of Health (2000) *The NHS plan*. The Stationery Office, London.

Diderichsen, F., Varde, E. and Whitehead, M. (1997) Resource allocation to health authorities: the quest for an equitable formula in Britain and Sweden. *British Medical Journal*, **315**, 875–8.

Drummond, N., McConnachie, A., O'Donnell, C. A., Moffat, K. J., Wilson, P. and Ross, S. (2000) Social variation in reasons for contacting general practice out-of-hours: implications for daytime service provision? *British Journal of General Practice*, **50**, 460–4.

Dunlop, S., Coyte, P. C. and McIsaac, W. (2000) Socio-economic status and the utilisation of physicians' services: results from the Canadian National Population Health Survey. *Social Science and Medicine*, **51**, 123–33.

Essex, C., Counsell, A. M. and Geddis, D. C. (1993) Immunization status and demographic characteristics of New Zealand infants in the first 6 months of life. *Journal of Paediatrics and Child Health*, **29**, 379–83.

Fraser, S., Bunce, C., Wormald, R. and Brunner, E. (2001) Deprivation and late presentation of glaucoma: case-control study. *British Medical Journal*, **322**, 639–43.

Gillam, S. (1992) Provision of heath promotion clinics in relation to population need: another example of the Inverse Care Law. *British Journal of General Practice*, **42**, 54–6.

Graham, H. (1993) *Hardship and health in women's lives*. Harvester/Wheatsheaf, Hemel Hempstead.

Haglund, B. (1994) Equity in care. *EpC-rapport Socialstyrelsen, Stockholm* (in Swedish), **3**.

Hahn, R., Eaker, E., Barker, N., Teutsch, S. M., Sosniak, W. A. and Krieger, N. (1995) Poverty and death in the United States – 1973 and 1991. *Epidemiology*, **6**, 490–7.

Hastings, A. and Rao, M. (2001) Doctoring deprived areas. *British Medical Journal*, **323**, 409–10.

Hemmingway, H. and Marmot, M. (1999) Psychosocial factors in the aetiology and prognosis of coronary heart disease: systematic review of prospective cohort studies. *British Medical Journal*, **318**, 1460–7.

Hippisley-Cox, J., Hardy, C., Pringle, M., Fielding, K., Carlisle, R. and Chilvers, C. (1997) The effect of deprivation on variations in general practitioners' referral rates: a cross sectional study of computerised data on new medical and surgical outpatient referrals in Nottinghamshire. *British Medical Journal*, **314**, 1458–61.

Hippisley-Cox, J. and Pringle, M. (2000) Inequalities in access to coronary angiography and revascularisation: the association of deprivation and location of primary care services. *British Journal of General Practice*, **50**, 449–54.

Hull, B. P., McIntyre, P. B. and Sayer, G. P. (2001) Factors associated with low uptake of measles and pertussis vaccines-an ecologic study based on the Australian Childhood Immunisation Register. *Australian and New Zealand Journal of Public Health*, **25**, 405–10.

Jimenez, J. (2001) Vaccines – a wonderful tool for equity in health. *Vaccine*, **19**, 2201–5.

Joint Health Surveys Unit (1999) *Health Survey for England 1998*. The Stationery Office, London.

Judge, K. (2000) Testing evaluation to the limits: the case of the English health action zones. *Journal of Health Services Research Policy*, **5** (1), 3–5.

Keskimaki, I., Koskinen, S., Salinto, M. and Aro, S. (1997) Socioeconomic and gender inequities in access to coronary artery bypass grafting in Finland. *European Journal of Public Health*, **7**, 392–7.

Keskimaki, I., Salinto, M. and Aro, S. (1995) Socioeconomic equity in Finnish hospital care in relation to need. *Social Science and Medicine*, **41**, 425–31.

Le Grand, J. (1978) The distribution of public expenditure: the case of health care. *Economica*, **45**, 125–42.

Leese, B. and Bosanquet, N. (1995) Change in general practice and its effects on service provision in areas with different socioeconomic characteristics. *British Medical Journal*, **311**, 546–50.

Mackenbach, J. P., Cavelaars, A. E., Kunst, A. E. and Groenhof, F. (2000) Socioeconomic inequalities in cardiovascular disease mortality; an international study. *European Heart Journal*, **21**, 1141–51.

MacLeod, M. C., Finlayson, A. R., Pell, J. P. and Findlay, I. N. (1999) Geographic, demographic, and socioeconomic variations in the investigation and management of coronary heart disease in Scotland. *Heart*, **81**, 252–6.

Majeed, A., Bardsley, M., Morgan, D., O'Sullivan, C. and Bindman, A. B. (2000) Cross sectional study of primary care groups in London: association of measures of socioeconomic and health status with hospital admission rates. *British Medical Journal*, **321**, 1057–60.

McMahon, L. F., Wolfe, R. A., Griffith, J. R. and Cuthbertson, D. (1993) Socioeconomic influences on small area hospital utilization. *Medical Care*, **31** (5), Suppl. YS29–YS36.

Mitchell, R., Shaw, M. and Dorling, D. (2000) *Inequalities in life and death: what if Britain were more equal?* The Policy Press in association with Joseph Rowntree Foundation, Bristol.

Murphy, A. W. (1998) 'Inappropriate' attenders at accident and emergency departments I: definition, incidence and reasons for attendance. *Family Practice*, **15**, 23–32.

Navarro, V. and Benach, J. (1997) *Social inequalities in health in Spain: report of the Scientific Commission to Study Social Health Inequalities in Spain* (in Spanish). Ministerio de Sanidad y Consumo, Madrid.

O'Donnell, C. A. (2000) Variation in GP referral rates: what can we learn from the literature? *Family Practice*, **17**, 462–71.

O'Donnell, O. and Propper, C. (1991) Equity and the distribution of UK NHS resources. *Journal of Health Economics*, **10**, 1–19.

Office for National Statistics (1997) *Mortality statistics: perinatal and infant: social and biological factors*, Series DH3. The Stationery Office, London.

Paris, J. and Player, D. (1993) Citizens' advice in general practice. *British Medical Journal*, **306**, 1518–20.

Payne, N. and Saul, C. (1997) Variations in use of cardiology services in a health authority: comparison of coronary artery revascularization rates with prevalence of angina and coronary mortality. *British Medical Journal*, **314**, 257–61.

Pearson, M., Dawson, C., Moore, H. and Spencer, S. (1992) Health on borrowed time? Prioritizing and meeting needs in low-income households. *Health and Social Care*, **1**, 45–54.

Pell, J. P., Pell, A. C. H., Norrie, J., Ford, I. and Cobbe, S. M. (2000) Effect of socioeconomic deprivation on waiting time for cardiac surgery: retrospective cohort study. *British Medical Journal*, **320**, 15–19.

Reid, F. D., Cook, D. G. and Majeed, A. (1999) Explaining variation in hospital admission rates between general practices: cross sectional study. *British Medical Journal*, **319**, 98–103.

Rice, N. and Smith, P. C. (2002) Strategic resource allocation and funding decisions. In E. Mossialos, A. Dixon, J. Figueras and J. Kutzin (eds) *Funding health care: options for Europe*. Open University Press, Buckingham.

Rogers, A., Hassell, K., Noyce, P. and Harris, J. (1998) Advice giving in community pharmacy: variations between pharmacies in different locations. *Health and Place*, **4**, 365–73.

Roos, N. P. and Mustard, C. A. (1997) Variation in health and health care use by socioeconomic status in Winnipeg, Canada: does the system work well? Yes and no. *The Milbank Quarterly*, **75**, 89–111.

Sen, A. (2000) *Development as freedom*. Oxford University Press, Oxford.

Shaw, M., Dorling, D., Gordon, D. and Davey Smith, G. (1999) *The widening gap: health inequalities and policy in Britain*. The Policy Press, Bristol.

Simonetti, A., Adamo, B., Tancredi, F., Triassi, M. and Grandolfo, M. E. (2002) Evaluation of immunization practices in Naples, Italy. *Vaccine*, **20**, 1046–9.

Sooman, A. and Macintyre, S. (1995) Health and perceptions of the local environment in socially contrasting neighbourhoods in Glasgow. *Health and Place*, **1**, 15–26.

Stirling, A. M., Wilson, P. and McConnachie, A. (2001) Deprivation, psychological distress, and consultation length in general practice. *British Journal of General Practice*, **51**, 456–60.

Titmuss, R. (1968) *Commitment to welfare*. Pantheon, New York.

Townsend, P. (1979) *Poverty in the United Kingdom*. Penguin, Harmondsworth.

Tudor Hart, J. (1971) The inverse care law. *Lancet*, **1**, 405–12.

Valkonen, T., Martelin, T., Rimpela, A., Notkola, V. and Savela, S. (1993) *Socio-economic differences in mortality, 1981–90*. Population, 1. Central Statistical Office of Finland, Helsinki.

Van-Ingen, F. (2002) *Universal health insurance: reaching the poorest communities in France. A series in poverty and health case Study 2*. Venice, World Health Organization Venice Centre on Investment for Health and Development.

Watt, R. and Sheiham, A. (1999) Inequalities in oral health: a review of the evidence and recommendations for action. *British Dental Journal*, **187**, 6–12.

Whitehead, M., Dahlgren, G. and Evans, T. (2001) Equity and health sector reform: can low-income countries escape the medical poverty trap? *Lancet*, **358**, 833–6.

Whitehead, M. and Diderichsen, F. (1997) International evidence on social inequalities in health. In F. Drever and M. Whitehead (eds) *Health inequalities – Decennial Supplement. Office for National Statistics* Series DS No. 15. The Stationery Office, London.

Whitehead, M., Evandrou, M., Haglund, B. and Diderichsen, F. (1997) As the health divide widens in Sweden and Britain, what's happening to access to care? *British Medical Journal*, **315**, 1006–9.

Wiggers, J. H. and Sanson-Fisher, R. (1997) Practitioner provision of preventive care in general practice consultations: association with patient educational and occupational status. *Social Science and Medicine*, **44**, 137–46.

Wilkinson, R. (1996) *Unhealthy societies the afflictions of inequality*. Routledge, London.

Yuen, P. (1999) *Office of Health Economics Compendium of Health Statistics*, 11th edition. Office of Health Economics, London.

Chapter 6

Access and Equity in Australian Rural Health Services

John S. Humphreys and Jane Dixon

Introduction

Despite unrelenting urbanization, rural dwellers still comprise a significant minority in many western countries – 30 per cent in Australia, 25 per cent in the United States and 16 per cent in Canada (Hugo 2002). 'Rurality' does not, however, imply uniformity; in fact, rural areas are often extremely diverse, comprising a complex mosaic of activities and communities differentiated by geography, economic activity, environment, population characteristics and social organization. From such diversity derive community needs, expectations, health status and well-being levels that are often significantly different from those experienced in urban regions.

The focus of this chapter is rural Australia. While recognizing that rural areas are integral parts of larger national structures, there are nonetheless justifiable reasons for focusing on the rural, not just because of differences with metropolitan regions, but importantly because there is ample evidence of increasing disadvantage and inequity of access to social provisions for rural relative to metropolitan dwellers, and of their increasing economic dependence on government (Haberkorn *et al.* 1999).

What follows is a review of Australian efforts to ensure equitable life-chances and resource allocation for rural areas, whose residents are often both socially and geographically disadvantaged. We begin by describing relevant population characteristics and recent data showing significant rural–metropolitan health status discrepancies. We then summarize the shifting relationship between the state and civil society over the last quarter of a century, draw out implicit assumptions about the politically instituted basis of claims, and comment on how rural Australia has fared under different governance regimes. Several examples then follow of how rural Australia's claims-making efforts have been translated into health service provision. In particular, we identify innovative models of delivering health care to rural populations, which seek to address the difficulties of ensuring equitable service provision to disadvantaged rural areas. While innovative health services assist to overcome, or at least in part ameliorate, geographical disadvantages, without a comprehensive inter-sectoral approach that addresses the broader determinants of health, many rural–urban health outcome inequalities will persist and may even be exacerbated. We conclude by asking what rural Australians might reasonably expect from a publicly funded health system.

The distinctive demography of rural Australia

In 2001, Australia's population reached 19.5 million, 2.5 per cent of whom were Aborigines and Torres Strait Islanders. Although Australia covers a land area about the size of the continental United States, over 60 per cent of the population live in half a dozen capital cities, the majority living within fifty kilometres of the eastern seaboard; the remainder live in rural regions. Rural Australia therefore runs the gamut from major provincial centres (with generally fewer than 100,000 residents) to small country towns, isolated mining communities and indigenous outstations, and includes both the closely settled coastal farming regions as well as the sparsely settled areas of northern and inland Australia.

In recent years, population growth has been concentrated mostly around the largest cities and coastal communities, with population decline the hallmark of many small inland settlements and farming regions. Compounding the general ageing process resulting from fertility decline over than last fifty years, internal migration is contributing to a shift in age structure in both metropolitan and non-metropolitan Australia – and most notably to ageing in rural regions. At the same time that younger and higher income individuals migrate to major centres for education and lifestyle opportunities, many low-income households migrate to rural towns where costs are lower. Retirees are leaving farms and small rural communities and gravitating towards coastal towns and regional centres that have a wider range of health care services. In short, many rural regions are becoming depopulated, characterized by an ageing, less affluent population.

While the proportion of retirement age population still is greater in the major cities than the non-metropolitan area, the proportion dependent on social services is significantly higher in non-metropolitan Australia – 36.5 per cent compared to 29.5 per cent (Hugo 2002). Higher proportions of single parent families and disabled people, together with a significant percentage of the population on very low incomes from paid employment, contribute to average weekly incomes for rural dwellers being approximately two-thirds the level of city inhabitants (Glover *et al.* 1999).

These contrasting population characteristics result in considerable social diversity. Coastal towns have age and socio-economic profiles quite different from those of towns only fifty kilometres further inland. The health service needs of large regional towns (with base hospitals and choice of resident doctors) are very different from those of small rural communities lacking these services. Some regions, based, for example, on wine growing and tourism, are relatively economically advantaged, while once-prosperous service towns in the wheat and sheep belts have below average incomes (Haberkorn *et al.* 1999; Hugo 2002).

By comparison with many major urban centres, however, rural areas generally are significantly worse-off in terms of the distribution of wealth and levels of well-being, as revealed by social indicators such as employment and education (Haberkorn *et al.* 1999). Since 1980 there have been dramatic shifts in the geographic relativities of wealth and income since global economic processes have largely benefited urban and educated populations. As a result, farming districts now dominate the list of postcodes with lowest mean incomes (Australian Taxation Office 1998), with the remote outback and northern Australia figuring large among the worst 10 per cent of localities. Rural regions have also experienced a worsening in levels of well-being over recent years (Walmsley and Weinand 1997).

Rural Australia is also home to a large number of Australia's multiply disadvantaged Aboriginal and Torres Strait people, a group that is growing more rapidly than the rest of the population, but which still accounts for only approximately 450,000 persons. Overall, 70 per cent of indigenous Australians live outside the major cities, with more than half of these people living in parts of the country classified as 'remote' (Phillips 2002). Since in some states, the numbers of indigenous Australians living in the metropolitan centres outnumber those in outlying areas, some have argued that what is special about Aborigines is not their geographic location but their Aboriginality, a matter that is dealt with elsewhere in this book.

Given the diversity just described, it is reasonable to conclude that relative economic and educational disadvantage are features of rural and remote Australia and that the pattern of disadvantage increases with distance from major urban centres. Typically, as disadvantage grows, access to the whole range of public and commercial services diminishes and community capacity to press a claim for these services declines (Hugo 2002).

Health status relativities

Given that rural Australia is characterized by socio-economic and environmental diversity, it is hardly surprising that health status is similarly diverse, ranging from indigenous communities with appalling levels of morbidity and mortality to communities whose health status is arguably as good as that of the 'healthiest' suburbs in metropolitan areas. The spatial heterogeneity of disease becomes even more apparent when one disaggregates the data of indigenous from non-indigenous Australians. For some conditions, such as respiratory disease, the rates for non-indigenous Australians living in remote areas are worse than for those living in rural towns and cities, but for others, including ischaemic heart disease and male cancers, residents in remote areas do better than those in rural and metropolitan Australia (Phillips 2002). In general, however, the health of Australians living in rural and remote regions is 'worse than those living in capital cities and other metropolitan areas' (Australian Institute of Health and Welfare 1998). These health inequalities typically exhibit a gradient of health disadvantage that displays consistent increments in mortality and morbidity as one travels away from capital cities and other metropolitan areas (Rolley 2000).

Although rural–urban health status data are patchy, the evidence suggests a pattern of health status differentials with considerable scope for improvement. Based on available health indicators and recognized risk factors, the health of Australians living in rural and remote areas compares unfavourably with those living in capital cities. The following generalizations can be drawn from national data collections and other cross-sectional surveys:

◆ Based on standardized death ratios, the death rate for men in capital cities is 6 per cent lower than for men in large rural centres and 20 per cent less than in remote centres.

◆ The health of indigenous Australians is significantly worse than that of other Australians, with death rates for indigenous people being five to seven times those of non-indigenous people aged 25–54 years (Australian Institute of Health and Welfare 2000; McLennan and Madden 1999).

◆ Hospital separation rates for diabetes in remote areas are twice that of the metropolitan zone, while in rural areas, the rates are 50 per cent higher for males and 25 per cent higher for females.

◆ The population-wide improvements in coronary heart disease over the last decade have stalled among blue-collar males in New South Wales country towns and rural Victoria (Burnley 1998; Peach and Bath 1999).

◆ Since the 1960s, per capita rates of suicide have continued to increase among young men aged 15–24 years, doubling in metropolitan areas, but with a twelve fold increase in communities with fewer than 4000 people (National Rural Health Alliance 2000).

◆ Rural employees continue to suffer a disproportionate number of work-related deaths and injuries (Phillips 2002). Respiratory problems, like 'farmers lung' (including bagassosis), problems resulting from the extensive use of agricultural herbicides and pesticides, allergies relating to dust and pollens, skin cancers, brucellosis and hydatids, are essentially outcomes of rural living (Humphreys and Rolley 1991). For males, hospital separation rates for injury are 39 per cent higher than capital cities in rural areas and 145 per cent higher in remote areas.

♦ Road trauma, mental illness and alcohol and substance abuse are more prevalent in rural and remote areas than in urban areas (Auditor General 1998).

♦ The dental health of Australians living in rural and remote areas is significantly inferior to that of other Australians (Australian Institute of Health and Welfare 2002).

♦ Smoking rates and alcohol consumption are both significantly higher in non-metropolitan areas (Australian Institute of Health and Welfare 2002).

While the extent of a specifically rural epidemiology is difficult to ascertain (Humphreys 1998), preliminary evidence suggests the existence of inequalities in the prevalence and incidence of many diseases, significantly higher death rates overall in rural areas, and even more extreme disadvantage in remote areas (Fragar *et al.* 1997). Furthermore, there is growing consensus as to the major social determinants that lie behind the generally inferior health status of those living outside the cities. The first determinant concerns features of geography, in particular distance, the physical environment, sparse infrastructure and harsh climates. The second involves the nature of economic activity, occupation and lifestyles of rural inhabitants, with low incomes, low educational achievement and particular occupational categories contributing to a clustering of attitudes to health and illness and risk-taking behaviours. Finally, access to services is compromised by geographical location. The 'tyranny of distance' and lack of transport remain major impediments to accessing health care for many rural Australians. While it is often difficult to disentangle the effects of socio-economic from locational disadvantage, and locational disadvantage from the effects of the physical environment, there is little doubt that the coincidence between the three creates the worst of all possible health environments.

In short, the data offer an objective insight into the distinctive health needs of rural Australia, and in an era of evidence-based health care, provide a strong basis for claims upon governments for appropriate remedial and preventive services. Although need has been espoused as the main determinant of 'who *should* get what where', and remains a necessary distributional principle underpinning the resource allocation process, by itself the concept has proven problematic to operationalize and is in any event insufficient (Culyer 1995). Indeed, Harvey identified need as only one of eight possible grounds supporting a population's claims upon the society in which they 'have their being' (Harvey 1973); others include inherent equality, valuation of services in terms of supply and demand, inherited rights, merit, contribution to the common good, actual productive contribution and efforts and sacrifices. However, the emphasis that is placed on these factors will alter with changing community expectations and aspirations and these in turn must influence the precise nature of the relationship between the state and civil society. An understanding of the nature of the claims for rural Australia for health services can therefore only be appreciated when they are seen against the broader background of the changing role of the state and its continual realignment with civil society.

State–civil society relationships and claims-making

Like some other industrialized countries, Australia is in a protracted phase of 'rolling back' its Welfare State ethos and provisions. From the 1950s to 1970s the Australian government assumed a leading role in providing financial support at vulnerable transition points (such as childhood, old age, unemployment and sickness) and accepted that needs assessment should drive program development and implementation (Hoatson et al. 1996). Regional programs (including those covering rural areas), a highlight of government in the mid 1970s, were pursued as a means of bringing together spatial equity issues with fiscal crisis concerns. The issues of whether the state should provide universal or targeted services, and whether service planning was best fulfilled at a local or central level, revolved around cost considerations as well as social justice considerations – specifically utilitarianism. In this period, rural Australia benefited from government transfers, mainly in the form of farm subsidies and the regulation of producer boards. This was the major special concession to the 40 per cent of the population who then lived outside the major cities but it was limited in its reach beyond the agricultural sector.

With the widespread adoption of neo-liberal policies of privatization of government services, of privileging the individual over the social unit, and of stressing efficiencies that involved doing more with less, the so-called 'Contract State' came into being in the 1980s (Hoatson et al. 1996). National and state governments took on the role of enabling rather than doing, of directing policy rather than program delivery, and of purchasing but not providing services. Notions of achieving fairness through government provision gave way to ideas of individual choice in the marketplace. However, a lack of marketplace providers in areas characterized by small, fragmented and poor populations (many rural communities) proved troublesome to the advocates of smaller government and their espousal of a market orientation towards everyday life.

The failures associated with dependence on the market place as the mechanism for delivering health care services, particularly in sparsely populated rural areas, are all too apparent (Hancock 1999). Research has highlighted how competition policy and compulsory competitive tendering in the state of Victoria led to 'the economic hollowing of country Victoria; where metropolitan Melbourne and half a dozen regional centres will in future service the needs of ever-declining rural population, bereft of local services, local opportunities and local control' (Ernst *et al.* 1998). The problems of favouring privatization of rural health services over their public provision were further exemplified in the 1990s by the shortcomings associated with the introduction of case mix funding for small rural hospitals in Victoria (Department of Health and Community Services 1994) and the recently aborted experiment of privatising the Gippsland Base Hospital.

The Third Way political philosophy, adopted by the Australian Labor Party and practised to varying degrees over the last four years by state and territory Labor governments, has had a paradoxical impact: not only has it legitimized further the market's involvement in the delivery of the public good, but it has reinserted normative considerations into political discourse. Anthony Giddens, the architect of this approach, stressed the fundamental step of ensuring equality of access to material resources at the same time as emphasizing freedom or autonomy of action within a social contract that there be 'no rights without responsibilities' (Giddens 1998). But Giddens' formulation of rights, obligations and responsibilities has been criticized for the way in which the duty of care that Welfare States previously assumed for themselves has been transferred to individuals: under the new social democratic way of thinking care for self dominates care for others (Sevenhuijsen 2000). Indeed, Australia's flirtation with care for self through the market has revealed, at the very least, that rural Australia is not an attractive environment for private, competitive health care providers. Furthermore, the market will not yield a socially just or equitable distribution of goods and services unless every member of society competes from a fair and equal basis, a fundamental tenet of Rawls' notion of social justice.

Throughout this changing policy context, one constant has remained. Undoubtedly the defining characteristic distinguishing 'rural' health continues to be that of access. While many think immediately of access in terms of geographical proximity and the ease with which distance can be transcended, access must be viewed more broadly to encompass that bundle of factors contributing directly or indirectly to meeting health needs, for example, access to employment and education.

Translating claims into service provision

The challenge of how best to provide accessible and effective health care services over vast, thinly populated and highly diverse rural areas (traditionally an arena that has attracted little private provision of health services) must be evaluated against government policy in which an overriding supply side consideration is the containment of health costs within affordable limits (Podger and Hagen 1999). Hence health service models have focused more than ever on promoting cost-effective health interventions, minimizing inappropriate or unnecessary care, and identifying priority areas. In short, health services rationing is taking place implicitly and without the debate about how much to spend in total; what general services are to be publicly funded; and which groups are entitled to what care (Hancock 1999).

In broad terms, the Australian health system can be conceptualized as a three-tiered pyramid. The bottom layer, representing the largest proportion of health care, comprises health professionals such as general practitioners, public health workers, midwives and community health nurses. These people provide primary health care, encompassing essential health and medical services for common problems as well as health promotion and illness prevention activities. Most health care takes place at this first point of contact with the health care system. The middle tier comprises generalized hospital care and the specialist doctor providing specialized care for more technical health problems, such as 'at risk' obstetrics and orthopaedics. At the top of the pyramid, highly specialized hospitals and clinics provide advanced tertiary health care, including organ transplants, neurosurgery and *in vitro*-fertilization programs. While there is some overlap between each level, the hierarchical organization of services frequently mirrors the geographical distribution of facilities. In terms of availability of services, numbers decrease and locations become more distant as the degree of specialization increases. Hence very small communities have limited health care facilities and personnel, even at the most basic primary care level, usually requiring residents to travel to larger centres for most secondary and tertiary health care.

Responding to rural and regional diversity is not easy for health systems that operate largely around mainstream programs.

> It is in practice unrealistic to expect that all citizens can be offered identical levels of access to identical modes of health care delivered at identical standards. The ethical principle of equal treatment for equal need is likely to be tempered by a recognition that health care in (say) highly rural areas must be qualitatively different from its counterpart in urban areas.
>
> Rice and Smith 2001

What is clear is the need for a distinctive rural health approach, while at the same time avoiding the failures associated with adopting a 'one-coat-fits-all' mentality (Wakerman and Humphreys 2002).

Confronted with the many demographic, technological and changing requirements of the health system (Podger and Hagen 1999), including central-ization of many health facilities in metropolitan and major regional centres, the traditional model of rural health care service delivery is gradually changing. Many small isolated communities lack sufficient people to sustain a local serv-ice, so residents are required to seek health care from other larger centres. The distances they must travel to access and obtain health care places heavy cost burdens on consumers of health care services. Indeed, for many people the time and costs involved in such travel are a major barrier to health care.

The particular combination of health care services and facilities available to any rural community reflects its particular geographical circumstances and mix of health care needs. A range of specifically rural health programs and services – including discrete, integrated and outreach models – has evolved to counter the problem of locational disadvantage (Humphreys 2002). An inven-tory of alternative models of rural and remote health service provision in Australia is set out in Table 6.1.

Innovative health services are found especially in areas where both distance and small, dispersed population numbers combine to highlight locational disadvantage – namely the outreach programs. These aim to minimize the long distances rural residents must travel by taking services to people in the form of scheduled clinics, on request, or for emergencies, thereby increasing their access and reducing inequities in the supply of services. Many forms of outreach arrangements have evolved to meet the health needs of residents of small isolated communities. Such arrangements encompass mobile services, visiting services, satellite and other networking facilities. National examples include the Royal Flying Doctor Service (*www.rfds.org.au*) that from its 21 bases provides primary health care services and evacuation for residents of remote Australia; the Medical Specialist Outreach Assistance program aims to improve access of rural and remote Australians to specialist health care serv-ices; and the Rural Women's General Practice service offers 'fly-in fly-out' women general practitioners to, so far, 90 localities around Australia that are without regular access to women doctors. In recognition of the importance of the 'golden hour' for acute and emergency care, a range of training programs for the emergency management of severe trauma target regional providers of health care. A variety of other arrangements such as the Patient Assistance Travel Schemes provided by States and Territories also exist to offset patient travel and accommodation expenses for health care purposes.

Table 6.1 Typology of rural and remote health services

Framework	Health service models
Discrete service providers (general practice and nursing)	Models for sustainable rural and remote general practice services Case management model for rural communities Remote area nurse management model Sole nurse practitioner health service model
Integrated services	Multipurpose centre and multipurpose services Regional Health Service Centres Shared resources Coordinated care trials Primary health care and participatory management
Outreach arrangements	Mobile services – Royal Flying Doctor Service Mobile intensive care services Visiting specialist paediatric service Visiting specialist surgeon Visiting specialist psychiatric/mental health service Fly-in fly-out female general practitioners Oral health services Satellite services and networking
Information technology	Telemedicine Allied health education Oral health education and training Neonatology education

Source: after Humphreys (2002).

Local examples of outreach arrangements abound in the form of roadside services (such as Life Education and Breast Screening vans), home services (such as domiciliary services, including meals of wheels), and visiting or rotating services where allied health teams visit isolated communities on a regular basis. The success of these services depends on good management to minimize their cost burden, avoid worker 'burn-out' and ensure close coordination among health care providers and services. Despite their sporadic nature, evidence suggests that the needs of residents of small isolated rural and remote communities can be well served by the face-to-face care provided by outreach workers operating from a regional centre (Humphreys *et al.* 1996).

Advances in information technology have also helped to bridge the gap between distance and health care. Increased information not only assists consumers to access services but also enhances the scope for self-care. For providers, better access to information reduces professional isolation, improves education and training opportunities, assists in service delivery, and facilitates improved coordination and collaboration between service providers.

In its most advanced form, telehealth or telemedicine, based on interactive audio-visual communication systems, enables effective diagnosis, treatment and other health care activities across vast distances, thereby helping to overcome the spatial inequities associated with rural health workforce maldistribution. Ideally, telehealth or telemedicine provides a cost-effective way of delivering effective health care without the need for excessive travel by remote patients, while at the same time enhancing interaction between health workers and specialist consultants.

In order to take into account specific local needs and circumstances, education, training and research programs have been devolved to rural and remote regional centres through a network of Regional Clinical Schools and University Departments of Rural Health. These Commonwealth government funded units have a mandate to increase the local capacity and skill base and to maximize rural health workforce recruitment and retention.

Matching rural health needs and entitlements

The inherent difficulties associated with how to distribute scarce resources equitably are exacerbated by the limited appreciation by city-folk of the different social, philosophical and political values and needs of those living in rural areas. The day-to-day life of those who live on rural properties or in the numerous smaller communities that service them remains hidden from the mass of Australia's population (63 per cent of whom live in six metropolitan capital cities). The perceived lack of national attention to rural and regional development issues and the failure of the rural based National Country Party to adequately represent their interests in government, have led to considerable rural disquiet and electoral volatility. This dissatisfaction climaxed at the 1996 Federal government election when rural Australians showed that they could no longer be taken for granted politically. Instead of voting for the National Country Party, they voted for a radical conservative party that was only a few years old (McManus and Pritchard 2000). Governments subsequently initiated rural 'summits' at which the inadequacy of rural health services loomed large on the agenda (Department of Transport and Regional Services 2000).

In particular, emphasis was placed on the rural population's disproportionate burden of efforts and sacrifices due to living away from the opportunities and services offered in the cities. Renewed claims for improved resource allocation and service provision for rural areas based on principles of equality and equity were at the forefront, arguments often crudely expressed in the form that the 30 per cent of Australia's population living in rural areas 'should' receive 30 per cent of the national resources. The concern with equity in providing rural health care services does not imply that such resources should be uniformly or equally distributed, as illustrated in the concepts of horizontal and vertical equity. Horizontal equity requires equal access and treatment for equal needs, and in rural areas, much attention has focused on this aspect in order to ensure that consumers are not disadvantaged just because they reside in a non-metropolitan area. Vertical equity, on the other hand, requires different treatment to produce equal outcomes, so that access may vary proportionately in accord with variations in need (Mooney and Jan 1997).

Although some health services and programs specifically target people in rural and remote areas, most health services in these areas are funded through the major Commonwealth and State programs and hence come under health financing arrangements for Australia as a whole. In general, the Commonwealth government is responsible for the funding of health services; the States are responsible for the provision of services; while local government provides virtually no health care but undertakes environmental control measures and a broad range of community-based and home-care service (Palmer and Short 1994).

To overcome the financial imbalance within the Australian federal system, money is transferred from the Commonwealth to the states with a view to ensuring a just allocation of resources with respect to states' needs (Humphreys 1988). The purpose of this process of fiscal equalization, which takes account of the differential revenue-raising capacity as well as their differential costs in providing standard services (including population dispersion), is to enable each state to provide services at standards not appreciably different from those prevailing elsewhere. Despite this revenue sharing arrangement, the states and territories continue to argue that existing health financing arrangements limit the ability of rural and remote health services to respond to local health needs, work against equity of access to affordable health services, limit collaboration between providers of services, and fail to encourage workforce recruitment and retention.

Recently, in an attempt to expand the range of health care services to small rural and remote communities, a number of models of health service provision for rural areas, based on innovative 'pooled funding' arrangements, have come into existence. Most significant has been the establishment of Multipurpose Centres, Multipurpose Services, Health Streams, and the more recent Regional Health Services Program. In contrast to discrete service models, these aim to maximize efficiency and coordination across health services, particularly through sharing resources, geographical co-location and simple management structures (Department of Health and Aged Care 2000; Humphreys et al. 1996). In these models, Commonwealth funds for aged care and State government health and community service funds are pooled, with a view to preserving locally valued hospitals, while at the same time increasing the capacity to better meet the community's broader health and aged care needs. The idea is that the economies gained will enable service providers to increase the range and mix of local health care. Hence, core services such as disease prevention, health promotion, comprehensive primary care, emergency medical care and some inpatient care can be supplemented by other services such as home health care, hospice care, community based aged care, long-term care and mental health services, where population size is sufficient to support them.

The Co-ordinated Care Trials have experimented with ways of funding and providing health services for people with complex and chronic care needs (Department of Health and Aged Care 1999). With funding pooled from both Commonwealth (including the Medicare Benefit Fund and the Pharmaceutical Benefits Scheme) and State programs, these trials purchase appropriate health services for clients from a range of health and community services and estimate costs compared to non-participation. The rationale for these trials has been to reorientate services around consumers' care needs rather than around providers, with case-managed care to overcome problems associated with poor coordination between health services funded from disparate channels.

While Australia's publicly funded Medicare program – providing universal doctor and hospital coverage for all Australians (regardless of where they live) – remains the backbone of the health care system, it often fails to ensure that the health care entitlements of rural residents are met in situations where rural communities do not have the services of a general practitioner, the cornerstone of access to the health system. This contributes to continuing problems of access for rural communities as well as to the perceived lack of territorial justice and the ongoing inequitable distribution of rural health resources. Many community-based and health service provider-driven initiatives designed to improve access to, and to ensure more effective delivery of, health care services throughout rural and remote regions have foundered for want of appropriate resource allocation to underpin their implementation.

Research undertaken by the National Rural Health Alliance (NRHA), in partnership with the Commonwealth, identified some key differences in the patterns and levels of availability and utilization of health services between capital city and rural residents (Australian Institute of Health and Welfare 2000; Department of Health & Aged Care 2000). In terms of primary medical care, for example, rural and remote residents are characterized by fewer medical practitioners (general practitioners and specialists) per 100,000 population and less services per capita, with more patients required to travel outside their region to access medical care. In rural areas, the level of direct-billing for medical care and private health insurance participation is significantly lower, the number of hospital beds per 100,000 is lower despite higher numbers of acute hospital separations per 100,000 population, and a greater proportion of nursing home type patients are treated in public hospitals. Although nursing employment is higher in rural areas, more rural nurses have only minimum training when compared with those in capital cities.

In terms of health care funding, according to the National Rural Health Alliance, on average, people in rural communities receive $92 (€51) per year in Medicare services compared with $145 (€81) in urban areas (National Rural Health Alliance 2001). The difference is even starker in remote areas. According to the Australian Institute of Health and Welfare (Australian Institute of Health and Welfare 1998), the per capita rate of GP consultations in 'other remote areas' is less than 50 per cent of that in 'capital cities'. In New South Wales, the average person uses $363 (€202) of Medicare benefits per year, whereas someone in the remote Kimberley or Pilbara areas uses only $66 (€37) per year. It is important to recognize that some of this gap may be offset, however, by the increased use of other services in rural and remote areas, for example, hospital services, salaried community medical services (including the Aboriginal Medical Services), Aboriginal Health Workers and remote area nurses.

Even so, the availability and use of non-Medicare services does not fully compensate for the discrepancy between rural/remote and urban benefits from Medicare. Based on the above 92 : 145 spending ratio, rural people are $250 (€139) million worse off in terms of Medicare rebates for GP services. Lack of access to a GP is the most significant factor explaining this difference. Rural people receive $460 (€256) million (19.6 per cent) of the total $2.3 (€1.3) billion of Medicare rebates for non-referred consultations. An additional $250 (€139) million in Medicare funds would achieve the '30 per cent fair share' for rural people on this measure alone.

Recent reforms in the Northern Territory have been designed in part to redress this problem. Under a plan agreed to by the Federal and Territory governments, the Commonwealth Government has agreed to treat remote area Territorians the same as urban Australians by allocating previously unavailable funds from the Medicare Benefit Fund and the Pharmaceutical Benefits Scheme. The money will be pooled to attract doctors and nurses to undersupplied areas. In the words of the Federal Aboriginal Affairs Minister, 'Here you have a situation in which the Commonwealth and Northern Territory governments are making available funding on the basis that any Australian is *entitled* to expect' (*The Australian*, 22 May 2002 p. 1) (authors' emphasis).

Reduced geographic access to health care resulting from living in a rural location is compensated for, to some extent, by the innovative enhanced referral and access mechanisms outlined above. Nonetheless, since the national review of the state of rural health in Australia 25 years ago (Hospitals and Health Services Commission 1976), there has been ample evidence to substantiate the continuing relevance of Tudor Hart's 'inverse care' law when it comes to rural health care (Hart 1971). Those whose needs are greatest (invariably the socio-economically marginalized and transport-poor) face the greatest difficulties in access to care. In the case of the elderly, this has not been helped by the move from institutional to community-based care, at a time when local services have been withdrawn and insufficient institutional resources have flowed to support the needs for patient care in the community.

Relevant, too, is the debate about whether rural health issues should be incorporated into all mainstream programs, as recommended by the Federal Auditor-General, or should fall within a specific rural portfolio. The pros and cons advanced by advocates of each strategy have been outlined in the introductory chapter to this book. Whatever the approach adopted by governments, it is clear that we cannot return to the neglect of rural health issues that characterized the pre-1990 period, a neglect that resulted from the failure to recognize the specific needs and circumstances of rural and remote Australians and those responsible for the delivery of services into their communities (Humphreys *et al.* 2002).

The changing role of the state and reasonable expectations

Reappraisal of the role of the state in relation to rural service provision is long overdue. The shortcomings of the recent period in which we have seen a rolling back of the role of the state are all too apparent. Not only has excessive dependence on market forces exacerbated socio-economic and geographical circumstances (since capital knows no allegiance to place), but considerations of equity and justice have also been minimized. However, for small, marginalized and fragmented minority populations in most rural regions, marketplace providers are scarce or uninterested. In this situation, many rural places are 'at risk' or unable to provide sustainable services. The result is often that the already poorer health status and associated disadvantaged set of life-chances are further diminished.

The recently adopted principles that underpin health care activity with respect to rural and remote communities by Commonwealth, State and Territory governments, lack an explicit acceptance of principles of fairness and equity. Instead, reflecting the Third Way and pluralist thinking, minus the social justice element, these principles were built around:

♦ an orientation to *primary health* care and public health;
♦ increased *consumer participation* and community involvement in health care planning;

- *accessibility* to ensure that health care and health services are actually available at times of need;

- *flexibility* in order to cope with the diverse health needs, demographic and workforce changes, and the unique local circumstances characterizing many rural communities;

- *intersectoral coordination* and multidisciplinary collaboration in order to maximize the limited resources available to service the health needs of the community; and

- enhancing community capability and ensuring *sustainability* of the health care system. (Australian Health Ministers' Conference 1999).

Only the principle of 'accessibility' addresses the distributional rules that relate to one's entitlement to society's scarce resources. The remainder focus on attributes of the health system.

With the demise of the role of the state in judging the claims of competing populations, there is no alternative institution capable of objectively managing reasonable expectations to health services. While Australia leads the world on a number of rural health initiatives, the dearth of coordinated and consultative planning, and the plethora of glossy brochures describing rural health services, breeds suspicion that the better deal for 'the bush' is politically driven. The concern with perceived inequities and lack of territorial justice is left to the rural lobby groups to pursue. In this situation their very self-interest negates any claims to be impartial judges of what is just. For this reason, we believe it is time to return to more systematic and explicit approaches to adjudicating territorial justice. In Harvey's (1973) formulation, the extent to which a distribution was considered to be 'territorially just' required correlating the actual allocation of resources (against the criteria of need, contribution to the common good, and merit). Such a procedure allows the identification of geographic areas that depart most from the norms suggested by standards of social justice.

Revisiting this formula would be a good start. However, in the context of health inequities, it is not sufficient to have territorial justice only in health services because many of the determinants of health lie outside the health arena. If health equity concerns 'health disparities that are particularly unfair because they are associated with underlying social characteristics, such as wealth . . .' (Zwi and Yach 2002), then territorial justice must extend to include opportunities for employment, education and safety in the physical environment. It is in the area of 'mitigating structural inequality' that the Third Way has been found most wanting (Taylor-Gooby 2000).

In the interests of both social and territorial equity and justice, governments must reclaim the ground they have relinquished to the marketplace, in which corporate society has been able to use its economic clout excessively to drive the political agenda in terms of 'who gets what where'. It is not sufficient to exhort rural communities to pursue collaborative development based on local initiative and leadership, without any assistance from the public cavalry. Many small rural communities have seen their employment opportunities diminish or effectively disappear, local infrastructure and services gutted, and have been depopulated by the youngest and often most resourceful families who seek more favourable educational and employment opportunities in the larger metropolitan centres. Only when these socio-economic determinants of health are addressed, can we expect to see sustained improvements in the health status of rural and remote Australia.

Acknowledgements

The assistance and constructive comments of Professor Murray Wilson and Dr Fran Rolley on an earlier draft of this chapter are gratefully acknowledged.

References

Auditor General (1998) *Planning for rural health.* Australian National Audit Office, Canberra.

Australian Health Ministers' Conference (1999) *Healthy horizons.* National Rural Health Policy Forum and the National Rural Health Alliance, Canberra.

Australian Institute of Health and Welfare (2000) *Australia's health 2000.* AIHW, Canberra.

Australian Institute of Health and Welfare (2002) *Chronic diseases and associated risk factors 2001,* AIHW Cat. No. PHE 33. AIHW, Canberra.

Australian Institute of Health and Welfare (1998) *Health in rural and remote Australia,* AIHW Cat. No. PHE 6. AIHW, Canberra.

Australian Taxation Office (1998) *Taxation statistics 1996–96.* Australian Government Publishing Service, Canberra.

Burnley, I. (1998) Inequalities in the transition of ischaemic heart disease mortality in New South Wales, Australia, 1969–1994. *Social Science & Medicine,* **47,** 1209–22.

Culyer, A. (1995) Need: the idea won't do – but we still need it. *Social Science & Medicine,* **40,** 727–30.

Department of Health and Aged Care (1999) *The Australian co-ordinated care trials: background and trial descriptions.* Commonwealth Department of Health and Aged Care, Canberra.

Department of Health and Aged Care (2000) *Portfolio budget statement 2000–01, budget related paper No. 1.11.* Commonwealth Department of Health and Aged Care, Canberra.

Department of Health and Community Services (1994) *Small rural hospitals task force report.* Department of Health and Community Services, Melbourne.

Department of Transport and Regional Services (2000) *Final report of the Regional Australia summit steering committee.* Department of Transport and Regional Services, Canberra.

Ernst, J., Glanville, L. and Murfitt, P. (1998) Issues in the implementation of compulsory competitive tendering in local government in Victoria. *Urban Futures*, **24**, 1–6.

Fragar, L. J., Gray, E. J., Franklin, R. J. and Petrauskas, V. (1997) *A picture of health*. The Australian Agricultural Health Unit, Moree.

Giddens, A. (1998) *The third way. The renewal of social democracy*. Polity, Cambridge.

Glover, J., Harris, K. and Tennant, S. (1999) *A social health atlas of Australia, Vol 1: Australia*, second edition. Public Health Information Development Unit, University of Adelaide, Adelaide.

Haberkorn, G., Hugo, G., M, F. and Aylward, R. (1999) *Country matter: social atlas of rural and regional Australia*. Bureau of Rural Sciences, Canberra.

Hancock, L. (1999) *Health policy in a market place*. Allen & Unwin, St. Leonards, NSW.

Hart, J. (1971) The inverse care law. *Lancet*, **1**, 405–12.

Harvey, D. (1973) *Social justice and the city*. Edward Arnold, London.

Hoatson, L., Dixon, J. and Sloman, D. (1996) Community development, citizenship and the Contract State. *Community Development Journal*, **31**, 126–36.

Hospitals and Health Services Commission (1976) *Rural health in Australia*. Australian Government Publishing Service, Canberra.

Hugo, G. (2002) Australia's changing non-metropolitan population. In D. Wilkinson and I. Blue (eds) *The new rural health: an Australian text*. Oxford University Press, Melbourne.

Humphreys, J. S. (1988) Social provision and service delivery: problems of equity, health, and health care in rural Australia. *Geoforum*, **19**, 323–38.

Humphreys, J. S. (1998) *Rural health and the health of rural communities*. Latrobe University, Bendigo.

Humphreys, J. S. (2002) Health service models in rural and remote Australia. In D. Wilkinson and I. Blue (eds) *The new rural health: an Australian text*. Oxford University Press, Melbourne.

Humphreys, J. S., Hegney, D., Lipscombe, J. M., Gregory, G. and Chater, A. B. (2002) Whither rural health? Reviewing a decade of progress in rural health. *Australian Journal of Rural Health*, **10**, 2–14.

Humphreys, J. S., Mathews-Cowey, S. and Rolley, F. (1996) *Health service frameworks for small rural and remote communities – issues and options*. University of New England, Armidale.

Humphreys, J. S. and Rolley, F. (1991) *Health and health care in rural Australia*. University of New England, Armidale.

McLennan, W. and Madden, R. (1999) *The health and welfare of Australia's Aboriginal and Torres Strait Islander peoples*. Australian Bureau of Statistics, Canberra.

McManus, P. and Pritchard, B. (2000) Geography and the emergence of rural and regional Australia. *Australian Geographer*, **31**, 383–91.

Mooney, G. and Jan, S. (1997) Vertical equity: weighing outcomes? or establishing procedures? *Health Policy*, **39**, 79–87.

National Rural Health Alliance (2000) *Suicide prevention in rural areas. Discussion notes*. National Rural Health Alliance, Canberra.

National Rural Health Alliance (2001) *Position papers 2000–2001*. National Rural Health Alliance, Canberra.

Palmer, G. R. and Short, S. D. (1994) *Health care and public policy.* Macmillan Education Australia, Melbourne.

Peach, H. and Bath, N. (1999) Prevalence and socio demographic determinants of cardiovascular risk in a rural area. *Australian Journal of Rural Health,* 7, 23–27.

Phillips, A. (2002) Health status and utilisation of health services in rural Australia: a comparison with urban status and utilisation using national data sets. In D. Wilkinson and I. Blue (eds) *The new rural health: an Australian text.* Oxford University Press, Melbourne.

Podger, A. and Hagen, P. (1999) *Reforming the Australian health care system: the role of government.* Department of health and aged care Occasional Papers: New Series No. 1. Commonwealth Department of Health and Aged Care, Canberra.

Rice, N. and Smith, P. (2001) Ethics and geographical equity in health care. *Journal of Medical Ethics,* 27, 1–7.

Rolley, F. (2000) *Establishing research priorities for healthy rural communities.* Discussion Paper prepared for the Health Inequalities research Collaboration Workshop, 12 July, Canberra.

Sevenhuijsen, S. (2000) Caring in the third way: the relation between obligation, responsibility and care in Third Way discourse. *Critical Social Policy,* 20, 5–37.

Taylor-Gooby, P. (2000) Blair's scars. *Critical Social Policy,* 20, 331–48.

Wakerman, J. and Humphreys, J. S. (2002) Rural health: why it matters. *The Medical Journal of Australia,* 176, 457–8.

Walmsley, D. J. and Weinand, H. C. (1997) Is Australian becoming more unequal? *Australian Geographer,* 28, 69–88.

Zwi, A. and Yach, D. (2002) International health in the twenty-first century: trends and challenges. *Social Science & Medicine,* 54, 1615–20.

Chapter 7

Captive Populations

Prison health care

Andrew Coyle and Vivien Stern

Prisons and ill-health

Of the eighty-five corpses investigated by the London coroner in 1315–16, nearly three-quarters came from Newgate Prison. It was, essentially, a 'house of death' (Ackroyd 2000 p.66). In the seventeenth century it was a matter of anxiety that those involved with prisoners, for example judges and jurymen, became infected through their contact with prisoners. Some judges in the Central Criminal Court died from gaol fever caught from prisoners in London prisons (Harding *et al.* 1985). In Russia today one in three of those actively infected with tuberculosis is in prison (ICPS 2002). It is estimated that 40 per cent of prisoners in New York State may be infected with hepatitis C (Correctional Association of New York 1999). HIV infection is up to 30 times more common in women prisoners than in women in the civilian population (Stöver 2002). Prisons and ill-health have, for centuries, gone hand in hand. Prison medicine as a specialism has a long and not very glorious history.

In this chapter we look at what is known about the health of prisoners as a group and set out the basis of their entitlement to health care. We then consider the different ways in which health services are provided to prisoners. There are three main options: a prison health service organizationally part of the overall prison administration, prison health care provided by the public health services, or a middle way in which the responsibility for the administration of prison health services is shared between the prison administration and the public health services. We then look at three case studies of systems that have changed their methods of health care delivery. Finally, we consider the evidence, scant as it is, of the effectiveness of these different methods of providing prison health care and reach some very tentative conclusions about the best system of health care provision, both for incarcerated populations themselves and for broader public health. Prison systems in the West and in Eastern Europe and Central Asia are the main focus for consideration, although we also draw on our knowledge of prison systems worldwide.

The health of prisoners as a group

The reasons for people being in prison are many. In some countries the majority of prisoners are awaiting trial, in some instances for several years. The charges that they face can vary from serious acts of violence to offences against property, such as burglary, major embezzlement or stealing food in order to assuage hunger. A minority may have been accused of terrorist or organized crime.

Prison populations are very far from representative of the population as a whole. It is true that people from across different social classes are to be found in prison. However, in almost all countries the majority of people in prison are likely to come from the marginalized and socially excluded groups in society.

For many, being sent to prison can be a one-off experience of perhaps six weeks, never to be repeated. For others imprisonment is more of a fact of life, with more years spent as a prisoner than as a free person.

Prison populations are also unrepresentative of the population as a whole in their gender balance. In all countries prisoners are overwhelmingly male. The

Table 7.1 Prisoners compared with the general population in England and Wales on various indices of disadvantage

Characteristic	General population	Prisoners
Ran away from home as a child	11%	47% of sentenced men and 50% of sentenced women
Taken into care as a child	2%	27%
Lone parenthood	9%	21% of women prisoners
Regularly truanted from school	3%	30%
Excluded from school	2%	49% of men and 33% of women
Suffer from three or more mental disorders	1% men, 0% women	44% sentenced men, 62% sentenced women
Drug use in previous year	13% men, 8% women	66% sentenced men, 55% sentenced women
Long-standing illness or disability	29% men aged 18–49	46% of sentenced men aged 18–49
Hepatitis	0.3% hepatitis B 0.4% hepatitis C	8% men, 12% women, 4% young offenders tested hepatitis B positive 9% men, 11% women, 0.6% young offenders tested hepatitis C positive

Adapted from *Report from the Office of the Deputy Prime Minister* (2002).

proportion of female prisoners in any country varies between 2–8 per cent, with the average around 5 per cent (World Prison Brief 2002). An important consequence of this for our present interest is that prison health care tends to be focused on the needs of the majority population and the specific needs of women prisoners are frequently overlooked.

The age profile of prisoners is younger than the age distribution in the population as a whole. However, in some countries, such as the United States of America, the needs of prisoners who will grow old and die in prison are an increasingly important issue. In some prisons in the United States, units in prisons have been converted into hospices for the dying (*Journal of Law* 1999).

Minorities who face discrimination in the wider society are likely to be disproportionately represented in the prison population. This is true of black people in countries such as the United States, the United Kingdom, France and the Netherlands. It is also true of Roma people in many Central European countries, of Aboriginal people in Australia and of Mäori in New Zealand (Stern 1998).

The disadvantaged nature of the prison population gives some pointers to the likely health status of prisoners. In health terms they are a very problematic group – they are more likely not to be registered with a general practitioner; many have untreated health conditions and a high proportion has addictions. Estimates of the proportion of drug-users in European prisons vary, with 47 per cent in Sweden, 32 per cent in France, 15–29 per cent in England and Wales and between 38 per cent and 70 per cent in Portugal (Stöver 2002 pp. 24–5). Rates of infection with hepatitis B and C, tuberculosis or HIV are much higher than in the community. In some systems the level of mental health problems amongst prisoners is very high (Corrections Health Service 2001; Department of Health 1999; Ministère de la Justice 1999; Office for National Statistics 2000; Vasseur 2000). The high rate of mental illness raises the question of how far prisons are being used to deal with people who should be in the health system but are shunted down the criminal justice route because of shortage of resources.

As well as arriving in prison in an unhealthy state, for prisoners in many countries the prison experience itself is unhealthy. Prison conditions are often conducive to the spread of infections. Overcrowding is common and can encompass a wide range of conditions. In England, for example, overcrowding means two people living in a small cell measuring say six square metres with an unscreened lavatory. In many countries in Eastern Europe and Central Asia it will usually mean living in a dormitory with only one square metre per prisoner and more prisoners than beds, so that prisoners have to sleep in shifts. In many of these dormitories metal grilles and shutters cover the windows so that very little light or air penetrates the room (Council of Europe 2002;

Stern 1999). Prisoners spend up to 23 hours a day in these conditions, leading a Russian Deputy Minister of Justice to describe a prison sentence in Russia as a potential death sentence (Penal Reform International 1998). Clearly, mental illness can be worsened by the experience of prison conditions such as these and the attraction of drug-taking can increase. Research from Western European prisons suggests that the proportion of drug-using prisoners who first started to inject drugs whilst in prison ranges from 7 per cent to 24 per cent (Stöver 2002 p. 33). Overcrowded single sex prisons can also be places of great violence. In many instances this violence can lead to injury and rape (Heilpern 1998). In addition to the trauma of this violence, the result can also be a spread of HIV and other infections. HIV transmission in prisons has been widely reported (Dolan and Wodak 1999) and juveniles are particularly at risk. Research carried out into the spread of HIV in prisons in Malawi revealed that staff can be bribed by wealthier prisoners to allow juvenile prisoners to be abducted into the adult male dormitory where they are then rented out for sexual purposes. The prisoner who bribed the guard pockets the proceeds (Penal Reform International 1998). In Mozambique diarrhoea and skin diseases are 'almost endemic' because of the poor living conditions (African Commission on Human and Peoples' Rights 2001). In some poor countries prisons have no transport to take very sick prisoners to hospital (African Commission on Human and Peoples' Rights 1999 p. 26).

It is not inevitable, however, that being in prison leads to health deterioration. There can be some unintended benefits. People from the marginalized and disadvantaged sections of society might for the first time receive adequate health care that can identify and begin to deal with their chronic health problems. For example in New South Wales a greater percentage of women prisoners have been screened for breast and cervical cancer than women in the community (Corrections Health Service 2001). In New York State prisons the availability of the latest HIV drugs has reduced AIDS-related deaths by 85 per cent since 1995 (Correctional Association of New York 2002 p. 21).

What prisoners are entitled to expect

There has been considerable debate over the last fifty years about which rights prisoners should lose by the fact of their imprisonment and which they should retain as human beings. By definition, anyone who is sent to prison loses the right to freedom of movement. But what about other rights such as contact with family, religious observance and access to lawyers? In respect of our present interest, what about access to health care?

The most useful starting point for any discussion of these matters is the extensive set of human rights instruments governing the treatment of all those who have lost their liberty. This has been developed over the last sixty years, principally by the United Nations (United Nations 1988). It is noteworthy that the provision of health care and the role of health care workers is a major element in this international human rights framework. This corpus of standards and norms developed by the United Nations and regional human rights bodies can be summarized under a few main principles. Prisoners should receive the same standard of health care as people not in prison; their care should be free of charge and lack of resources is no defence for inadequate care. Once a state has made the decision to deprive someone of their liberty then a duty of care rests on the state to provide proper medical care even when access to health services outside is limited (Council of Europe 2002). The role of medical workers in places of captivity is the subject of a range of requirements. Doctors in prisons must never take part in administering cruel, inhuman or degrading treatment or punishments. Prisoners should never be used for medical experiments (British Medical Association 2001; Council of Europe 1998; Reyes 2001).

It is all very well to have an impressive set of international standards but this means little unless they are implemented. How far are these expectations met in practice? In many countries, unfortunately, the answer is, not very far. In many jurisdictions the provision of prison health care is at best patchy. Resources are scarce. Medical personnel are very poorly paid or sometimes not paid at all. In such circumstances corruption flourishes and everything can be bought or sold, including medicines, a bed in the prison hospital where the conditions will be better than in the rest of the prison, and even a diagnosis of tuberculosis infection that can provide access to better food and a less crowded cell (World Health Organization 2000).

Delivery of health services in the prison setting

The debate about models of delivery of health services in the prison setting has for many years centred on whether health care should be provided by a specialist prison health care service responsible to the prison authorities, or by the national health service that provides care for other members of the community. A range of arguments is deployed in the debate.

The human rights strand is very important in the argument that prison health care should be integrated into public health care. Medical staff who are independent of the prison authorities as far as their employment, conditions of service and promotion are concerned may well be in a better position to put the interests of their patients first. It will be easier for them to report suspicious injuries, to protest when prison conditions are leading to the dangers of infection, when the treatment of individuals is likely to injure their health or when prisoners are being punished for behaviour caused not by recalcitrance but by mental illness. It may be easier for independent medical staff to handle any conflict that might arise between their duty to the patient and issues of security or prison management. This might occur, for example, when the prison doctor is faced with a request from the prison management to help in dealing with a difficult prisoner by using methods of sedation or isolation that will benefit the prison rather than the prisoner. Independent medical staff will find it easier to argue that condoms and other harm reduction materials are essential for public health and that public health imperatives are at least as strong as security considerations. They are more likely to be able to express a strong view on the propriety or otherwise of shackling prisoners when they are taken to outside hospitals and of strapping them to the beds whilst they are there.

It is inevitable that the doctor/patient relationship will be affected in a negative way in situations where prison health workers are employed by the same authority that runs the prison, disciplines the prisoners and controls their access to a better life in the prison and perhaps even their chances of leaving it through parole. Prisoners will be uncertain whether the medical staff see them as primarily prisoners, or as patients. They will not be sure that they can trust the medical staff with information that they wish to keep confidential.

There is also a strong public health argument for integrating the provision of health care in prisons with that provided in civil society. The separation of prison health care from public health care is inefficient because, although prisons are closed and are sometimes far from centres of population, they are in fact places of considerable traffic. Staff normally go in to prison every day and return home to their families at the end of their shift. Families and friends of prisoners visit the prison. Professionals, such as social workers and lawyers, enter and leave. In England and Wales, in 1997, 201,000 people entered prison (HM Prison Service and NHS Executive 1999). Many prisoners may only stay a short time in prison. Those involved with petty crime may come into and go out of prison frequently; this is the so-called 'revolving door' syndrome.

For all these reasons the infections of the prison cannot be kept within its walls for long. Researchers in the USA studied the effects on the community of an outbreak of tuberculosis that occurred in the prison in Memphis and affected 38 prisoners and five staff. The researchers studied cases of tuberculosis in the county where Memphis is situated. Of the 156 infected people in the county the researchers were able to take genetic fingerprints of the strain of mycobacterium from 81. Results showed that the strain first found in the jail spread through an ever-widening circle of people and went on to infect people who had not had any association with the prison or with people directly connected with the prison (Corrections Journal 2001).

In addition, many of the conditions from which prisoners suffer are chronic and need long-term attention. They came into prison with these conditions and will leave with them. Continuity of care before, during and after the prison sentence is thus essential.

The conclusion to be drawn from all these considerations is that the general community health services should regard prisoners as part of their responsibility. Having a separate prison health service contributes to the view that prisoners are a group who are separate, out of society and someone else's responsibility.

The separation of prison health care from public health care may also affect the careers of those medical professionals who choose to work in the prison setting. This kind of work is not likely to be held in high regard by professional colleagues. As a result prison medical staff can become inward-looking and fail to keep in touch with developments in their field. A lack of peer respect can also make it difficult to recruit high quality staff in prison health care.

The contrary position, that the prison authorities are best placed to provide the care in prisons, is based on pragmatic rather than principled arguments. There may be a genuine fear that prisoners would lose out if their health care was not specifically defined, with budgets protected and staff specifically employed for work in prisons. Prisoners are, after all, unpopular patients, presenting a range of difficult problems which might be costly to treat, and who might constitute a physical threat to health care staff. As far as medical staff are concerned, the prison environment can be a stressful and unattractive workplace. Thus, it is argued, the national health authorities would not be prepared to make an effort to provide care for prisoners, who would be disadvantaged in any political competition about resources. A separate prison health service ensures that prisoners get proper and dedicated care, not the crumbs remaining in the national health service after those seen as more deserving have been dealt with.

Second, it is argued that prison health care is a genuine specialism. Providing health care to people who have been detained against their will is very different from treating those in free society. The ability to work professionally in an environment where security has to be a constant feature involves considerations that are not included in the training of most medical staff. According to this argument, prisoners are likely to get better treatment from medical staff who have had special training and who understand the environment, the population and the pressures that come into play.

It also needs to be acknowledged that there are attractions for the prison authorities in controlling the totality of the prison institution. Professionals coming from outside who do not owe direct allegiance to the prison authorities can seem challenging and difficult in the eyes of the administration.

Both models of health care provision are to be found (Stöver 2002; Tomascevski 1992). In many countries there is a specialist prison health care service under the control of the prison authorities. This model was taken to the extreme in the countries of the former Soviet Union. Until the fall of communism the penitentiary system in these countries was a closed world run by the Ministry of the Interior with its own enterprises, business managers, education service and medical service. The medical system was so separate from the public medical service that two different sets of statistics of infectious disease prevalence were kept by the government, one for prisoners and one for non-prisoners. In Norway, on the other hand, where the philosophy is to integrate prisons as far as possible into the community, the responsibility for prison health was transferred to the Ministry of Health in 1988 (Tomascevski 1992). The Norwegian approach is, however, unusual.

Case studies

The majority opinion among those involved in prison reform is that the responsibility for prison health care should lie with public health authorities, or at least there should be a mixed economy, in which there is very close collaboration between the prison and the public health authorities. In recent years three jurisdictions, France, England and Wales, and New South Wales in Australia, have undertaken reforms of their prison health care arrangements with the objective of raising prison health care standards. These reforms are worth looking at in a little more detail.

France

Reforms in prison health care in France have been called 'the greatest change in the field of prisons in France in the last ten years' (Combessie 2001). Following a report from the High Committee on Public Health (Haut Comité de la Santé Public) in 1993 highlighting health problems in prisons, responsibility for prison health care was transferred, under a law of January 1994, from the Ministry of Justice, which runs French prisons, to the public hospital sector. The aim of the transfer was to meet the requirement to provide the same standard of health care for prisoners as was available to the population outside prisons. As a first step, and to ensure eligibility for care, all prisoners were automatically given membership of the social security, general health and maternity insurance scheme.

Under the new system every prison has agreed a protocol with the nearest public hospital, which is required to set up a consultation and health care unit in the prison. If the hospital cannot provide the psychiatric service a separate protocol is drawn up with another hospital. In each prison this unit is responsible for providing all health services to prisoners including medical examination on admission into prison, nursing and distribution of medicines, screening for communicable diseases, dental care, health education, specialist medical care and 24 hour health cover. The unit also organizes continuity of medical care on release from prison.

The reform was accompanied by a substantial increase in resources. For example, at Fleury-Mérogis, the biggest prison in western Europe, which held 4000 prisoners on 1 January 1999 and with a throughput of 12,000 prisoners a year, the number of nurses increased from 15 to 29 and the number of medical secretaries from one to ten after the reform.

The new system applied to all the prisons wholly in the public sector and covered 149 prisons holding at the time of implementation 45,000 prisoners. The 10,000 prisoners held in the 21 prisons where the private sector provides all services except management, surveillance and welfare continued after the reform to receive their health care from private medical providers (Ministère de la Justice 1999). However, in a move that suggests that the change had positive outcomes, the government decided in 2000 to bring the 21 prisons where the private sector provides all services into the public prison health care scheme from March 2001 (Ministère de la Justice 2001).

Little information is available as yet on the impact of these reforms. Research carried out for the Ministry of Justice in two prison institutions and published in 1997 suggests that prison health care had become more professional, with prisoners being cared for as if they were in hospital. However, the researchers noted that there had been limited impact on the state of prisoners' health. A further study also published in 1997 noted that harm reduction policies had begun in prisons since the reform. In some prisons, but not all, condoms were distributed and there were also prisons with needle exchanges. Programmes for tracing and dealing with tuberculosis and sexually transmitted diseases had been introduced (Combessie 2001). A further longitudinal study in two prisons produced in 2000 (Bessin and Lechien 2000) is mainly concerned with the interaction between the various players in prison health care and, especially, the role of prison guards as an intermediary in the relationship between health care staff and their prisoner-patients. The study notes that access to medical care is strictly regulated. Some prisoners are inhibited by having to submit written requests for appointments through the guards. Some prisoners refuse hospital treatment because they have to appear in public handcuffed to a guard and they have no confidentiality because the guards are present at the doctor-patient consultation. Prisoners often saw medical staff working in prisons as less competent ('they're only working in prison because no-one wants them on the outside'). They suspected that the supply of medicines to prisoners was rationed. On the other hand medical staff were suspicious of the demands of prisoners ('they're very demanding', 'they want everything straightaway').

The prison guards saw the arrival of external medical staff as an intrusion. Conflicts occurred in the early stages mainly over the independent medical status of the new practitioners and the identification of the health care staff with humanity and the guards with repression. Medical confidentiality was at the heart of a great deal of the conflict between health care staff and guards. Health care staff were unsure of their role in the maintenance of order and pursuit of the prison objectives.

In 2001 the findings of a joint evaluation by the Judicial Inspectorate and the Social Affairs Inspectorate were published (Ministère de la Justice and Ministère de l'Emploi et de la Solidarité 2001). The report stresses the undeniable progress made since the 1994 reforms. Benefits include more frequent access to specialist and inpatient care, the professionalization of prison health care teams and setting professional standards for matters such as the distribution of drugs and disinfectant. A new ethics of prison health care affirms a genuine right to health care whatever the conditions of imprisonment, allows a strict demarcation between the roles of doctors and guards and assures greater respect for medical confidentiality. However, the successes are limited by a number of factors. The reality of health care needs at the time of the reforms was little understood and difficult to evaluate, and the new reforms have brought an increase and diversification in the demand for health care. The acceleration in ageing of the prison population (e.g. because of longer sentences) triggers new needs. There is conflict, misunderstanding and mistrust between medical and prison staff and territorial conflict between medical and psychiatric units. Relationships with external medical and judicial authorities are complex and this works against the interests of the prisoner, as seen in the lack of a multidisciplinary approach to, for example, suicide prevention. Problems over resources available to supervise prisoners whilst they are in outside hospitals (called 'bed-watches') means police and prison authorities may set quotas so that medical staff have to triage between urgent and non-urgent cases.

England and Wales

The provision of health care in prisons in England and Wales has been controversial for many years. Concerns have frequently been raised about its quality, the secrecy of its administration, the overuse of psychotropic drugs and deaths in custody due to negligence (British Medical Association 1990; Health Advisory Committee for the Prison Service England and Wales 1997; Prison Reform Trust 1985; Smith 1984). One of us (AC) was Governor of Brixton

Prison in London in the early 1990s and remembers part of the prison called F Wing where 230 men were living whilst remanded to the prison so that medical reports, usually of a psychiatric nature, could be prepared for the courts. These prisoner/patients spent 23 hours a day in standard cells with a bed, a table, a chair and a chamber pot. The most disturbed of the prisoners were held in strip cells, concrete cells with no furniture, wearing tear-proof smocks, and sleeping in tear-proof sleeping bags on the concrete floor. The walls in F wing were bottle green and, as there was so little natural light, the lights were on all day. The air smelt of urine, faeces and stale food and the noise of wailing, shouting and banging went on day and night (Coyle 1994).

Against this background the preferred solution for many outside observers has been to incorporate the Prison Medical Service into the National Health Service and in the 1990s a growing impetus was given to the movement for more integration by pressure from the independent Inspectorate of Prisons. In annual reports as well as in reports on individual prisons, successive Chief Inspectors found much to criticize about the health care provision they saw in the course of their inspections. In 1996 the then Chief Inspector, Sir David Ramsbotham, published a discussion paper arguing that the NHS should take over responsibility for prison health care (HM Inspectorate of Prisons 1996). The new Labour Government elected in May 1997 responded quickly and in November of that year a joint working group of the Prison Service and the National Health Service Executive, jointly chaired, was established.

The Working Group carried out a detailed study of the health care arrangements in 38 prisons and undertook extensive interviews. Its report gave considerable comfort to those who had been campaigning for two decades for a better Prison Medical Service. It accepted that that were serious weaknesses in the provision of prison health care with 'less than optimal', 'overmedicalized', reactive rather than proactive health care delivery. It accepted that the structure was inappropriate. The service was isolated from the NHS, and suffered from 'lack of direction, poor lines of communication and confused accountability'. It accepted that the staff suffered 'skill decay', 'professional isolation' and low morale (HM Prison Service and NHS Executive 1999). Some succumbed to a traditional prison culture which put emphasis on security rather than nursing practice and health improvement. Continuing staff training and performance measurement were inadequate (HM Prison Service and NHS Executive 1999).

The report went on to recommend substantial changes. A formal partnership between the Prison Service and the NHS was to be set up but without changes in funding and departmental accountability mechanisms. The objectives of the partnership would be first to ensure that 'care is distinct from custody' (HM Prison Service and NHS Executive 1999). Second, it would aim to establish health care standards in prisons at the same level as in the NHS with comparable outcomes. The isolation of prison health staff should be ended by enabling moves in and out of the NHS, training and professional supervision. Arrangements to enable continuity of care from the moment prisoners come into custody through to the day they are released should be set up.

The changes were to be implemented over a period of five years. The machinery to achieve the changes was to be a new Task Force that would drive forward changes on the ground and a Policy Unit to drive forward the changes at the centre. The new Policy Unit would replace the former Prison Service Directorate of Healthcare and should in the view of the Working Group be located within the NHS Executive.

The question of the NHS taking over prison health care completely was rejected at the time in a clear statement of the arguments for the joint model of provision, but the report recommended that this should be reconsidered after its proposals had been implemented and their effects assessed. The report concluded that the two organizations needed to learn to work together without the major disruption that a transfer of responsibility would bring. Giving control to one or the other would result in perverse incentives.

The government accepted the recommendations in the report. The Task Force and Policy Unit were set up and a process of radical change was initiated. Prison Health Plans for each prison were required to be drawn up. Clinical governance approaches, as a means to improve quality of care, were introduced. Measures to improve screening on first reception into prison were introduced, particularly aimed at detecting mental health problems. Fourteen projects were established aiming at different areas that need to change. The first training post for a doctor training in general practice was established in a prison. NHS 'in-reach' teams for mental health started working in prisons. Models of good practice in primary care in prisons were devised. An assessment of the effects of Prison Service policies on maintaining contact with families on health was set up as well as ensuring that prison concerns were taken into account when new Department of Health policies were being considered. A strategy for a hepatitis B vaccination programme was drawn up. Since then a report on doctors working in prisons has been produced and substantial changes in doctors' employment conditions are being introduced (HM Prison Service and Department of Health 2001b). A policy paper Seeking Consent: Working with People in Prison was produced in 2002. It deals with the difficult questions that often arise in prison, such as restraining violent prisoners and hunger strikes (HM Prison Service and Department of Health 2002).

The first Annual Report notes that some improvements in delivery are already measurable. Some prisons have developed new contracts for primary care and other services. Prison health care staff are getting access to NHS training and development programmes. The number of prison health services presenting serious problems has reduced. Recruitment of staff has become easier (HM Prison Service and Department of Health 2001a).

New South Wales, Australia

In New South Wales changes were introduced in 1997. Under the Health Services Act of 1997 a new statutory health corporation, the Corrections Health Service, was set up (Corrections Health Service 2001). It provides the health care to all 25 prisons in New South Wales, to the centres where offenders are sent to undertake community work and to the police cells in the courts. There are five major clinical programmes: Drug and Alcohol, Mental Health, Population Health, Primary Health, and Clinical Services. The service works through a memorandum of understanding with the Department of Corrective Services: 16,000 men and women went through the system in 2000–2001 and in mid 2001 the Corrections Health Service was responsible for nearly 8000 prisoners.

The New South Wales model is trying to deal with the problems with prison health care that have been widely identified internationally. First, it is tackling the isolation of prison health services through its close professional links with the health world. The service is responsible to a Board chaired by a distinguished Professor of Public Health. The Minister for Health showed support by attending the 2000 Annual General Meeting of the Corrections Health Service.

Second, it is addressing the poor performance and status of prison health care staff. High-level training is being developed. A Graduate Certificate in Corrections Health Nursing was launched in 2000. A chair of Corrections Health Nursing was created by the service with a local university. In 2001 the Corrections Health Service received its first accreditation from the Australian Council on Health Care Standards. A quality improvement plan is in place. Plans for 2001–2002 include development of work on sexual health including sexual assault and a major emphasis on hepatitis C and hypertension. Some prisoners are being allowed to take control of their own medication and administer it themselves.

Third, it is dealing with the problem of detained people getting access to the services they need. A consultation with prisoners showed that they were not always aware that the prison health services were independent of the prison authorities. The prison clinics were therefore given new signs that made it clear that they were run by the health services of New South Wales and not the corrections services.

Fourth, it is facing up to the need for continuity of care by establishing a programme to provide care on release for prisoners with addictions. There is liaison between community methadone clinics and pharmacies about prisoners on methadone.

Key issues remain, however, such as the nature of the relationship with the prison service and prison staff and whether the prisoners see a difference in the health care available to them.

Conclusions

Can we learn from these three different models of change? Have the radical organizational changes in our three case study jurisdictions dealt with the problems identified earlier? First, are prisoners assured of easy access to care? The evidence from France suggests that access is somewhat better than it was. The New South Wales project on improving access is a promising sign. Second, has the quality of the health care that prisoners receive improved? There is some evidence from all three jurisdictions that it has, but the starting point was very low and much more needs to be done. Third, is isolation being reduced? The evidence from all three reforms suggests bringing the services from outside into prison does reduce the isolation of prison health care. Also the continuity of care between inside and outside health care seems to have been improved by the reforms. Lastly, the ethical conflicts, which are probably irresolvable, have been understood and taken into account in the provision.

When the reforms are assessed on a wider question, what effect have they had on the prison as an institution that produces ill-health, the jury is still out. We do not know how far they have changed the prevailing attitudes in the system, attitudes first of all to prisoners who are ill; second, attitudes to prisoners as equal citizens entitled to equal medical care; and third, to the prison as a place that should not increase ill-health but reduce it. To achieve such attitudinal changes two issues are important. One is the state of the relationships between the medical staff and the other prison staff. The other is the level of input of the medical department into prison policy more generally. If a large number of prisoners are committing suicide, for instance, by hanging themselves from their upturned beds, is the response going to be to screw the beds to the floor or to look for the causes of the despair that leads to suicide and try to deal with them?

The evidence from the three change programmes is mixed. In France the question of the relationships between the medical and the custodial staff has been much studied but no conclusions have emerged. Little in the literature about New South Wales indicates how far the prison medical unit is an island of care and respect in a less respecting environment. The reformers in England and Wales seem at least to have grasped this nettle with the Policy Unit and the new structures that aim to integrate the two kinds of staff. The idea of 'health impact assessments', looking at particular areas of prison service policy for their 'health-friendliness' is a promising development.

However, the examples of England and Wales and France suggest that turning system change into actual delivery is demanding and can take some years. The prison environment militates against planned, well-organized, strategically delivered programmes because it is constantly being hit by crises. In England and Wales these are usually crises of overcrowding, which disrupt all activities save those of finding beds for prisoners, who may be taken hundreds of miles from their home area. In France, where the prison population is more under control through regular amnesties and a less prison-oriented sentencing framework, the crises come from frequent industrial action by prison staff (Michaels and Rozenman 2002; Stern 1998).

The final conclusion is that prison health care can certainly be improved by reducing its isolation and exposing the prison world to the values of the world of medical practice. However, whatever improvements are made it is worth reaffirming that the prison environment will be an environment that is bad for health for the foreseeable future in almost all countries of the world. Locking up hundreds, sometimes thousands, of human beings in one relatively small location, which is very often grossly overcrowded, in which hygiene and sewage facilities are frequently unsatisfactory, in which there is limited access to light, fresh air and exercise, in which diet is insufficient and there is limited access to water for drinking and washing, and in which there is limited opportunity for physical or mental stimulation cannot do other than place the health of those imprisoned at risk. There will inevitably be a threat to general public health if imprisonment is used more than is strictly necessary for public safety. Reducing the use of prison should be a public health aim.

Acknowledgements

We would like to thank Femke van der Meulen of the International Centre for Prison Studies (ICPS) for her help with this chapter. We are also grateful to ICPS Associate Jim Haines for his help in translating and analysing the French source material.

References

Ackroyd, P. (2000) *London: The Biography*. The Chatto and Windus, London.

African Commission on Human and Peoples' Rights (1999) *Report of the Special Rapporteur on Prisons and Conditions of Detention in Africa – Mali Prisons Revisited*. African Commission on Human and Peoples' Rights, Banjul.

African Commission on Human and Peoples' Rights (2001) *Report of the Special Rapporteur on Prisons and Conditions of Detention in Africa – Prisons in Mozambique: Report on a Second Visit*. African Commission on Human and Peoples' Rights, Banjul.

Bessin, M. and Lechien, M. (2000) *Soignants et Malades Incarcérés: Conditions, pratiques et usages des soins en prison*. EHESS, Paris.

British Medical Association (1990) *Working Party report on the health care of remand prisoners*. HMSO, London.

British Medical Association (2001) *The medical profession and human rights: a handbook*. Zed Books in association with the BMA, London.

Combessie, P. (2001) France. In D. van zyl Smit and F. Dünkel (eds) *Imprisonment today and tomorrow: international perspectives on prisoners' rights and prison conditions*. Kluwer Law International, The Hague.

Correctional Association of New York (1999) *Prisons and jails – hospitals of last resort: the need for diversion and discharge planning for incarcerated people with mental illness in New York*. Correctional Association of New York, New York.

Correctional Association of New York (2002) *State of the prisons: conditions of confinement in 25 New York Correctional Facilities*. Correctional Association of New York, New York.

Corrections Health Service (2001) *Corrections Health Service annual report 2000–2001*. Corrections Health Service, Sydney.

Corrections Journal (2001) Study documents TB's spread from jail to nearby community. *Corrections Journal*, **5** (10), 1–6.

Council of Europe (1998) *Recommendation No R (98) 7 of the Committee of Ministers to Member States concerning the ethical and organisational aspects of health care in prison*. Council of Europe, Strasbourg.

Council of Europe (2002) *Rapport au gouvernement de la République de Moldova relatif a la visite effectuée en Moldova par le Comité européen pour la prévention de la torture et des peines ou traitements inhumains ou dégradants, du 10 au 22 juin 200*. Council of Europe, Strasbourg.

Coyle, A. (1994) *The prisons we deserve*. Harper Collins, London.

Department of Health (1999) *The future organisation of prison health care*. Joint Prison Service and National Health Service Executive Working Party, London.

Dolan, K. and Wodak, A. (1999) HIV transmission in a prison system in an Australian State. *Medical Journal of Australia*, **171**, 5 July, 14–17.

Harding, C., Hines, B., Ireland, R. and Rawlings, P. (1985) *Imprisonment in England and Wales: a concise history*. Croom Helm, London.

Health Advisory Committee for the Prison Service England and Wales (1997) *The provision of mental health care in prisons*. Health Advisory Committee for the Prison Service England and Wales, London.

Heilpern, D. (1998) *Fear or favour: sexual assault of young prisoners*. Southern Cross University Press, Lismore.

HM Inspectorate of Prisons (1996) *Patient or prisoner?: a new strategy for healthcare in prisons*. Home Office, London.

HM Prison Service and Department of Health (2001a) *Prison Health Policy Unit and Task Force Annual Report 2000/2001*. HM Prison Service and Department of Health, London.

HM Prison Service and Department of Health (2001b) *Report of the Working Group on doctors working in prisons.* HM Prison Service and Department of Health, London.

HM Prison Service and Department of Health (2002) *Seeking consent: working with people in prison.* HM Prison Service and Department of Health, London.

HM Prison Service and the NHS Executive (1999) *The future organisation of prison health care.* Joint Prison Service and National Health Service Executive Working Group, London.

ICPS (2002) *Prison Healthcare News,* 2, Summer, 1.

Journal of Law, Medicine and Ethics, The (1999) Death and dying behind bars – cross-cutting themes and policy imperatives. *The Journal of Law, Medicine and Ethics,* 27 (3), 238–239.

Michaels, D. and Rozenman, M. (2002) Feeling insecure: in France, getting into prison is harder than getting out. *Wall Street Journal,* New York, 20 August.

Ministère de la Justice (1999) *Reforme de la justice, Responsibility for the health care of inmates.* Available at www.justice.gouv.fr.

Ministère de la Justice (2001) *Rapport annuel d'activité de l'administration pénitentiaire.* Ministère de la Justice, Paris.

Ministère de la Justice and Ministère de l'Emploi et de la Solidarité (2001) *L'organisation des soins aux detenus: rapport d'evaluation.* Ministères de la Justice et la Solidarité, Paris.

Office for National Statistics (2000) *Psychiatric morbidity among young offenders in England and Wales.* Office for National Statistics, London.

Office of the Deputy Prime Minister (2002) *Reducing re-offending by ex-prisoners.* Report by the Social Exclusion Unit. Office for the Deputy Prime Minister, London.

Penal Reform International (1998) *Interview with Yuri Ivanovitch Kalinin 21 August 1998 in Information Pack 1: Measures to Reduce Prison Overcrowding.* Penal Reform International, London.

Prison Reform Trust (1985) *Prison medicine: ideas on health care in penal establishments.* HMSO, London.

Reyes, H. (2001) Health and human rights in prisons. *In HIV in prisons: A reader with particular relevance to the newly independent states.* World Health Organization Europe, Copenhagen.

Smith, R. (1984) *Prison health care.* BMA, London.

Stern, V. (1998) *A sin against the future.* Northeastern University Press, Boston, MA.

Stern, V. (1999) Introduction: an overview and some issues. In V. Stern (ed.) *Sentenced to die? The problem of TB in prisons in Eastern Europe and Central Asia.* International Centre for Prison Studies, Kings College London, London.

Stöver, H. (2002) *Drugs and HIV/AIDS services in European prisons.* Bibliotheks und Informationssystem der Carl von Ossietzky Universität Oldenburg, Oldenburg.

Tomascevski, K. (1992) *Prison health; international standards and national practices in Europe.* HEUNI, Helsinki.

United Nations (1988) *Human rights: a compilation of international instruments.* United Nations, New York.

Vasseur, V. (2000) *Médecin-Chef Á la Prison de la Santé.* le cherche midi éditeur, Paris.

World Health Organization (2000) *Tuberculosis control in prisons: a manual for programme managers.* World Health Organization, Geneva.

World Prison Brief (2002) *International centre for prison studies.* Available at www.prisonstudies.org.

Chapter 8

New Citizens

East Germans in a United Germany

Reinhard Busse and Ellen Nolte

Introduction

In 1989, the fall of the Berlin Wall ended the post-war division of Germany. In a decade during which Europe was characterized by immense social and political transition, the experience of the people of the former German Democratic Republic (GDR) was unique. Within a few months it became a fully fledged market economy: part of the west German monetary system on 1 July 1990, and part of the Federal Republic of Germany (FRG) on 3 October 1990. With unification east Germany also became part of the European Union (Blacksell 1995). While other eastern European countries in transition were engaged in a major process of state building, enacting new constitutions and establishing new institutions and laws on health care and safety, these already existed in the Federal Republic and were simply extended to the territory of the former GDR when they became the new *Länder*. Within this context of a 'ready-made state' (Rose and Haerpfer 1997) the Soviet-style health care system was replaced by a pluralist insurance-based system of medical care of high technological standard.

This chapter revisits the process of transforming health care in East Germany in the course of political transition. It specifically looks at the context within which this process took place, explores reasons for the policy decision to adopt the west German model of health care and analyses the events that followed. Its importance for the topic of this book is that it raises some questions about how a country deals with the existence of two different health systems, each reflecting different sets of inherited traditions and institutional frameworks.

The east German health care system

After 1945 the three western allied forces maintained the health care system as it existed in their zones of occupation, adding only some pre-1933 features, often with the same personnel, leading to the re-establishment of a social health insurance (SHI)-based system with a high degree of decision-making powers for both sickness funds and health care providers. In contrast, the Soviets adopted a strong interventionist role within their zone from the beginning. They took an authoritarian approach, initially in order to control infectious diseases, and despite the protests of physicians gradually introduced a centralized state-operated health care system. They called together 60 health experts to advise them on the design for a new model, which came to be influenced by the traditions of social hygiene in the community health care services of the Weimar period, and by emigrants who had returned from Britain, Sweden and the Soviet Union (Busse 2000).

The resulting health care system in the GDR differed from its Soviet counterpart, however, by establishing a structural division between ambulatory and hospital services, although in practice they often operated from the same premises. In addition, the principle of social insurance was *de jure* maintained, with workers and employers sharing contributions, but with administration concentrated in only two large sickness funds, one for workers (89 per cent) and one for professionals, members of agricultural cooperatives, artists and the self-employed (11 per cent). De facto, however, the role of the social insurance system was extremely limited and the system was funded mainly through general government revenues.

As in most socialist countries, the majority of health care personnel in the GDR were employed by the state, with a few delivering ambulatory care in solo practices but mostly through community-based or company-based health care centres, which usually were staffed by a range of medical specialists and other health care professionals. Unlike the neighbouring Soviet bloc countries, not all health care institutions were formally nationalized. Instead, independent institutions could continue to exist but faced increasing difficulties when exercising their role as health care providers. As a result, the number of not-for-profit hospitals decreased from 88 to 75 between 1960 and 1989, and the number of private hospitals fell from 55 to 2 in the same period (Deutsche Krankenhaus-Gesellschaft 2000). However, in 1989 about 7 per cent of all hospital beds were still not state-owned and a few physicians were still in private practice.

Local communities provided preventive services, encompassing health education, child and maternity health and specialist care for chronic diseases such as diabetes or psychiatric disorders. These health care services were complemented by comprehensive social support provided by the state, such as housing, child day-care and crèches, which also contributed to the policy imperatives of increasing the population and so the active workforce. Thus, they soon achieved a type of health care system to which the political left in West Germany and many other western countries aspired until at least the 1960s (Busse 2000).

However, due to under-financing and under-investment, a shortage of personnel and lack of access to modern technologies, the GDR health care system gradually began to fall behind the standards of western industrialized countries, beginning in the 1970s but becoming visibly worse in the second half of the 1980s. In the hospital sector, East Germany had about a quarter fewer hospital cases per 1000 population than in the west, yet hospital occupancy fell below 75 per cent in the 1980s (Table 8.1).

This lack of modern medical care has been associated with poor population health. Available evidence suggests that, for example, shortages in surgical capacity may have been related to higher infant death rates due to congenital anomalies of the heart and cardiovascular diseases in the GDR compared to the west in the 1980s (Bundesminister für Gesundheit 1993). Other data indicate under-treatment or less effective treatment of hypertension as the prevalence of recognized but untreated hypertension was lower, while rates of treated but uncontrolled hypertension were higher than in the old FRG (Heinemann and Greiser 1993). Further evidence suggests possible under-treatment of elderly stroke patients in the former GDR, which was reflected in a high case fatality, especially among those over 65 (Eisenblätter et al. 1994). A recent study of fatal outcomes after hip fractures in 1989 in the former GDR reported a case-fatality rate of about 20 per cent, considerably higher than in the west (Wildner et al. 1998). Although other factors such as case mix have to be considered, these findings point to the possible contribution differences in medical care may have made to the widening mortality gap between the two parts of Germany pre-unification (Nolte et al. 2000b). However, this relative disadvantage in the east had only developed since the mid-1970s. Before this, life expectancy had improved almost equally, with even a slight advantage for men in the east during the 1960s and early 1970s (Figure 8.1).

In 1989, a National Health Conference had decided to introduce major health care reforms and to increase investment, but shortly afterwards the opening of the Berlin Wall in November that year brought an end to the entity of East Germany.

Transforming health care

The events following the fall of the Berlin Wall unfolded at a tremendous speed, with the ten-point plan 'for overcoming the division of Germany and Europe' announced by the west German Chancellor Helmut Kohl by the end of November 1989 leading, eventually, to unification. It is within this context

Table 8.1 Inpatient structure and utilization: general and psychiatric hospitals in western and eastern parts of Germany 1970–1998

	Beds/1000			Cases/1000			Length of stay (days)			Occupancy rate (%)		
	West	East	E/W ratio	West	East	E/W ratio	West	East	E/W ratio	West	East	E/W ratio
1970	11.20	11.13	0.99	146.3	135.6	0.93	24.9	23.3	0.94	88.5	81.2	0.92
1980	11.48	10.27	0.89	181.6	140.9	0.76	19.7	19.1	0.97	84.9	74.8	0.88
1989	10.69	9.94	0.93	208.6	152.9	0.73	16.2	17.3	1.07	86.0	74.6	0.87
1991	8.19	8.89	1.09	179.3	151.1	0.84	14.3	16.1	1.09	86.0	74.9	0.87
1992	8.02	8.08	1.01	180.4	159.4	0.88	13.9	14.2	1.02	85.3	76.0	0.89
1993	7.80	7.50	0.96	180.3	162.9	0.90	13.2	13.0	0.98	83.9	77.4	0.92
1994	7.68	7.16	0.93	181.9	169.0	0.93	12.7	12.2	0.96	82.7	79.0	0.95
1995	7.55	7.03	0.93	185.4	175.9	0.95	12.2	11.7	0.96	82.0	80.1	0.98
1996	7.30	6.98	0.96	186.8	181.9	0.97	11.5	11.2	0.97	80.3	79.6	0.99
1997	7.12	6.87	0.96	189.4	187.5	0.99	11.1	10.8	0.97	80.7	80.5	1.00
1998	7.01	6.78	0.97	194.4	194.9	1.00	10.8	10.5	0.97	81.8	82.3	1.01

Source: authors' calculations based on data from the Federal Statistical Office.

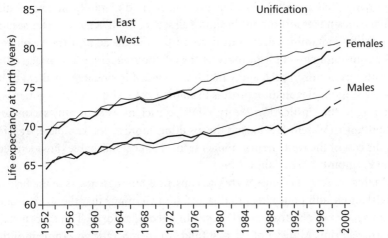

Figure 8.1 Life expectancy at birth in east and west Germany, 1952–1999 [from 1998, data for east Berlin are included in 'west'].
Source: adapted from Nolte *et al.* (2000b); Statistisches Bundesamt (2001).

of strong dynamics of political unification that health care reform in east Germany was to be achieved (Manow 1994, 1997; Nolte 2002; Wasem 1997a).

> In the first phase after the autumn of 1989, health politicians and corporatist actors in the health field assumed that their task would be to reform the East German health system with the perspective of an independent East German state in mind. Then it became apparent that a reformed East German health care system would have to be integrated into the West German sector later. Finally the actors realised that most parts of an East German health reform would not occur before the accession to West Germany.
>
> Wasem 1997

The decision to adopt the west German statutory insurance system

The speed with which the unification of the two states was driven required 'pragmatic solutions' (Stone 1994) with virtually no space for innovations or experiments in reforming east Germany's health care sector. The pace of polit- ical developments following the resignation of the GDR's former leader Erich Honecker in October 1989 rapidly led to disintegration of political authority with a breakdown of order, which in turn placed the east in a very weak bar- gaining position compared with the west (Lehmbruch 1994; Manow 1994). The almost complete discrediting of the GDR administrative (civil) service during this process also contributed to the weak negotiating role of east

Germany (Lehmbruch 1994). The previously rigid hierarchy and party discipline meant that institutions in almost all sectors of GDR society were seen as politically contaminated, causing deep mistrust in the administrative bodies. The continuing loss of legitimacy of the GDR bureaucracy also affected the health care sector in such a way that it was almost impossible for them to be involved in the negotiation process (Manow 1994). Thus, in the negotiations leading to the Unification Treaty, GDR politicians were of only secondary importance (Wasem 1997a), and the resulting, more or less complete, transfer to the east of the west German model seemed almost inevitable (Freudenstein and Borgwardt 1992; Manow 1994).

In this context of change, there was consensus amongst actors in the field of social and health policy in both east and west Germany that the social insurance system of the former GDR was in need of reform. Thus, Lothar de Maizière, Prime Minister of the first (and last) democratic government of the GDR declared in the first government statement in spring 1990 that the 'centralized administration of the social insurance run by the FDGB (Free German Trade Union Association) does not meet the demands of a democratic welfare state' (Spree 1994). Whilst reorganization was perceived as essential, the structure and content of this reorganization, especially in relation to health care, were less clear. In fact, there was much controversy among west German governmental and non-governmental actors, interest groups and even the administration itself. The main areas of conflict concerned the structure of the new health insurance system, funding mechanisms and the survival of the outpatient policlinic system (Wasem 1997a).

Importantly, however, although the proposed reorganization was of the east German health care system, those shaping the reform were exclusively west German (Manow 1997). Initially, the Social Democratic Party and the Federal Association of General Regional Sickness Funds (*AOK Bundesverband*) were very successful in introducing their proposals into the coalition agreement of the newly elected GDR government in spring 1990 (Robischon *et al.* 1994). However, their suggestions to preserve some basic features of east Germany's health care sector, namely some form of unified health insurance (in the form of one insurance fund for each of the 15 regions of the GDR), and retaining the policlinic system as the main institutional setting for providing outpatient care, faced strong opposition. The associations of substitute funds lobbied hard to transfer the highly fragmented west German health insurance system to east Germany (not the least out of fear that monopolistic funds would strengthen the position of the AOK in a united Germany), an effort supported by the chambers of physicians, who traditionally favour a pluralistic health insurance structure (Lehmbruch 1994). This alliance gained decisive support not only from the governing coalition party but also from the Federal Republic's Chancellor Helmut Kohl, who then had strong negotiating power (Wasem 1997a). As a result of the negotiations on the Unification Treaty, the east German health care system was to be put on the same financial and organizational basis as that of the west from 1 January 1991.

Once substitute sickness funds were given free rein to compete in the east they began intensive marketing campaigns to persuade east German citizens to leave their regional sickness funds. Both regional and substitute sickness funds put a great deal of effort into training staff and offering ongoing technical support for their 'adopted' area in the east. Regional as well as substitute sickness funds soon established offices in the east and were able to start work by January 1991 (Spree 1994).

The fight to dismantle the policlinics

Even more fiercely disputed was the 'policlinic issue'. Initially, there was consensus among the east German actors that this particular aspect of ambulatory care provision should remain in parallel with private practices. It was argued that,

> [d]espite chronic financing shortfalls, incomplete reforms, spreading environmental hazards, and mounting personnel shortages, East Germany's policlinic system delivered a quality of care that compared favourably with West Germany on some health indicators. Because most shortcomings were identified as financial rather than structural, a post-unity increase in capital outlays promised significantly improved results. Consequently, East German officials and some West German Social Democrats urged that the policlinics be retained as part of a 'pluralistic' approach to health care delivery in the new *Länder*.
>
> Scharf 1999

This, however, was perceived as a substantial threat by west German physician organizations to their monopoly in ambulatory care (*Sicherstellungsauftrag*) (Stone 1994; Wasem 1997a) and they decided to lobby hard against policlinics, declaring the free exercise of private medical practice as a 'basic right'.

In the negotiations leading to the State Treaty on Monetary, Economic and Social Union in July 1990, the organizational aspects of medical care provision were left relatively imprecise although 'those in favour of radical change managed to insert a clause' (Wasem 1997a) requiring the east German government to transform ambulatory care provision towards private practice. Eventually, a compromise was found that, first, granted every east German physician the freedom of establishment in private practice, and second, authorized policlinics and related facilities to provide services at least until the end of 1995 (Stone 1994; Wasem 1997a). This time limit was removed later through the Health Care Reform Structure Act (GSG) in 1992.

However, despite this compromise 'corporatist power coalesced to conquer the policlinic challenge' (Robischon *et al.* 1994). The most vigorous opposition to a continuing role for the policlinics came from the Federal Association of SHI Physicians (*Kassenärztliche Bundesvereinigung*) which regarded them as a potential threat both to medical autonomy and to the system of fee-for-service reimbursement that was the basis of their relatively high incomes.

'The frontal assault on the policlinics took the form of publicly ridiculing their lack of modern equipment and their 'outmoded' forms of treatment. The more extreme view condemned them as a Soviet invention' (Robischon *et al.* 1994), although policlinics had begun to emerge before 1933. A more devastating blow to the policlinics resulted from their ambiguous financial situation, which was deliberately planned by the physicians associations. Given the mammoth infrastructure needs and uncertain revenues of local government, public investment plans for policlinics were slow and, in any case, hospitals took priority. Of course, private financing was available in principle, but because of the five-year transition period (and possibly also for ideological reasons) banks were reluctant to grant long-term credits. On the other hand, for a physician willing to set up an independent practice, the regional physicians' association could assure the bank of the applicant's creditworthiness. The federal government supported establishment of private practices through special loans (Bundesministerium für Gesundheit 1998).

The time limit imposed on the survival of policlinics and, more importantly, the remuneration method negotiated between the sickness funds and the Federal Association of Social Health Insurance Physicians that favoured private practice, put substantial pressure on physicians to become self-employed (Freudenstein and Borgwardt 1992; Robischon *et al.* 1994). The major discrepancy in physicians' incomes resulted from the fact that fee-for-service was used to remunerate services delivered in private practice while the capitation method was used to compensate policlinics. Regional and local governments in the east, now owning the majority of policlinics and fearing substantial deficits in their budgets, placed additional pressure on physicians to set up private practices.

As a consequence, more than 80 per cent of outpatient physicians had become office-based by the end of 1991. While on 31 December 1990, only 12.6 per cent of physicians in ambulatory care worked in private practice, this figure jumped to 35.5 per cent on 1 January 1991, reached 56.8 per cent on 1 April, 66.2 per cent on 1 July and 83.6 per cent by 31 December, i.e. within one year the vast majority had moved to private practice. Initially, the speed differed between the six regions (including the eastern part of Berlin) with Berlin lagging behind and Saxony-Anhalt and Thuringia in the lead. In the end, however, the change was almost complete, independent of the governing party in the respective Land or the initial intention of the physicians to stay with the policlinics (Wasem 1997b).

Almost two years after unification, around 70 per cent of the former policlinic facilities were either removed or transferred into other forms of health care provision. By 1998 about 96 per cent of all physicians in east Germany were established in private practice while only 4 per cent were still based in policlinics (Bundesministerium für Gesundheit 1998).

Continuing adaptation to western standards

The health care system in the new *Länder* was not only legally put on a completely new financial and organizational basis, but converged quite rapidly in terms of infrastructure, utilization and spending patterns with the western part of Germany.

In the hospital sector, the need to overhaul the infrastructure facilitated a rapid decrease in the number of hospital beds. Between 1991 and 1994, more than 20 per cent of all acute care beds were closed while in the west the respective figure was only 6 per cent. By the late 1990s, figures were, however, quite similar (Table 8.1). While bed numbers were reduced, the east experienced a rapid increase in hospital cases of almost 30 per cent between 1991 and 1998, resulting in the same per capita level as in the west. Length of stay and occupancy rates also converged. These trends led to drastically increasing costs per hospital day, case and bed, though overall expenditure remained somewhat below the western figures until the end of 1990s due to the lower wages in the east (Table 8.2).

In ambulatory care, the income of the office-based physicians had reached, on average, 85 per cent of that of their western colleagues. Their persisting lower income was due mainly to having fewer privately insured patients. The average figure of 85 per cent hides huge variation between specialties, with radiologists and surgeons doing even better than in the west mainly because of the continuing lower numbers in relation to the population (Table 8.3).

While total sickness fund expenditure per capita was only 57 per cent of that in the west in 1991, it rapidly increased to 74 per cent in 1992 and 87 per cent in 1994. By the end of the 1990s, it almost equalled that in the west (Table 8.4). Costs for pharmaceuticals (which are not influenced by the lower wages in the east) have been higher in the east since 1993, due to both higher prescription rates and a more liberal use of newer and more expensive drugs (Table 8.4).

As the gross domestic product (GDP) has remained considerably lower in the east, health care expenditure as a percentage of GDP in east Germany was, at least according to one calculation (Schneider 1999), higher than in the

Table 8.2 Expenditure data for general and psychiatric hospitals in western and eastern parts of Germany 1991–2000

	Expenditure/bed			Expenditure/day			Expenditure/case		
	West (€)	East (€)	E/W ratio	West (€)	East (€)	E/W ratio	West (€)	East (€)	E/W ratio
1991	62 309	31 160	0.50	199	114	0.60	2 849	1 833	0.64
1992	68 232 +9.5%	43 571 +39.8%	0.64	219 +10.0%	157 +37.3%	0.72	3 032 +6.5%	2 210 +20.5%	0.73
1993	72 158 +5.8%	52 708 +21.0%	0.73	236 +7.8%	187 +19.2%	0.79	3 120 +2.9%	2 429 +9.9%	0.78
1994	75 477 +4.6%	61 672 +17.0%	0.82	250 +6.1%	214 +14.6%	0.85	3 188 +2.2%	2 614 +7.6%	0.82
1995	80 569 +6.7	68 249 +10.7%	0.85	269 +7.6%	233 +9.2%	0.87	3 281 +2.9%	2 729 +4.4%	0.83
1996	83 368 +3.5%	71 834 +5.3%	0.86	284 +5.4%	246 +5.6%	0.87	3 260 −0.7%	2 758 +1.1%	0.85
1997	85 624 +2.7%	75 174 +4.7%	0.88	291 +2.5%	256 +3.8%	0.88	3 218 −1.3%	2 755 −0.1%	0.86
1998	88 395 +3.2%	78 955 +5.0%	0.89	296 +1.8%	263 +2.7%	0.89	3 187 −1.0%	2 747 −0.3%	0.86
1999	91 181 +3.2%	81 218 +2.9%	0.89	306 +3.3%	269 +2.4%	0.88	3 191 +0.1%	2 731 −0.6%	0.86
2000	93 769 +2.8%	84 343 +3.9%	0.90	315 +3.1%	278 +3.3%	0.88	3 207 +0.5%	2 762 +1.1%	0.86

Source: authors' calculations based on data from the Federal Statistical Office.

United States. As health care in Germany is largely funded through statutory health insurance, which in turn is financed almost exclusively through wage- or social benefits-related contributions, this high expenditure increased the contribution rate (i.e. the percentage to be paid for health insurance) in the east above the level in the west after the mid-1990s. This contributed to a downturn in economic growth in the east. In response to these developments the Act to Equalise the Law in Statutory Health Insurance (*Gesetz zur Rechtsangleichung in der gesetzlichen Krankenversicherung*) was introduced to put the Risk Structure Compensation Mechanism (*Risikostrukturausgleich*), which redistributes money among sickness funds to compensate for different income and, to some extent, expenditure levels of their members (Busse 2001), on a uniform basis for the whole of Germany from 2000.

Table 8.3 Remuneration/income of SHI-affiliated physicians in private practice in 1998 (partly averaged for 1996–98)

	Ratio (East/West)			
	SHI remuneration	Total remuneration (incl. private patients etc.)	Costs for personnel and equipment	Surplus = income before tax
Dermatologists	0.81	0.63	0.58	0.72
ENT physicians	0.80	0.65	0.68	0.62
Gynaecologists	0.84	0.75	0.76	0.75
Internists (general and subspecialists)	1.02	0.88	0.84	0.93
Neurologists	0.98	0.85	0.93	0.77
Ophthalmologists	0.91	0.80	0.74	0.88
Orthopaedists	0.88	0.80	0.73	0.91
Paediatricians	0.71	0.67	0.64	0.71
Radiologists	1.21	1.24	1.22	1.32
Surgeons	0.93	0.98	0.95	1.03
Urologists	1.08	0.89	0.91	0.86
All specialists (incl. other)	0.94	0.85	0.83	0.87
General practitioners	0.88	0.80	0.76	0.85
TOTAL	**0.90**	**0.81**	**0.78**	**0.85**

Source: authors' calculations based on data from the Federal Association of SHI Physicians.

In spite of this considerable financial burden borne by Germany as a whole, east Germans feel left behind: in 1998, 44 per cent of east Germans were not satisfied with their social protection in case of illness – compared with only 34 per cent in the west (Statistisches Bundesamt 1999). The physicians themselves emphasize how they continue to receive less remuneration for work in ambulatory care, which has remained at around 77 per cent of that in the west (Table 8.4). They claim that this also makes it difficult for retiring general practitioners to find successors, especially in rural areas. Since 1998, east German physicians in ambulatory care have conducted their own separate *Ärztetage* (physicians' congregation) four times, an event that is otherwise

Table 8.4 Per capita expenditure in eastern areas of Germany compared to western areas, 1991–1999

	East/West ratio per SHI-insured person								
	1991	**1992**	**1993**	**1994**	**1995**	**1996**	**1997**	**1998**	**1999**
Hospitals	0.64	0.74	0.79	0.86	0.89	0.96	0.97	0.98	1.02
Ambulatory physicians	0.49	0.59	0.68	0.75	0.79	0.76	0.78	0.78	0.77
Pharmaceuticals	0.64	0.78	1.02	1.10	1.14	1.13	1.10	1.07	1.07
Devices and services by other health professions	0.43	0.63	0.74	0.77	0.79	0.82	0.80	0.82	0.84
Dentists	0.68	0.90	0.94	0.98	1.03	1.01	1.01	1.00	1.01
Maternity	0.41	0.43	0.44	0.46	0.52	0.52	0.56	0.59	0.61
TOTAL	**0.57**	**0.73**	**0.80**	**0.87**	**0.91**	**0.92**	**0.93**	**0.92**	**0.94**

Source: authors' calculations based on data from the Federal Ministry of Health.

reserved for the annual meetings of the representatives of all physicians in Germany. An indication that some physicians may well have regretted their initial support for opening a private practice can be found in the highly surprising, and quite positive, cover story of the *Deutsches Ärzteblatt* (German Medical Journal', published jointly by the Federal Physicians' Chamber and the Federal Association of SHI Physicians) on policlinics with the title *Vom Auslaufmodell zur Alternative* ('From an obsolescent model to an alternative') (Richter 2001).

The changing pattern of population health

Considering the substantial transformation of the east German health care system since unification, one might expect some impact on changing mortality in the former GDR. For example, Becker and Boyle noted a fall in mortality from testicular cancer among east German men of 50 per cent between 1990 and 1995, suggesting that the rapid increase in the availability of modern pharmaceuticals may be the most likely explanation for this decline (Becker and Boyle 1997). Nolte *et al.* reported that since unification there was a substantial decline in neonatal mortality despite a slight worsening of the birth weight distribution with an increasing proportion of very low-birth weight infants in both east and west (Nolte *et al.* 2000a). They further demonstrated that, in the east, the net effect of the change in the birth weight distribution would, in the absence of other factors, have led to an increase in neonatal mortality or, at least, kept mortality at the 1991 level. Instead, neonatal mortality fell markedly by over 30 per cent. This was due to an improvement in survival at all birth weights, but in particular, among those with low and very low birth weight. Differences in survival in this group are closely linked to effective medical interventions.

Subsequent analyses showed that, in terms of mortality, medical care did not only benefit infants but also adults. A study on the potential impact of medical care on changes in mortality in east Germany estimated that of an increase in life expectancy between birth and age 75 of 1.4 years in men and 0.9 years in women between 1992 and 1997 (west Germany: 0.6 and 0.3 years), 14–23 per cent was accounted for by declining mortality from conditions amenable to medical intervention (Nolte et al. 2002). Falling death rates from hypertension and cerebrovascular diseases and, among women, from cervical cancer and breast cancer have been important contributors. Along with the finding of a substantial decline in birth weight specific neonatal mortality, this identifies medical care as one important component in the post-unification mortality decline in east Germany.

These findings are in line with other, albeit indirect, evidence of improved medical care in east Germany. For example, a study on provision of dialysis demonstrated that between 1989 and 1994 there was a two- to three-fold increase in dialysis facilities in east Germany, which was accompanied by a 2.5 fold increase in the number of patients receiving regular treatment (Thieler et al. 1994, 1995). This was due, largely, to increased treatment of elderly and diabetic patients who had been given lower priority because of shortage of funds in the former GDR (Knox 1993). Other evidence suggests that in the 1990s there was a also substantial increase in indicators reflecting intensified treatment of cardiovascular disease in east Germany, for example, an increase in ischaemic heart disease-related surgery, by 530 per cent between 1993 and 1997 (Brenner et al. 2000). The number of coronary catheterization units increased from 7 in 1990 to 42 in 1997 (Bundesministerium für Gesundhert 1998). There was also a considerable increase in the number of primary pace-maker implantations after unification, from 220 per million population in 1986/87 to 450–490 in 1993/95 (Spitzer 1999).

Yet while life expectancy at birth in east Germany improved substantially after unification, by about 2.4 years between 1992 and 1997 (Nolte et al. 2000c), by the end of the 1990s there was still a mortality differential between the two parts of Germany (see Figure 8.1). Looking specifically at the potential role of medical care it was estimated that about 16 per cent of the gap in male life expectancy between birth and age 75 was attributable to higher mortality from conditions amenable to medical care in the east (Table 8.5) (Nolte et al. 2002).

Table 8.5 Cause specific contribution to differences in temporary life expectancy (e $_{0-75}$), in years by cause group between East and West Germany: 1992 and 1997

	Contribution in years to differences in life expectancy by age group											
	0		1–14		15–39		40–64		65–74		All	
	Male	Female	Male	Female	Male	Female	Male	Female	Male	Female	Male	Female
1992												
Conditions amenable to medical care	0.055	0.047	0.004	0.011	0.060	0.033	0.146	0.069	0.056	0.060	0.321	0.220
Conditions amenable to health policy measures	0.003	0.003	0.016	0.031	0.405	0.081	0.348	0.063	0.012	−0.004	0.784	0.174
Ischaemic heart disease	0.000	0.000	0.000	0.000	0.023	0.007	0.266	0.091	0.086	0.071	0.375	0.168
Non-amenable conditions	−0.025	−0.003	0.014	0.011	0.133	0.020	0.412	0.186	0.032	0.059	0.566	0.273
Total	0.033	0.048	0.034	0.053	0.621	0.140	1.173	0.409	0.186	0.187	2.046	0.836
1997												
Conditions amenable to medical care	0.054	0.030	0.022	0.002	0.021	0.014	0.084	−0.013	0.050	0.022	0.201	0.055
Conditions amenable to health policy measures	0.001	0.005	0.030	0.012	0.287	0.076	0.235	0.023	0.031	0.003	0.577	0.120
Ischaemic heart disease	0.000	0.000	0.000	0.000	0.015	0.002	0.170	0.040	0.075	0.060	0.260	0.101
Non-amenable conditions	−0.032	−0.048	0.030	0.011	0.098	−0.021	0.170	0.011	−0.036	0.010	0.231	−0.037
Total	0.023	0.014	0.045	0.026	0.421	0.071	0.659	0.061	0.120	0.095	1.268	0.239

Among women, the corresponding figure was 25 per cent. Importantly, although the overall differential became smaller during the 1990s, the relative contribution of these conditions to the remaining gap remained fairly stable. It would thus appear that, despite the major achievements in rebuilding the health care system in the former GDR, health outcomes continue to lag behind those in west Germany. This is also illustrated by the finding that, despite a considerable improvement since 1991, neonatal mortality in east Germany in 1996 could have been lowered by a further 15 per cent if birth weight specific neonatal mortality rates seen in the west had applied (Nolte *et al.* 2000a).

There are several possible explanations for these findings, such as data arte-facts, differences in underlying morbidity and differences in access to and/or quality of health care. Whilst a possible bias due to variation in data quality or comparability may be assumed to be of minor importance, available evidence suggests that some conditions where premature death is 'avoidable' by timely and effective medical care are more frequent in the adult east German population, such as hypertension and diabetes (Thamm 1999; Thefeld 1999). Thus, the burden of cardiovascular and endocrine morbidity appears to be higher in the east, which in turn could explain some of the higher mortality from these diseases. However, limited evidence also suggests a possible undersupply of some health services in east Germany. Thus it was noted that the higher prevalence of hyper-tension partly reflects a true east–west difference, but may also indicate possible under-treatment of this condition in the east (Bundesregierung 2001). There is also some evidence of east-west variation in certain diagnostic and therapeutic interventions for ischaemic heart disease (Perleth *et al.* 1999). However, how these differences impact on population health remains to be investigated.

Conclusions

Since unification, both the health care system in the former GDR and the health status of the population in this part of unified Germany has changed dramatically. The eastern part of the country has experienced one of the most remarkable increases in life expectancy in recent years. While many factors have contributed to this success, health care is definitely one of the major fac-tors. Yet neither the improvement in health status for east Germans or the role of the health care system have really been appreciated as a success story within Germany. Rather, the high costs of unification and the disappointment that the economic situation has not improved as much as initially promised have tended to be the focus of debate.

There may, however, be a reluctance to address these issues because of the negative connotations among the population (at least in the east) of how the reform of the health care system (as in most aspects of life) was dominated by west German actors and west German interests. Any acceptance of the uniform health insurance or the policlinic system in east Germany would have posed a considerable threat to the interests and corporatist identities of west German actors (Stone 1994; Wasem 1997a). Consequently, the east German model was never given a serious chance. We therefore do not know whether it might have produced outcomes as good – or even better – than those achieved under the current system. However, the fact that east German actors were of so little importance in shaping the reform because of their weak position might be a factor contributing to the limited sense of public ownership of the new system, despite its considerable successes.

However, the circle continues to turn and current German discussions on health policy and, in particular, how to provide 'integrated care', or 'disease management programmes', which have been found to be difficult to implement in the existing model of delivery, raises the interesting question of whether a policlinic or dispensary-type structures might be (re-) established, and whether such a development would produce some satisfaction in the east that not every characteristic of the GDR health care system was as bad as it was made out to be.

References

Becker, N. and Boyle, P. (1997) Decline in mortality from testicular cancer in West Germany after reunification. *Lancet*, **350**, 744.

Blacksell, M. (1995) Germany as a European power. In D. Lewis and J. R. P. McKenzie (eds) *The new Germany. Social, political and cultural challenges of unification*, pp. 78–100. University of Exeter Press, Exeter.

Brenner, G., Altenhoten, L., Bogumil, W., Heuer, J., Kerek-Bodden, H., *et al.* (2000) *Gesundheitszustand und ambulante medizinische Versorgung der Bevölkerung in Deutschland im Ost-West-Vergleich*. Zentralinstitut für die kassenärztliche Versorgung, Köln.

Bundesminister für Gesundheit (1993) *Indikatoren zum Gesundheitszustand der Bevölkerung in der ehemaligen DDR. Schriftenreihe des Bundesministeriums für Gesundheit Band 23*. Nomos Verlagsgesellschaft, Baden-Baden.

Bundesministerium für Gesundheit (1998) *Das Gesundheitswesen in den neuen Ländern*. Bundesministerium für Gesundheit, Bonn.

Bundesregierung (2001) *Gutachten 2000/2001 des Sachverständigenrates für die Konzertierte Aktion im Gesundheitswesen*. Bedarfsgerechtigkeit und Wirtschaftlichkeit. Drucksache 14/6871. Deutscher Bundestag, Berlin.

Busse, R. (2000) *Health care systems in transition: Germany*. European Observatory on Health Care Systems, Copenhagen.

Busse, R. (2001) Risk structure compensation in Germany's statutory health insurance. *European Journal of Public Health*, **11**, 74–7.

Deutsche Krankenhaus-Gesellschaft (2000) *Zahlen daten fakten 2002*. Deutsche Krankenhaus-Gesellschaft, Düsseldorf.

Eisenblätter, D., Claßen, E., Schädlich, H. and Heinemann, L. (1994) Häufigkeit und Prognose von Schlaganfallerkrankungen in der Bevölkerung Ostdeutschlands. Ergebnisse von Schlaganfallregistern in den Jahren 1985–1988. *Nervenarzt*, **65**, 95–100.

Freudenstein, U. and Borgwardt, G. (1992) Primary medical care in former East Germany: the frosty winds of change. *British Medical Journal*, **304**, 827–9.

Heinemann, L. and Greiser, E. M. (1993) Blood pressure, hypertension, and other risk factors in East and West Germany. *Annals of Epidemiology*, 3 Suppl., S90–5.

Knox, R. A. (1993) *Germany: one nation with health care for all*. Faulkner & Gray, New York.

Lehmbruch, G. (1994) The process of regime change in East Germany: an institutionalist scenario for German unification. *Journal of European Public Policy*, **1**, 1350–63.

Manow, P. (1997) Entwicklungslinien ost- und westdeutscher Gesundheitspolitik zwischen doppelter Staatsgründung, deutscher Einigung und europäischer Integration. *Z Sozialreform*, **43**, 101–31.

Manow, P. (1994) *Gesundheitspolitik im Eingungsprozeß*. Campus Verlag, Frankfurt/ New York.

Nolte, E. (2002) The transformation of the East German health care system. Lessons for enlargement? *Eurohealth*, **8**, 42–4.

Nolte, E., Brand, A., Koupilova, I and McKee, M. (2000) Neonatal and postneonatal mortality in Germany since unification. *Journal of Epidemiology and Community Health*, **54**, 84–90.

Nolte, E., Shkolnikov, V. and McKee, M. (2000a) Changing mortality patterns in east and west Germany and Poland: I. Long-term trends (1960–1997). *Journal of Epidemiology and Community Health*, **54**, 890–8.

Nolte, E., Shkolnikov, V. and McKee, M. (2000b) Changing mortality patterns in east and west Germany and Poland: II. Short-term trends during transition and in the 1990s. *Journal of Epidemiology and Community Health*, **54**, 899–906.

Nolte, E., Scholz, R., Shkolnikov, V. and McKee, M. (2002c) The contribution of medical care to changing life expectancy in Germany and Poland. *Social Science and Medicine*, **55**, 1905–21.

Perleth, M., Mannebach, H., Busse, R., Gleichmann, U. and Schwartz, F. W. (1999) Cardiac catheterization in Germany. *Internation Journal of Technology Assessment in Health Care*, **15**, 756–66.

Richter, E. A. (2001) Vom Auslaufmodell zur Alternative. *Deutsches Ärzteblatt*, **98**, A2784–8.

Robischon, T., Stucke, A., Wasem, J. and Wolf, H.-G. (1994) Die politische Logik der deutschen Vereinigung un der Institutionentransfer: Eine Untersuchung am Beispiel von Gesundheitswesen, Forschungssystem und Telekommunikation. MPIFG Discussion Paper 94/3. Max Planck Institut für Gesellschaftsforschung, Köln.

Rose, R. and Haerpfer, C. (1997) The impact of a ready-made state: east Germans in comparative perspective. *German Politics*, **6**, 100–21.

Scharf, B. (1999) German unity and health care reform. In F. D. Powell and A. F. Wessen (eds) *Health care systems in transition – an international perspective*, pp. 101–12. Sage, Thousand Oaks, CA, London, New Delhi.

Schneider, M. (1999) *Gesundheitssysteme im internationalen Vergleich – Übersichten 1997*. BASYS, Augsburg.

Spitzer, S. G. (1999) Pacing and ICD therapy in Germany (west and east) before and after reunification in 1989. *Pace*, **22**, 1248–52.

Spree, H.-U. (1994) *Der Sozialstaat eint.* Nomos Verlagsgesellschaft, Baden-Baden.

Statistisches Bundesamt (1999) *Datenreport 1999 – Zahlen und Fakten über die Bundesrepublik Deutschland.* Bundeszentrale für politische Bildung, Bonn.

Statistisches Bundesamt (2001) Todesuvsadienstatistik. Statistisches Bundesamt, Wiesbaden.

Stone, D. A. (1994) German unification: East meets West in the doctor's office. *Journal of Health Politics and Policy Law,* **16,** 401–12.

Thamm, M. (1999) Blutdruck in Deutschland – Zustandsbeschreibung und Trends. *Gesundheitswesen,* **61** Suppl. 2, S90–3.

Thefeld, W. (1999) Prävalenz des Diabetes mellitus in der erwachsenen Bevölkerung Deutschlands. *Gesundheitswesen,* **61** Suppl. 2, S85–9.

Thieler, H., Achenbach, H., Bischoff, J., Koall, W., Kraatz, G., *et al.* (1994) Evolution of renal replacement therapy in East Germany from 1989 to 1992. *Nephrology Dialysis Transplantation,* **9,** 238–41.

Thieler, H., Kohler, I., Achenbach, H., Goetz, K. H., Kraatz, G., *et al.* (1995) Further advances of chronic renal replacement therapy in eastern Germany, 1994 versus 1989. *Clinical Nephrology,* **44,** 108–12.

Wasem, J. (1997a) Health care reform in the Federal Republic of Germany: the new and the old Länder. In C. Altenstetter and B. J. W (eds) *Health policy reform, national variations and globalization,* pp. 161–74. Macmillan, London.

Wasem, J. (1997b) *Vom staatlichen zum kassenärztlichen System: Eine Untersuchung des Transformationsprozesses der ambulanten ärztlichen Versorgung in Ostdeutschland.* Campus, Frankfurt.

Wildner, M., Markuzzi, A., Casper, W. and Bergmann, K. E. (1998) Disparitäten der Krankenhaus-Fatalität nach proximalen Femurfrakturen in der DDR 1989. *Soz Präventivmed,* **43,** 80–9.

Chapter 9

Overseas Citizens

Citoyens de France

Virginie Halley des Fontaines

Oh God! please forgive France
which indeed says where the right way is
and goes along oblique lines
Senghor 1945

In France, health and social welfare benefits are now officially available to all legal residents: it is not necessary to be a French citizen to claim them. This concept of legal residency represents a major change in the national health insurance system. Until 2000, social protection was linked to employment status rather than citizenship. Entitlement then shifted from participation in the labour market, although with state aid for the unemployed, to universal health cover is also covered for legal residents. It should, however, be noted that emergency care is also covered for illegal migrants, although their other needs are met by humanitarian organizations.

This chapter examines the situation of one group of residents of France, so-called 'overseas citizens'. These are French citizens who were born in the French overseas departments and thus are officially entitled to the full range of benefits of the French health care system.

As in many rich countries, France is undergoing several population shifts: from rural to urban areas, overseas departments and ex-colonies to metropolitan (continental) France, and from less developed countries to industrialized France. Many overseas citizens have moved to metropolitan France in recent years. They often have particular health needs reflecting their lack of resources and are also vulnerable to discrimination due to their place of birth or different ethnic or cultural background. However they are, to a considerable extent, officially invisible as few health and social statistics are gathered because since they are French citizens, and the collection of separate statistics on the basis of ethnicity is regarded as discriminatory. Further, since all legal residents of France are assumed to have equal access to universal health services, there are no attempts to offer types of health services that might reflect their particular needs. Notwithstanding these limitations, this chapter examines what is known about French health care policy in relation to its overseas citizens and their health status and access to health services.

A brief history of French health insurance

Social protection in seventeenth-century France was based on solidarity underpinned by religious values. Later, with industrialization from the end of the nineteenth century, charitable committees were established that evolved into mutual benefit societies for workers and their families. Organized social protection thus emerged in parallel with the rise of organized labour. When the French Social Security system was established formally in 1945 with universal access for the population, it was based on a patchwork of mutual societies, each seeking to retain its autonomous status. Funded mainly by employer and employee contributions, the insurance funds were managed jointly by employers and employees under Social Security supervision (and recently under Parliamentary supervision). By the late 1990s, public insurance accounted for 75 per cent of total health expenditure in France and private health insurance and out-of-pocket payments made up the remainder. In 1992, people on a low-income were paying more of their income for health costs, 16 per cent compared to 8 per cent for the population as a whole (Couffinhal 2000). Financial barriers to access to health care by the poor prompted reform of health insurance; for example, it was estimated that 14 per cent of poorer patients could not afford the necessary out-of-pocket payments and were often obliged to postpone seeking care (Bocognano *et al.* 2000). Subsequently, a policy of equitable access for all was introduced from January 2000 with the implementation of *Couverture Maladie Universelle* (CMU) or Universal Health Coverage (Boisguérin *et al.* 2001–2002). This compulsory national health insurance system, funded by a tax on income (above a certain amount) rather than through wage contributions, established the following principle: all residents of France should be reimbursed for health expenditure by one of the health insurance schemes. This regulation is a major departure from the earlier eligibility principle as it stresses residency rather than employment: health care is available to anyone living legally in France for more than three months. However, in practice, while legal status and residency are the main criteria, the long-established link between social insurance and employment continues to shape how people view health care claims.

In theory, the French social coverage system is now virtually universal. It covers foreigners and even illegal migrants if their health needs are urgent or cannot be treated in their own country, children whose foreign-born parents have no social insurance, and any person living officially with an insured person. In reality, those living illegally in any country find it difficult to deal with social institutions and public services. But the principle of equal access has been established in France, leading to a new concept that some commentators have described as 'social citizenship' (Fassin *et al.* 2001; Fassin and Gilloire 2000).

Post-colonial France: rich and guilty?

Is the French health system more generous than in other industrialized countries? Are French people eager to share the benefits of their national health service? Some of France's neighbours suggest that the nation feels a sense of guilt stemming from its colonial past, and so compensates by its stand against discrimination and xenophobia with humanitarian aid as a guiding principle. One way to explore these arguments is to look at the health status and health care services of French citizens in France's overseas regions and territories (four departments and their corresponding four regions), the Départements d'Outre Mer and Territoires d'Outre Mer (DOM-TOM), which are subject to the same laws and administrative constraints as the 'Metropole', that is, continental France (with its 106 departments and 22 regions).

In 1995, the Guadeloupe islands (including Saint Barthelemy and Saint Martin in the northern Caribbean) had an estimated population of 403,000, Martinique had 395,000, French Guyana in north-east South America had 145,000, and la Réunion, east of Madagascar in the Indian Ocean, had 666,000 inhabitants, a total of 1.7 million people in the four overseas departments.

In contrast, in 2001, there were 59 million inhabitants in continental France. The overseas citizens of France are extremely heterogeneous, of different ethnic backgrounds, belong to various cultures, some live in poor social conditions, and many want to migrate to continental France in order to earn a living.

Is there a difference between migrants who have a French passport, and others who do not, in terms of accessibility to health services? Is the quality of care in the French overseas territories the same as in continental France? The official response is that there is no point in asking this question: there should be no difference and there is no difference. The purpose of this chapter, however, is to explore whether the possession of a national identification card influences access to health care.

Citizenship and health

The first question to ask is whether lack of citizenship denies the right to health care? According to French regulations the answer is definitely 'no'.

A non-citizen or a low-income foreigner living in France for a minimum of three months is entitled to free access to the public hospital system and, if living in France for at least three years, to free access to any outpatient service, the bill being paid by the State. In reality, problems arise when officials are unfamiliar with the regulations or when some adopt discriminatory or inappropriate attitudes (Gisti 2001). Voluntary organizations specializing in the rights of immigrants suggest that discriminatory treatment often results from language barriers and lack of cultural awareness.

A second question is whether a 'new' French citizen has the same equal access to health care as an 'old' citizen? While a right to care might exist, the answer cannot be an unqualified 'yes'. One must take into account the extent to which the health problem is recognized by the individual and the level of understanding of the medical and administrative system. There is also scope for discriminatory attitudes, for instance, some physicians may be less likely to offer certain treatments to patients because of ethnic origin.

The third question is whether overseas French citizens suffer from discriminatory attitudes because of ethnic considerations? This question, as formulated, is taboo in all French departments, and perhaps especially in overseas French departments. It can only be answered by tracking the progress of an individual through the system, in order to explore whether there are differences in health needs and in access to and use of health services.

The health of French overseas citizens

Two decades ago, health data on overseas French regions were difficult to obtain, but since 1995, thanks to regulations that accompanied decentralization, regional health authorities are required to provide statistics on patterns of diseases. So far, however, only nine out of the 22 regions of France have fulfilled these requirements, including only one overseas region: French Guyana. The epidemiological services (Ministère de la Santé 2000) in French Guyana and the Caribbean islands of Guadeloupe and Martinique also collect data on infectious diseases by virtue of their membership in the Pan-American Health Organization (PAHO), which regularly reports on malaria, dengue fever, yellow fever and tuberculosis.

In practice, the epidemiological services have been unable to collect comprehensive data. Although local professionals confirm the serious scale of tropical diseases, these are not well recorded in official statistics. Surveillance and disease prevention activities are hampered by lack of funding and weak enforcement. Some specific problems have attracted research, however, such as the health impacts of volcanic gas in Guadeloupe and methyl mercury poisoning amongst French Guyana gold-washers (Cordier and Garel 1999; Fréry et al.

Table 9.1 Economic indicators by region in Euros

	Guadeloupe	Martinique	Guyana	la Réunion	Metropole
GNP per capita, 1995* thousands (a)	10.48	11.98	11.67	9.80	20.54
Income per family unit, 1995 thousands*	18.44	22.84	25.91	17.53	25.45
Total social security contributions, millions, 1993†	499.423	521.376	172.420	884.357	
Transfers from Metropole, 1993†	408.868	438.596	30.1849	894.86	

Source: adapted from * DREES. Directorate of Research, Analysis, Evaluation and Statistics (2001); † INSEE National Institute for Economical Studies (1993).

1999). The Guyana study, which took place in a remote area, also documented the lack of birth records and pre-natal care, and documented widespread threats to health, including malaria, alcoholism and poor health care, as well as methyl mercury poisoning which affects children's neurological development.

In 2001, following a World Health Organization commitment to report on the health status of populations in South America and the Caribbean islands, data were collected in four overseas regions (including la Réunion Island in the Indian Ocean). The study (Bazely and Catteau 2001) noted that these regions are officially part of France and that people are entitled to the same administrative and political benefits, including family allowances, minimum income regulations and housing benefits. Low income from employment is only partially compensated for by social transfers from continental France (Table 9.1).

The French Annual National Report on Public Health (2002) compares health indicators in overseas territories with continental France (Metropole) in a special chapter dealing with inequalities. Although life expectancy at birth for men and women in these four overseas territories has increased (Figure 9.1), it was still slightly lower for men (74.2 years in Metropole except Martinique with 74.9 years), and also for women (82.1 years in Metropole but only 78.7 in French Guyana). Infant mortality has improved markedly since the 1960s although it remains higher in the overseas regions (Figure 9.2), as has perinatal mortality (deaths the first few weeks of life). In 1998, infant mortality per 1000 live births was 10.9 in Guyana, 10.1 in Guadeloupe, 8.6 in Martinique and 8.2 in Réunion compared to 4.6 in Metropolitan France. This higher mortality is thought to be, in part, because of higher levels of premature births and low weight babies in the overseas regions than in continental France (Table 9.2).

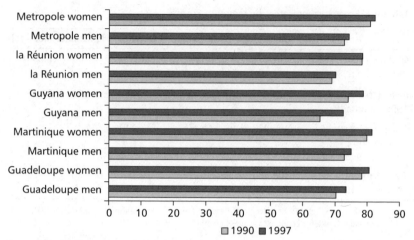

Figure 9.1 Life expectancy in DOMs and Metropolitan France, 1990 and 1997.
Source: adapted from Directorate of Research, Analysis, Evaluation and Statistics (DREES).

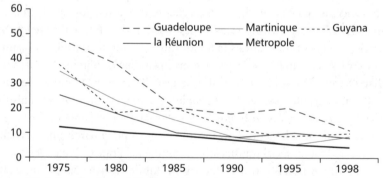

Figure 9.2 Infant deaths in DOM and Metropole (rate per 1000 live births).
Source: adapted from National Institute for Statistics and Economics Studies (INSEE).

Table 9.2 Premature births and low weight births per 1000 live births, 1998

	Guadeloupe	Martinique	Guyana	Réunion	Metropole
Premature birth (< 37 weeks)	11.4	10.3	14.0	10.2	6.8
Low weight at birth (< 2500 g)	11.4	11.1	13.7	10.7	7.2

Source: adapted from DREES, Directorate of Research, Analysis, Evaluation and Statistics, *National Perinatal Survey* 1998.

Potentially adverse social factors also appear more common in the overseas departments, as indicated by a range of measures. Single motherhood is more common, accounting for 40 per cent of pregnant women in Martinique and 28 per cent in Guyana, compared to only 7 per cent in continental France. Over 5 per cent of pregnancies in La Réunion were among adolescents compared to less than 1 per cent in continental France (DREES 2001). There are high levels of alcoholism and drug abuse, while liver cirrhosis is the fourth most common cause of death for women, and traffic injuries are responsible for a large amount of disability.

The immunization programme in the overseas regions is officially the same as in continental France, except for yellow fever campaigns in exposed areas such as Guyana. In 1991 and 1999, immunization coverage in Guyana was assessed. The main differences were between coastal zones and inland areas of Guyana, where very low figures were recorded for BCG and measles immunization – around 50 per cent to 30 per cent for pertussis and less than 10 per cent for yellow fever immunization (Chaud 2000). Despite extensive 'catch-up' campaigns in primary schools, immunization programmes remain largely unsuccessful in places where population density is low and French is not widely spoken.

In summarizing the tuberculosis (TB) surveillance programme, the French national surveillance agency (INVS) identifies the main risk factors for TB as poor social and economic conditions. TB incidence rates are higher in the overseas departments than continental France, particularly in Guyana, where they increased by 39 per cent between 1997 and 2000 (Table 9.3). The high figures in Guyana, however, are also partly attributed to better reporting.

The incidence of TB in continental France is much higher among people of foreign nationality than French nationality (Table 9.4), and mostly is

Table 9.3 Incidence rate per 100,000 persons, tuberculosis and HIV

	Guadeloupe	Martinique	Guyana	Réunion	Ile de France, Paris	France
TB 1993	7.2	10.6	68.8	21.5	–	
TB 1997	5.1	5.6	14.7	13.5	–	
TB 2000	3.6	2.9	39.4	12.3	–	
Average annual change 1997–2000	−12%	−20%	+39%	−3%	–	
HIV 1999	8.28	7.34	44.53	3.11	6.53	2.99

Source: adapted from *Weekly Health Report*, Number16–17/2002.

Table 9.4 Tuberculosis incidence rate per 100,000 persons, continental France, 1997–2000

	French nationality				Foreign nationality			
	1997		2000		1997		2000	
n	Incidence $/10^5$	n	Incidence $/10^5$	n	Incidence $/10^5$	n	Incidence $/10^5$
Total	4291	8.1	3778	6.8	1584	44.2	1728	53.0

Source: adapted from *Weekly Health Report* no16–17/2002.

attributed to lack of control at the European Union frontier. Place of birth is a better indicator than nationality in assessing the endemic source (Decludt 2000). The TB incidence rate is 7 per 100,000 for patients born in France, 32 for patients born in North Africa and 125 for patients born in sub-Saharan Africa. Young African adults have a very high TB incidence rate of over 170 per 100,000.

The HIV incidence rate varies considerably across France, with high rates in some areas of Paris such as the Ile de France, and high rates in some overseas regions and particularly in Guyana (Table 9.3). Decludt has advocated anonymous registration as a means of strengthening the surveillance system, with compulsory treatment to reduce the risks of transmission (Decludt 2000).

Overseas citizens in Metropolitan France

Since the 1960s, there has been large-scale migration from the French overseas territories to continental France. From its origins in a search for employment, migration from the overseas departments has become an ongoing process of resettlement. About 25 per cent of the French Caribbean population now lives in continental France, that is, about 98,000 families, most of them in Ile-de-France, the area around Paris, which is often called the 'fifth DOM'. There are more inhabitants from Guadeloupe in continental France than on the island itself. These families are often headed by a single mother living in social housing in the suburbs, most of whom have regular jobs, often within the public sector and mainly in health services. Educational attainment is low and many children experience racial discrimination (as do migrant children from Africa) with high levels (27 per cent) of youth unemployment compared to 'only' 16 per cent among other young French people (Marie 2002).

According to a famous Caribbean author, Aimé Cesaire, an army officer in Fort-de-France in Martinique, spoke of his 'compatriots' as these 'strange foreigners'. Overseas citizens report many examples of inappropriate treatment on grounds of ethnicity, and have experienced considerable social exclusion, although their widely held views have not been verified objectively. As noted earlier, since these are French citizens, equal treatment is assumed, while statistics are not kept on ethnicity since this is regarded as discriminatory.

A recent 600-page review by the National Observatory for Poverty and Social Exclusion provided extensive data on poverty and access to social benefits across France. But there is no specific mention of overseas citizens, and the report does not include data from overseas departments even though this is, in theory, available. At present, it is simply not possible to collect data on overseas citizens who live in continental France, since this would require permission from the National Commission for Individual Liberties (CNIL). Furthermore, it is not possible to link personal data across databases. Thus there is little research on the health needs of overseas citizens apart from some attempts to collect data on place of birth in specific epidemiological surveys.

Equal access to health services

French citizens have a right to equal treatment, which means that access to health care should reflect health needs. The concept of a basic package of health services, while discussed in France, has received little support, given adherence to the principles of equality and universality. Health priorities are decided at a local level but within a framework of national guidelines, while national funding allocations are intended to reduce regional disparities.

The *ODR*, the local newspaper in La Réunion, reported on 17 January 2001 that people of the island are spending more money on health care, which appears to be taken as a positive health development indicator. This view does not take into account whether people may be sicker than previously or are using more health services since the introduction of universal health insurance.

Turning to health care resources in overseas departments, the supply of acute hospital beds is higher in Martinique (2.7) than in continental France (2.2) but lower in other overseas departments (Table 9.5), while numbers of surgical beds are very low. The National Social Insurance system reported a 5 per cent drop in hospitalization days in overseas hospitals in 1996/1997 but no drop in continental France. Since no official explanation is given, one can only speculate that the drop may be due to lack of resources, lack of trust in local health care services, or perhaps people seeking more advanced health care in continental France. Overseas departments have fewer physicians, both general practitioners (half as many in Guyana) and specialists, than continental France (Table 9.5).

In the French welfare system, social income helps compensate for low wages, including maternity leave, child allowances and social security benefits, plus

Table 9.5 Health care resources and utilization by region

	Guadeloupe	Martinique	Guyana	Réunion	France
Acute hospital beds per 1000 persons, 2000 (a)	2.1	2.7	1.9	1.4	2.2
GPs per 1000 persons, 2000 (b)	1.8	1.9	1.4	2.2	2.8
Specialists per 1000 persons, 2000 (a)	1.4	1.4	0.9	1.4	2.6
Hospital medical and surgical admissions per 100 persons (1993) and extra care in continental France (estimation) (a)	17.4 +3.8%	15.44 +2.1%	14.27 +8.2%	17.22 +0.9%	20.3
Social allowances 1993, Euros (c) (d)	369.698	405.972	86.7435	623.821	
Health allowances 1993, Euros (c) (d)	499.575	511.162	111.288	953.721	

Sources: adapted from (a) DREES. Directorate of Research, Analysis, Evaluation and Statistics. (b) WHO Health For All Database; (c) CNAM. National Medical Insurance Services. (d) INSEE. National Institute for Statistics and Economics Studies.

health allowances for the unemployed (Table 9.5). In the overseas departments, social workers are important officials, either well regarded or feared, because they control the discretionary social welfare and health allowances. In some places the social benefits have a pejorative image of 'easy money'. Over the last decade social expenditure has increased five times in Guyana compared with less than twice in continental France, but these figures should be interpreted with caution as we do not have precise information on the levels of social and health needs.

In the decade prior to the 2000 implementation of national health insurance (CMU), those who could afford to purchase private health insurance did so in order to reduce their out-of-pocket payments for expensive items, such as dental prostheses or glasses prescriptions. These items are expensive and public insurance covered no more than one-third of the cost (Bocognano *et al.* 2000). Although the new insurance system (CMU) is meant to be universal, it is not yet clear whether the new regulations have been applied equally to all residents of France, since private complementary insurance reimbursements remain high (Gremy and Brixi 2002).

The principle of national solidarity aims to reduce disparities, but poverty levels are higher in the overseas departments than in continental France partly because there are larger families: families have 39 per cent more children in Guyana and 18 per cent more in Martinique. Large families are often regarded as poor families, which sometimes prompts discriminatory attitudes when these families are accused of having more children in order to increase their social benefits.

In contrast to these various poor social indicators, the overseas departments scored quite well in 1995 on the Human Development Index (a measure that adds life expectancy, adult literacy and cost-adjusted per capita income), and were only just below the national figure. France is among the highest-scoring countries, ranking number 13 in the world in 1999 (United Nations Development Programme 2001).

Are overseas citizens hidden victims of discrimination?

There is no research to confirm or refute this question other than claims from advocacy groups, since little is known about inequalities in access to health services or the extent of racial discrimination. Poor health status among overseas citizens may be explained by poor economic conditions, as in the general population. The distribution of health facilities is determined by historical, political and economic factors. Since the implementation of political decentralization there have been further developments in health services in all the overseas departments. Specific research is undertaken when necessary, and measures are implemented, such as screening for sickle cell disease or measures to prevent dengue fever in the Caribbean islands. Yet despite such initiatives, NGOs often accuse health professionals of being blind to instances of discrimination and to their own discriminatory practices.

How is it possible to help French citizens appreciate the extent of exclusion suffered by overseas citizens, new citizens and second-generation citizens? The long and often painful progression towards cultural mixing often fails to promote assimilation and instead stresses social differences. These differences are multiplied endlessly in health-related circumstances. The way that health professionals analyse specific health problems and disease states leads to intricate biological categorizations rather than to an appreciation of the total health status of an individual or group of people.

In the French tradition, which emphasizes a respect for human rights and equality of treatment, comments about social and health inequities between groups are not well received, because these are considered sensitive issues. Thus little is known about the health of the different immigrant groups. Few studies explore the adverse effects that racism and experiences of discriminatory attitudes may have upon an individual's health. In its national report (Haut Comité de la Santé Publique 2002) the Public Health National Committee argued that such taboos, which prevent debate, help to maintain prejudicial attitudes and are, in the long run, against the interests of the general population. The report goes on to argue that positive discrimination is a political choice which should be considered in order to compensate for disadvantages, disabilities and vulnerabilities.

Ambivalent feelings and persistent contradictions

Citizenship does not emerge merely from the adoption of a nationality. It is a long process, which includes nostalgia for and the idealization of a lost paradise, the dream of return to a place that has remained unchanged, a willingness to pass on traditional cultural practices, together with strong incentives to integrate new practices. The literature on migration emphasizes lifestyle differences, alienation from emotional ties, and more simply the difficulties of adjusting to a different climate as major factors in the loss of one's own identity. A person's new nationality is manifest in an Identity Number, which opens the door to the administrative offices of the Metropole. Once this number is obtained, the migration process is legally concluded. It becomes illegitimate to make a complaint.

For many years overseas citizens have internalized their resentment about the legacy of slavery. But each new piece of legislation raises social questions about exclusion and discrimination and offers an opportunity to bring these resentments among uncertain citizens into the open. France has been active recently in passing new laws, such as the July 1998 Law against Social Exclusion, the March 2000 Law for Health in a Democracy, and the March 2002 Law against Social Discrimination. In this context, changes in the relationships between France's continental and overseas citizens might be expected. Before the 2002 presidential election in France, the Government addressed the issue of overseas professionals working in Paris hospitals. The fifty hospitals in Paris belong to Assistance Publique – Hôpitaux de Paris, the largest employer in France, in which overseas citizens constitute 15 per cent of the employees. State Secretary Paul recalled in his talk the slavery and social discrimination of the past that had tainted the image of the French Republic. Quoting Franz Fanon, an anti-colonial medical doctor from Martinique, he proposed an 'optimistic choice' where citizens born overseas will represent a durable dimension of life in Metropolitan France.

References

Bazely, P. and Catteau, C. (2001) *Document de travail: Etat de santé, offre de soins dans les départements d'Outre-Mer: Guadeloupe, Guyane, Martinique, la Réunion.* DREES, Ministère de la Santé, Paris.

Bocognano, A., Couffinhal, A., Dumesnil, S. and Grignon, M. (2000) *In supplementary health insurance: who benefits from which reimbursements?* Résultats de l'enquête Santé Protection Sociale 1998, Rapport n° 1317. CREDES, Paris.

Boisguérin, B., Casès, C. and Gissot, C. (2001–2002) *La couverture maladie universelle: synthèse des résultats disponibles. Les travaux de l'Observatoire national de la pauvreté et de l'exclusion.* La Documentation Française, Paris.

Chaud, P. (2000) *La couverture vaccinale en Guyane.* Institut de Veille Sanitaire, Ministère de la Santé, Conseil Général de la Guyane, Paris.

Cordier, S. and Garel, M. (1999) *Risques neurotoxiques chez l'enfant liés à l'exposition au méthylmercure en Guyana française.* Institut de Veille Sanitaire, INSERM, Saint-Maurice.

Couffinhal, A. (2000) *The French health care system: a brief overview.* Report 1317. CREDES, Paris.

Decludt, B. (2000) Les cas de tuberculose déclarés en 2000. *BEH*, **16/17**, 68–70.

DREES (2001) *Document de travail: programme d'études et de statistiques des services déconcentrés.* DREES, Ministère de la Santé, Paris.

Fassin, D., Carde, E., Ferre, N. and Musso-Dimitrijevic, S. (2001) *Un traitement inégal. Les discriminations dans l'accès aux soins.* Rapport d'étude n°5. CRESP, Bobigny.

Fassin, D. and Gilloire, A. (2000) Santé, le traitement de la différence. Repenser les enjeux de santé autour de l'immigration. *Hommes et Migrations*, **1225**, 5–12.

Fréry, N., Maillot, E. and Deheeger, M. (1999) *Exposition au mercure de la population amérindienne Wayana de Guyane: enquête alimentaire.* Institut de Veille Sanitaire, Saint-Maurice.

Gisti (2001) *La situation juridique des etrangers dans les DOM.* Le Groupe d'information et de soutien des immigres, Paris.

Gremy, F. and Brixi, O. (2002) *Questionnement et propositions sur la politique de santé en France.* Société Française de Santé Publique, Nancy.

Haut Comité de la Santé Publique (2002) *La Santé en France.* Haut Comite de la Santé Publique,

Marie, C. V. (2002) Les Antillais en France, une nouvelle donne, diasporas caraïbéennes. *Hommes et Migrations*, **1237**, 26–39.

Ministère de la Santé (2000) *CIRE Annual report 2000.* Institute de Veille Sanitaire, Saint Maurice.

Senghor, L. S. (1945) *Prayer for peace, for Georges and Claude Pompidou.* Written in French and freely adapted by V. H. des Fontaines.

United Nations Development Programme (2001) *Human development report 2001: making new technologies work for human development.* Oxford University Press, Oxford.

Chapter 10

Migrants

Universal health services in Sweden

Solvig Ekblad

A multicultural challenge to a universal health service

Sweden, a monarchy in northern Europe with a parliamentary form of government, until recently had a relatively homogenous population, so the country has only just begun to confront the challenges of multiculturalism. Does the universal, high quality health care system in Sweden meet the needs of minority groups? Sweden's health care policy states that sub-populations such as ethnic groups should have equitable access to health care. Yet although equity is a key objective of the World Health Organization, Europe has made little progress towards equity in health over past decades (Bollini and Siem 1995; World Health Organization 1993). Although this chapter will consider the shortcomings of the Swedish health care system in relation to immigrant groups, its strong public health sector has produced more comprehensive mental health services for refugees than many other European countries (van Willigen 1992).

We will explore the difficulties experienced by asylum seekers and refugees in accessing and using Swedish health services, in particular, mental health services. The chapter summarizes the history of immigration to Sweden, the current health care system and related immigration policies, reviews the literature on the health needs of immigrants, then presents a theoretical framework for considering health care delivery. The chapter concludes that access mostly depends on being an official resident, that mainstream services seldom understand and respond to cultural differences among 'outsiders', and that more special interventions are required.

Waves of refugees

Sweden, with a relatively small population of nearly nine million people in 2002, of whom 84 per cent live in urban areas, remained rural and ethnically homogenous until the 1940s (except for Sami, Finns and Roma). A new phase in Sweden's immigration history occurred with the influx of Baltic and other refugees, during and after the Second World War, involving more than 200,000 people from neighbouring countries, including concentration camp survivors.

The concept 'migration' means the resettlement of people within countries or between countries and thus encompasses both movement from (emigration) and movement to (immigration) a country. (When Vilhelm Moberg wrote his famous trilogy about Karl Oskar and Kristina from Duvemåla, who settled in the United States, he called the first two books *The emigrants* (Moberg 1951) and *Unto a good land* (Moberg 1957).) 'Ethnicity' is a complex concept and is defined here as country of origin, i.e. country of birth. Although this definition has obvious limitations, it does provide some useful information concerning different ethnic groups in Sweden.

During the industrial boom of the 1950s and 1960s, the Swedish government recruited labourers from Yugoslavia, Italy, Greece, Turkey and Finland. In 1967, the government introduced immigration controls, except for residents from other Nordic countries, by restricting immigration to certain categories of labour. New waves of immigrants during the 1970s, mainly refugees and relatives of earlier immigrants, came from Latin America in the 1970s, from Eastern Africa and the Middle East in the 1980s, and during the 1990s were mainly refugees from the Balkan wars. Sweden has received a large number of refugees from the former Yugoslavia (among the highest proportion per population of any country). Despite Sweden's humanitarian policy of accepting refugees, the economic recession during the 1990s and reservations by the Swedish-born population mean that conditions for immigrants and refugees are not always welcoming.

Immigrants are a growing and heterogeneous group, having risen from 6.7 per cent of the total population of Sweden in 1970 to about 12 per cent in 2001. The latter figure is based on a narrow definition (born abroad) but rises to 20 per cent if we use a broader definition (having at least one parent born abroad). About one-third come from Nordic countries (mostly Finland), one-third from other parts of Europe and one-third from outside Europe, with the largest number of recent asylum seekers coming from Iraq.

Health care system in Sweden

Sweden has a comprehensive and universal public sector health care system, mainly funded and run by the 21 counties, and covering all official residents. Thus health services for resident immigrants are seen as the responsibility of the counties. This section presents a summary of Sweden's health care system (for a more detailed overview see Hjortsberg and Ghatnekar 2001) in order to put access issues for immigrants in context.

The Swedish health care system covers all official residents regardless of nationality. The county councils run most public sector health care, becoming responsible for hospital care in the 1880s and for various non-hospital services from the 1930s. The 1946 National Health Insurance Act took the first step towards universal cover for physician consultations, prescription drugs, and sickness compensation. Thereafter, the Swedish health care sector has expanded with county councils given responsibility for health care planning in the 1980s. Total expenditure on health in 1998 amounted to 7.9 per cent of GDP, slightly less than the EU average of 8.4 per cent (World Health Organization 2001). Sweden has a mainly tax-based universal health care system supplemented by national health insurance and private payments (the latter represented 16.2 per cent of total health care expenditure in 1999). Health services mostly are county-based and financed by county taxes, which accounted for almost 70 per cent of total public health care expenditure in 1999. The social insurance system, managed by the National Social Insurance Board, covers individual income losses due to illness and also pays about one-fifth of health care costs, with a significant contribution coming from the state. Central government also contributes directly to health financing (some 10 per cent of total health care expenditure), redistributing funds among regional and local governments through earmarked and general grants.

The health care system is organized on three levels. At the national level, the central government retains responsibility for policy development, legislation and supervision through the Ministry of Health and Social Affairs. The National Board of Health and Welfare (Socialstyrelsen) acts as the government's advisory and supervisory agency for health and social services, and there is a large array of other national-level bodies.

At the regional level, the 21 county councils provide comprehensive health services from primary care to hospital care, including public health and preventive care, and also regulate the private health care market. The county councils are divided into health care districts, which normally consist of one hospital and several primary health care units. The county councils are also grouped into six medical care regions to facilitate cooperation in tertiary care.

At the local level, municipalities are responsible for social welfare, which includes child care, school health services, services for long-term psychiatric patients, community care for dependent people, and from 1992 residential care for the elderly. For example, Stockholm has several care nursing homes for elderly immigrant groups.

Patient co-payments have increased and in 1999 represented 2 per cent of total public expenditure. Each county council determines its own fee schedule for out-of-pocket payments for ambulatory care, although the national parliament has set fee ceilings on the total amount any citizen pays in a 12-month period (currently €99). The public paid 23 per cent of total expenditure for prescribed drugs in 1999, adults make co-payments for dental care, and for inpatient care (€8.5 per day, with reductions for pensioners and low income groups and no charges for children under the age of 18).

An essential health care package has not been defined but there are three stated priority principles – human rights, need or solidarity, and cost-effectiveness.

Refugees

Sweden, like most European countries, applies the principle of first asylum country agreed at the Dublin Convention between European Union member states. In 1997, the Swedish law concerning aliens was changed to widen the concept of a refugee in line with the Geneva Convention. Refugees are persons who legitimately fear persecution due to their race, their nationality, their membership of a particular social group, or their religious or political beliefs. Other categories also may be granted sanctuary in Sweden, including persons who have left their country of origin for fear of the death penalty, torture or inhuman or degrading treatment of some other kind, external or internal armed conflict, an environmental disaster or persecution due to their gender or homosexuality.

According to statistics from the Migration Board, 23,515 asylum seekers applied for permission to stay in Sweden during 2001 and with a 40 per cent increase in 2002, to 33,016 (www.migrationsverket.se). During 2001, 44,505 persons were granted residence permits on various grounds: family ties (56 per cent), refugees (17 per cent), European Union member (15 per cent), guest students (9 per cent), adopted children (2 per cent) and for labour market reasons (1 per cent). Most of the successful 7941 asylum seekers in 2001 were decided on humanitarian grounds (72 per cent), followed by quota refugees (14 per cent), others in need of protection (10 per cent) and other refugees.

Immigrants are not spread evenly throughout the country but are geo-graphically concentrated in urban areas, so that immigrant health issues are more relevant to some county governments than others. In 2001 in Stockholm County, 329,100 residents were foreign-born (19.4 per cent of the popula-tion), and of these about 20 per cent were born in Finland, while among more recent immigrants, 5.8 per cent came from Iraq, 5.5 per cent from Iran and 5.2 per cent from Turkey (www.rtk.sll.se).

When asylum seekers are granted a residence permit in Sweden, they are entered in the civic registry and given a national registration number, which means they have the same rights and obligations as all other inhabitants.

Swedish immigrant policy since 1975 has been based on three principles: equality (providing immigrants with the same standard of living as Swedes); freedom of choice (giving members of ethnic minorities the opportunity to retain their cultural identity or adopt Swedish cultural identity); and partnership (promoting working together).

In 1997, the Integration Office published guidelines on how municipalities should assist the integration of refugees using individualized introduction plans. Their purpose is to provide the individual with the prerequisites needed to be economically independent and to become part of Swedish society. This and later documents state that any health problems experienced by newly-arrived adults or children should be identified and attended to through health care and/or social provisions (www.integrationsverket.se, May 2002).

Generally speaking, mainstream county services (that is, those provided for the general population) are responsible for providing services to immigrants, with no separate health services established (except some trauma services, as explained later), but with some special funding for asylum seekers not registered as residents, as explained below.

Asylum seekers are not registered as residents

Where asylum-seekers and other foreign citizens are not registered as residents of Sweden, county councils (or the equivalent) have only a limited obligation to provide health care (Allmänna råd från Socialstyrelsen 1995; Ekblad 2003). There is no charge for maternity care, preventive child and mother care, and care under the Swedish Communicable Diseases Act. If an adult is taken ill while waiting for registration he or she is entitled to free emergency medical care and dental care. Asylum-seekers lacking money may be granted a daily allowance by the Migration Board (for details, see www.migrationsverket.se). For other treatment, they must pay a fee of €5.4, and the same amount for medicine on prescription. They may obtain one medical examination free of charge for which the county council is subsidized by central government, as well as for interpreting, medical devices, patient transportations or travel to obtain medical care, and for special high-cost care. However, a government study of 100 refugee medical records found that only nine mentioned that a health examination had been performed (National Board of Health and Welfare 2000).

When considering children's applications, the Migration Board takes into account the UN Convention on the Rights of the Child and the Swedish Aliens Act on the best interests of the child. Asylum-seeking and 'hidden' children are entitled to health care in the same way as other children in Swedish society.

County councils receive a government grant so that they may give children the care they need to ensure their physical and mental well-being, including a medical examination before they start day care, preschool or school.

Special mental health services

Kirmayer and Minas (2000) have summarized some salient differences in cultural psychiatry and mental health services in several countries (including Sweden), which they argue reflect a country's history of migration and models of citizenship. Sweden has developed mental health services for this target group in several parts of the country.

Stockholm has a Red Cross Centre for tortured refugees with branches in several other cities. The Stockholm Centre has three eligibility criteria: to have been subject to torture (physical or mental), to have a residence permit in Sweden, and to live in the Stockholm County Council area (www.redcros.se/rkcstockholm). Stockholm also has another centre for tortured and war-wounded refugees (Kris-och Traumacentrum, Danderyds hospital). Throughout Sweden, there are eight psychiatric clinics for refugees with permission to stay and six special clinics for refugee children and adults. However, the lack of trained staff and money make it difficult to offer sufficient and appropriate services, as this chapter goes on to discuss. Stockholm County Council has, however, funded a Transcultural Centre (www.vsso.sll.se/tc) to conduct clinical consultations and training programmes to improve the quality and accessibility of mental health services for the immigrant and refugee population.

Literature review of research on refugees

There are many research gaps on war-related trauma and health, especially mental health, despite a significant increase in morbidity among affected populations, and despite the World Health Organization's (1948) definition of health: 'Health is a state of complete physical, mental and social well-being and not merely the absence of disease or infirmity', i.e. it gave somatic, psychological and social factors equal importance.

Early prevention is important in identifying refugees in need of special health and social services as well as in identifying those who have good coping resources (Roth and Ekblad 1993). Data about refugee trauma and health status are not always easy to interpret due to differences in methods of collection and analysis, methodological difficulties (e.g. cultural and translation differences), and inadequate resources. Better knowledge is needed in order to plan health care in a multicultural society.

International literature on refugee health

Two consistent risk factors have emerged from the cumulative international research on the determinants of mental disorder in refugees: past trauma (torture) and post-migration stress (Silove and Ekblad 2002). Today, many refugees and immigrants are faced by discrimination and hostility that is fuelled by fears of global terrorism. Other post-migration stresses include administrative obstacles to receiving health care and to achieving family reunion.

Refugees may experience multiple symptoms of post-traumatic stress and depression, such as grief, dissociation, anxiety, anger and hostility, and drug and alcohol abuse. Unexplained somatic symptoms not linked to specific medical conditions also are associated with low acculturation, high treatment seeking, psychiatric disorders, and self-identified medical problems. In addition to psychiatric morbidity, refugees have a high prevalence of dental, nutritional, infectious and paediatric illness, and have higher self-rated impairment and disability than the general population. Refugees and other traumatized populations have increased morbidity, decreased life expectancy, vulnerability to medical illness, and poor health habits (for a review see Hollifield *et al.* 2002).

Swedish literature on immigrant physical health

A national report on population health during the 1990s noted that the long-standing upward trend in health improvement among the Swedish population has been broken (National Board of Health and Welfare 1998a). Some groups who exhibited worse health than the general population in the 1980s, especially young people, single parents, the long-term sick and some immigrant groups, have experienced further deterioration during the 1990s. In deprived areas of Swedish cities, women's health has deteriorated since the middle of the 1980s, partly due to the concentration of newly arrived immigrants. Many social and health indicators are worse in large cities than in less densely populated areas, and immigrants are less healthy on most measures than the Swedish-born population.

A study of living conditions and health compared immigrant groups from Chile, Iran, Poland and Turkey with native-born Swedes (National Board of Health and Welfare 1998b). In an individual interview sample based on Statistic Sweden's survey of living conditions, personal interviews were conducted with 1980 persons, who were in the age range 20–44 on arrival in Sweden. The study showed large differences between the health of immigrant groups and the native-born population. The immigrant groups generally perceived their health as poor compared to native-born Swedes, and women from Chile and Turkey, and men and women from Iran, compared to native-born

Swedes, perceived more symptoms of mental illness. This result is confirmed by a study (Kjellin *et al.* 1992) of refugee women in Västerås, where their health had deteriorated after six years in Sweden, particularly with regard to somatic and/or psychosomatic symptoms.

Morbidity among foreign-born people is higher than among native-born Swedes, regardless of whether it is measured as number of sick-days, an early retirement pension, long-term illness, or self-reported health. The suicide rate among immigrants and refugees also is higher compared to Swedes (Bayard-Burfield 1999; Ferrada-Noli 1996; Johansson 1997). As immigrants are over-represented among manual professionals and the unemployed, these results may partly be explained by differences in working environment and socio-economic status, especially since clinical experience and research findings indicate that employment and other meaningful activities are essential factors for the quality of life of anyone, not least resettled refugees.

A government report showed that in the mid-1990s immigrants from non-European countries were over-represented regarding work accidents and injuries related to violence and threats (National Board of Health and Welfare 1997). The previously cited National Board of Health and Welfare study of four immigrants groups showed that one-fifth of adults from Chile, Iran and Turkey felt anxious for themselves or for relatives and felt exposed to threats and violence due to their ethnic or religious backgrounds (National Board of Health and Welfare 1998b).

When looking at specific health conditions, however, there is only patchy information, with differences between immigrant groups as well as between immigrants and the Swedish-born population. Sundquist and Johansson (1997) showed that Finnish immigrants in Sweden have a higher frequency of cardiovascular diseases (measured by blood pressure and cortisol levels), while immigrants from Mediterranean countries have a lower frequency despite higher rates of smoking (mainly men) and being overweight. Diabetes is a risk factor associated with cardiovascular disease among immigrants (Hjelm 1998), and there are different perceptions of diabetes, for example, between Swedish-born and Yugoslavian-born women diabetics.

Sweden's official statistics (www.scb.se) report that, in general, male immigrants from all countries are more likely to smoke than Swedish-born males. However, more immigrant women from other Nordic countries were smokers compared to Swedish-born, European and non-European women. Non-European immigrants consume less alcohol compared with Swedish-born, but are more likely to use drugs.

According to Livsmedelsverket (1998) the most important nutrition-related problems among immigrants are poor dental health, being overweight, adult-onset diabetes, low rates of breastfeeding, and poor nutrition among dependent elderly people. There may be several reasons for these nutrition-related problems. For instance, with regard to poor dental health, there may be fewer dentists in the home country, no cultural tradition of regular dental visits, traumatic life events (e.g. torture methods involving teeth), and difficulties with the host language.

Knowledge is lacking regarding immigrants' health beliefs and access to health information. In one of the few studies, Essén *et al.* (2000, 2002) studied the pregnancy and childbirth experiences of Somali women in Sweden, showing that some of their practices differ from Swedish women, such as controlling weight gain to have a small baby to make for easier delivery. They concluded that these practices should be seen as 'survival behaviors' related to high maternal morality in Somalia, and that the women are unlikely to change so long as health care providers are unaware of their motives and thus unable to provide more culturally sensitive perinatal care.

One of the few studies regarding the association between physical inactivity and illness among immigrants, done among four immigrant groups (National Board of Health and Welfare 1998b), showed large variations between the groups, although immigrants generally were less physically active than Swedes.

Rates of tuberculosis among immigrants and refugees in 1999 were similar to the level among the Swedish population 30 years ago, with the risk mainly among people coming from countries with a high prevalence of infection. An epidemiological programme is needed to screen high-risk newcomers, especially for antibiotic resistant strains. Among the 440 cases of tuberculosis during 2001 in Sweden, with information on country of birth for 311, 70 were born in Sweden and 248 abroad (Tärnvik 2002). Rates of HIV/AIDS are low in Sweden compared to other countries, but refugees who come from high endemic areas are a risk group. Thus the National Institute of Public Health and other agencies have targeted information on the prevention of HIV and other sexually transmitted diseases (STDs) to immigrants and refugees.

Hallsten *et al.* (2002) have studied burnout among a national sample of Swedes aged 18–64 years. In a sample of 4810 persons (response rate 69 per cent), 7.1 per cent of the total sample and 5.7 per cent of employees showed clear signs of burnout. Immigrants (11.9 per cent) had a particularly high rate of burnout (13.1 per cent and 9.9 per cent, respectively of total immigrants and employees). More immigrants are unemployed and worse-off economically compared with Swedish-born, and while there were no obvious differences in working conditions between immigrants and Swedes, the immigrants more often described feeling trapped in their work.

Swedish studies on immigrant mental health

Post-traumatic stress disorder (PTSD) and depression is a major refugee health issue, with an estimated 25–30 per cent of refugees in Sweden suffering from severe post-traumatic related disorders as a result of torture, war-related trauma, persecution and forced displacement (Söndergaard and Ekblad 1998). Bosnian refugees in Sweden were screened by questionnaire for PTSD and compared to primary health care visitors, with 18–33 per cent of refugees meeting a PTSD diagnosis compared to less than 1 per cent of Swedes (Thulesius and Håkansson 1999). When assessed for PTSD using the Diagnostic and Statistical Manual of Mental Disorders, DSM-IV (APA, 1994), 40 per cent of foreign-born outpatients of a Swedish community centre fulfilled the criteria (Ekblad and Roth 1997). A recent longitudinal study in Sweden (Roth and Ekblad 2002) showed a substantial increase in rates of PTSD among refugees evacuated from Kosavar, from 45 per cent at the baseline date to 78 per cent at an 18-month follow-up (using screening instruments, diagnostic screening DSM-IV and stress hormones in saliva). The biological changes in post-traumatic stress (Roth and Ekblad 2002; Söndergaard 2002) include abnormal sleep patterns; increased arousal of the nervous system; elevated levels of adrenalin (as in the fight or flight response), decreased levels of serotonin (as in depression), and lower cortisol levels (but higher levels in depression). A longitudinal study of refugees from Iraq found that the number of negative life events in Sweden was associated with self-rated deteriorated health (Söndergaard et al. 2001).

Ekblad and Wennström (1997) in their pilot study of immigrant patients on the relationship between traumatic life events and physical symptoms, found that a low score on a sense of coherence and meaningfulness subscale was associated with mental distress and impaired functioning. In a three-month follow-up of evacuated Kosovan adults in Sweden, Ekblad et al. (2002) found that torture was associated with post-traumatic stress disorder, such as poor coping (manageability), depression, anxiety and aggression.

The gulf between patient and professional interpretations of illness

The question of how health is expressed and perceived by refugee patients seeking health care has been neglected in the literature. A pilot qualitative study (Ekblad et al. 1999) examined perception of quality of life among Iranian refugees compared to Swedes with reference to the six WHO Quality of Life domains (Kuyken 1995), finding differences in three domains: level of independence, social relationships and environment. Among patients seeking health care, Iranians with war-related experiences perceived quality of life differently than Swedish patients. Swedes separated individual and environment in concepts of quality of life, whereas Iranians emphasized a holistic integration. Iranians regarded migration stress-related problems, such as health in the family, empowerment, perceived independence and integration in the Swedish society, as constituting a holistic dimension. In contrast, Swedes mentioned the dimensions of 'fitting in' with social relationships, an ordered lifestyle, being independent, and spending time out of doors, i.e., being in nature.

Bäärnhielm (2000) analysed the meaning of illness for Turkish and Swedish-born women compared to health professionals. 'Different interpretations of illness meaning by patient and caregiver constitute a situation of different realities according to the significance and social reality of the illness' (Bäärnhielm 2000 p. 4). The Turkish women rarely accepted psychiatric attribution, valued it as a tool for recovery, or found it helpful to link bodily symptoms to emotional distress. The results of the study point to the mutual need of exploring meaning in the clinical encounter to help patients make sense of different perspectives of illness and healing (Bäärnhielm and Ekblad 2000).

Bäärnhielm and Ekblad (manuscript) explored clinical experiences among health professionals in focus group interviews in a multicultural district of Stockholm, looking at how patients communicated mental ill health and social problems via physical symptoms. These professionals reported that patients commonly expressed emotional distress through bodily symptoms, but the professionals found it difficult to communicate with patients or to decode their language of suffering. The professionals tried to create coherence between their medical model and a patient's understanding of suffering. They lacked organizational support and also shared models for adapting their work to the multicultural population and for treating mental ill health outside psychiatry. Such shortcomings in primary care make 'somatization' a coping strategy by which immigrant patients receive attention and medical help.

Immigrant's use of mental health services

Psychological barriers to using health services among immigrant adults are heightened by mistrust, stigma, cost, and clinician bias. Cultural beliefs and values influence perceptions of the need for health care, particularly mental health care. Other common factors are the stigmatization of mental ill health, the perception of privacy about such problems, the desire to hide such complaints, mistrust of staff, and feeling unable to talk openly about some issues (i.e. taboos). Since immigrants tend to be disadvantaged socially and economically, they may find consultations too expensive, and may instead visit the hospital emergency department. Further, immigrants may use traditional medicine or religious/traditional ceremonies for treatment and healing in the host country or when visiting their home country, and be less familiar with the Western mental health interventions. Western approaches tend to emphasise the individual and minimise the importance of the sociocultural context and social networks. Thus public health services should stimulate mechanisms of adaptation and foster self-help to reduce and minimize helplessness, for example, by providing regular health information, and by recognizing the social context of migration stress symptoms and coping strategies (Ekblad *et al.* 1997; Wennström *et al.* 2000).

The few studies in Sweden concerning ethnicity and utilization of health services indicate major challenges for the health care system in meeting mental health needs among the immigrant population. Diderichsen and Varde (1999) found that in Stockholm County, migrants from non-Scandinavian countries had lower psychiatric utilization rates than the rest of the county's population. In a register study in Stockholm County, Oxenstierna (1998) found a diverse pattern of psychiatric service use among different groups with apparent under-use among some migrant groups.

Lindencrona *et al.* (2001) studied 670 medical records of psychiatric clinic outpatients in an immigrant southern suburb of Stockholm. Many patients had various unmet social, psychological and medical needs, particularly newly arrived refugees, who also were in the poorest circumstances, often lacking work and unable to speak Swedish. Many were young parents who had to combine attention to their children (who thus were at risk of transgenerational symptom effects), with attempts to establish themselves in a new society, a process made more difficult by earlier trauma. This community mental health centre is in the process of redesigning its services, seeking better inter-sectoral collaboration, and strengthening participation from community and patient representatives.

Mainstream professionals are thus confronting challenges without the benefit of training, supervision and experience, when treating newcomers – especially traumatized refugees. They need to draw upon a range of interventions including standard Western treatments and traditional healing, as well as health promotion strategies in the community. In selecting the appropriate intervention, it is useful to consider the major psychosocial stress systems (Silove 1999), at the individual, group and societal levels, which are influenced by the refugee experience. The model can help identify protective and risk factors, for example, in relation to reception programmes in the host country. The next section goes on to discuss such a theoretical framework.

Theoretical model and practice implications in a health care setting

In the theoretical framework presented here (Figure 10.1), Ekblad and Silove (1998) identified five fundamental psychosocial stress systems, in order to conceptualize the sources of stress experienced by refugees in camps, the model being developed later to include experiences in the host country (Lindencrona *et al.* 2002). The purpose was to conceptualize mental health in an ecological context, which allows the inclusion of pre-migration, migration and post-migration experiences. This model can also be applied when considering health service delivery in the host county.

An holistic framework

The levels of action in the model refer to the different levels in society (McLeroy *et al.* 1998), in this case the host country, where risk and protective factors for health care can be identified. The model identifies five fundamental 'systems' that are threatened or disrupted, as discussed below.

The attachment system

Many immigrants and refugees are affected by loss and separation from close attachment figures that may influence their health and need for help. Since the literature shows that a high level of social support reduces the risk for psychiatric disorder and impairment, it is relevant to ask about the person's social network now (as compared with the home country). Since an adult asylum seeker in Sweden has access only to emergency health services, such busy physicians are likely to consider that family reunion is out of their control and

Health system Level of action	Attachment	Security	Identity/roles	Human rights	Existential/meaning
Individual level					
Interpersonal level					
Organizational level					
Community level					
Policy level					

Figure 10.1 Mental health-promoting introduction to newly arrived refugees – a theoretical framework. Source: Lindencrona *et al.* 2002, with permission from Nordisk Psykologi.

a matter for the Swedish Migration Board. Thus when an asylum seeker attends emergency care, if not suicidal, such matters will not be addressed.

The security system

Since the literature shows that economic stress, material deprivation and insecurity are sources of perceived illness, health care staff should ask a refugee about current living conditions compared with their former situation in the home country. Also, refugees often have witnessed or encountered threats to their own or their family's physical safety and security, so that it is natural, not pathological, to be somewhat paranoid about their environment.

The identity/role system

The refugee experience involves a major threat to the sense of identity of the individual and the group. Loss of land, possessions and professions divest individuals of a sense of purpose and status in society. The literature shows that a sense of control over one's situation and one's role in a social network affects perceptions of health. For example, when attending health services, the husband may want to answer for or interpret for his wife, as is traditional in the home country. But it may be better for the wife if the health service arranges a neutral professional interpreter, while also asking about current identities, roles and ambitions compared to normal life in the home country.

The human rights system

Many refugees have experienced assaults upon their human rights, including arbitrary and unjust treatment, persecution, brutality, and in some instances, torture. The literature shows that tortured survivors are unwilling to tell their story of trauma before basic needs are solved and basic trust is developed. The problem is that this reluctance may adversely influence the asylum application and integration process, especially since traumatized people may with time forget the details of traumatic life events or else focus upon issues that do not help their residency application. The staff at the Migration Board and in community reception programmes need to understand the psychological effects of severe trauma and to communicate these to health professionals, with due regard for confidentiality and trust.

The existential-meaning system

Traumatic life experiences pose threats to a person's sense of coherence and meaning. The loss of meaning that a stable community used to provide leaves an asylum seeker in a state of bewilderment and uncertainty, perhaps questioning the meaning of life. Historical continuities linking past, present and future are radically disrupted by the upheavals associated with traumatic life events, and also reduce a person's capacity to live 'a normal life'. In searching for ways to re-establish a sense of coherence in life, a person may, for example, become more religious than before or else abandon religion. The host country may contribute to the loss of sense of coherence, for example, by not providing places for religious activities or by keeping people in long-term unemployment. Commitment to the social ideology of the threatened or oppressed group can serve as a protective factor.

Psychological dimensions affecting health

The psychological dimensions affecting health, according to Antonovsky (1987), include a 'sense of coherence':

(1) 'comprehensibility' or the extent to which a person can make sense of internal or external stimuli;

(2) 'manageability' or the extent to which one perceives that resources are available; and

(3) 'meaningfulness' or the perception that life is meaningful and worth living despite its hardships.

A review of research on coping with stress shows that it is difficult for people to develop extra coping strategies beyond the managing skills they have already learned (Somerfield and McCrae 2000). Coping behaviours differ from individual to individual, while some of life's problems cannot be solved only by the efforts of individuals. Post-traumatic development and maturation differs from theories about learned helplessness and posttraumatic stress disorder, and according to Moos, 'we need a fundamental paradigm shift in how to construe and examine the aftermath of life crises' (Moos 2002 p. 79).

When it comes to immigrants, the psychosocial stressors include, according to Jaranson et al. (2001) 'acculturation pressures, financial and employment disadvantages, dissonance between traditional sociocultural values and the host country, intergenerational stresses and social isolation' (p. 123). Further, the loss of, or separation from, family members or significant others may influence mental well-being (Ekblad et al. 1994). The traumatic stress experienced by refugees may induce a feeling of hopelessness and lack of control, partly due to the fact that coping mechanisms no longer work (Ekblad 1996), since there are 'additional psychological burdens and potential risk factors for mental illness not encountered in non-refugee immigrants or migrants' (Ekblad et al. 1998 p. 42).

These symptoms can be described using Harvey's ecological model of psychosocial trauma. This postulates that response and recovery depend upon the interaction between person, event and environmental factors. For example, every individual's reaction to violence and traumatic stress depends on person-specific factors such as age and personality, event factors such as the extent and frequency of violence or trauma, and an individual's identification with his or her environment. Thus 'the efficiency of trauma-focused interventions depends on the degree to which they enhance the person-community relationship and achieve "ecological fit" within individually varied recovery contexts' (Harvey 1996 p. 3).

At the individual level, health can be improved by supporting the individual in managing the challenges and problems that currently limit his or her life. However, a refugee may be unwilling to talk about their trauma experiences due to lack of confidence in health care staff, a feeling of shame, fear of increasing their symptoms, and a lack of knowledge about available help. Contact with health care staff offers opportunities for health care, and the literature shows the importance of emphasizing the possibilities for support in the community, rather than only symptom reduction. The combination of medical, psychological, social and juridical actions that are required depend upon intersectoral collaboration (organizational level and community level). At the policy level in Sweden, emergency care for traumatized adult asylum seekers is emphasized. This ignores the majority of refugees who react 'normally' to violence and traumatic life events, although counselling and help may reduce later psychiatric disorders and impairment.

Implications for health service delivery

This section discusses the main challenges in making health services, particularly mental health services, more accessible and responsive to refugees.

Training staff in transcultural health issues

In addition to other acculturation difficulties, newly arrived people in need of mental health care may have different attitudes towards the mentally ill and unfamiliar mental health systems. Mental health professionals usually have limited knowledge of an immigrant's language, culture, or attitudes about mental illness. Sweden can draw upon some resources, however, at least in Stockholm County, where about 20 per cent of the health workforce have immigrant backgrounds.

Additional training is required, however, in understanding risk and buffer factors for mental illness during pre migration, migration and post migration processes (for an overview, see (Ekblad *et al.* 1998). Further, health professionals need shared models of work and must be prepared to build upon local capacities in order to develop sustainability (Silove *et al.* 2000). Professional legitimation is required in order to provide mentoring, partnering and succession.

Preventing burnout among staff working with torture survivors requires regular supervision and the support of colleagues. Trans-cultural psychiatric training must extend traditional pedagogic methods. For example, the author has started teaching a trans-cultural psychiatric course for final-year medical students in a weekly video-conference together with colleagues from the United States and Australia (Ekblad *et al*, in press).

In spite of the increased knowledge on migration and mental health issues, there are many barriers to applying this knowledge in improving migrant reception and mental health programmes. Such barriers reflect failures of communication between researchers, policy makers and service providers, but also reflect limited resources, including the lack of transcultural training in university curricula and in professional development courses (Jaranson *et al.* 2001).

Making health services more responsive

Staff in reception programmes and primary health care need to recognize the early signs of distress among asylum-seekers and refugees in order to take preventive measures. A patient's idioms of distress might rely on a complex system of metaphors and proverbs giving rise to miscommunication and early termination of treatment. Once clients trust the staff, a helping alliance can be developed and maintained. Three principles should underlie treatment decisions with asylum seekers.

> First, refugees, like all other human beings, have the right to adequate health care, including mental health care. Second, mental health services should aim to normalise the experience of psychological disturbance and aim to actively reduce stigma, marginalisation and the exclusion of the mentally ill. Third, wherever possible efforts should be made to integrate indigenous methods of health with Western interventions.
>
> Ekblad 2000 p. 65

Integrating health and community services

The policy document outlining the introduction programme for refugees and other immigrants (Överenskommelsen om utveckling av introduktionen för flyktingar och andra invandrare 2001) states that this should be tailored to the needs of the individual and the family. The document aimed for an intersectoral approach and was signed by the Swedish Integration Board, the Swedish Migration Board, the National Agency for Education, the Swedish Association of Local Authorities and the National Labour Market Board. In January 2003 the authorities reached an agreement with representatives from the health sector, such as the National Board of Health and Welfare, the Federation of Swedish County Councils, the National Social Insurance Board, the National Institute of Psychosocial Factors and Health (the author of this chapter) and the Karolinska Institutet to create a working group entitled Integration and Health. A national evaluation of the introduction programme for incoming refugees made several recommendations, including strengthening the links between health services and the community (Riksrevisionsverket/The Swedish National Audit Office 2002).

Resourcing transcultural research

Funding research on asylum seekers and refugees is construed by some as a threat to universal health services. Thus a refugee mental health policy must be based upon scientific analysis and empirical evidence if it is to receive national and international attention (Mollica *et al.* 2002). Cross-cultural research enhances our understanding of psychopathology in three ways (Canino *et al.* 1997). First, cross-cultural comparisons are useful in developing hypotheses about the aetiology of particular disorders. Second, cross-cultural studies help us to distinguish between aetiological factors susceptible to cultural and contextual influences and those more related to biological factors. Third, the identification of risk and protective factors associated with specific disorders can have important implications for prevention. The basic challenge is how to develop a mental health research approach that searches for common themes across different cultures while at the same time being flexible enough to register significant local differences in psychopathology.

Turning to research on immigrants in Sweden, Ekblad (2001) is running a four-year research project titled 'Health promoting introduction for newcoming refugees' funded by the Swedish Integration Board and the European Refugee Fund, which addresses for example, the following questions. How should the municipality organize health services for refugees and what type of interventions are needed? What policies are in place to prevent further loss of identity/role in the society?

National research councils should consider funding long-term research programmes in the field of refugee mental health. Although migration patterns vary across the world, many recipient countries receive displaced persons from similar areas. Thus it should be possible for collaborating international centres to develop a computerized software program for a core assessment of trauma and mental health for national and cross-national studies.

Conclusions

The universal health care system, which was designed for a relatively homogeneous Swedish population that values social solidarity, does not optimally fit the health and mental health needs of people from different cultures, who have often been traumatized by events in their home countries and by their experiences as asylum seekers and refugees. Health services should reflect the cultural multiplicity of a society. According to Ginsburg (1994 p. 107) 'ethnically specific public services should not be regarded as a privilege for certain groups but to protect minorities from hidden discrimination'. Sweden, as a welfare society, faces several challenges regarding the integration of newcomers. Immigrants, especially refugees and asylum-seekers, have health care needs that are not fully met by existing universal services. Their psychosocial and health needs may result from life crises and involve more than the provision of health services. The consequences of war, mass violence and social and political upheaval constitute a major public health issue. Refugees are at particular risk, not only for developing mental disorders and impairment, but also for failing to receive treatment. Early assessment of, and intervention with, psychosocial and health needs among asylum-seekers, as well as among those not permitted to stay in the host country, may prevent further impairment and mental illness.

Many newcomers to Sweden other than asylum seekers or refugees may also have experienced traumatic life events that affect their physical and mental health, while other migrants may also have special needs. The physical and mental health of all immigrants are closely interconnected and thus are of particular concern to mental health professionals. This calls for the strengthening of transcultural psychiatry and transcultural psychology as a relevant academic field.

References

Allmänna råd från Socialstyrelsen (1995) Hälso-och sjukvård för asylsökande och flyktingar. **4**, 1–51.

Antonovsky, A. (1987) *Unraveling the mystery of health.* Jossey Bass Publishers, San Francisco, CA.

American Psychiatric Association (1994) *Diagnostic and Statistical Manual of Mental Disorder, 4th ed.* American Psychiatric Press, Washington D.C.

Bäärnhielm, S. (2000) *Clinical encounters with different illness realities. Qualitative studies of somatization and illness meaning among Swedish and Turkish-born women encountering local health care services in Western Stockholm.* Licentiate thesis. Sweden, Karolinska Institutet, Department of Public Health Sciences, Division of Psychosocial Factors and Health, Stockholm.

Bäärnhielm, S. and Ekblad, S. (manuscript) In unfamiliar territory: caregivers' encounter with somatic communication of mental ill health in a multicultural community.

Bäärnhielm, S. and Ekblad, S. (2000) Turkish migrant women encountering health care in Stockholm. A qualitative study of somatization and illness meaning. *Culture, Medicine and Psychiatry*, **24**, 431–52.

Bayard-Burfield, L. (1999) *Migration and mental health. Epidemiological studies of immigrants in Sweden.* Dissertation. Department of Community Medicine. University of Lund, Malmö University, Lund.

Bollini, P. and Siem, H. (1995) No real progress towards equity: health of migrants and ethnic minorities on the eve of the year 2000. *Social Science and Medicine*, **41**, 819–28.

Canino, G., Lewis Fernandez, R. and Bravo, M. (1997) Methodological challenges in cross-cultural mental health research. *Transcultural psychiatry*, **2**, 163–84.

Diderichsen, F. and Varde, E. (1999) Konsten att fördela resurser efter behov. Stockholmsmodellens kriterier. *Läkartidningen*, **93**, 3677–83.

Ekblad, S. (1996) *Diagnostik och behandlig av patienter med invandrarbakgrund. En ettårsuppföljning på en psykiatrisk öppenvårdsmottagning.* Institutet för Psykoscial Medicin (IPM) Avdelningen för stressforskning, Karolinska Institutet, WHO's Psykosociala Center, Stressforskningsrapporter nr **262**.

Ekblad, S. (2000) *A survey of somatic, psychological and social needs of mass displaced refugees from the Kosova province while in Sweden.* National Institute of Psychosocial Factors and Health (IPM), Division of Psychosocial Factors and Health, Department of Public Health Sciences, Karolinska Institutet, WHO's Psychosocial Center, Stress Research Reports, Nr **293**, Stockholm.

Ekblad, S. (2001) *Health Promoting Introduction.* Grants from Swedish Integration Board and European Refugee Fund. Karolinska Institutet, Neurotec Department, Section of Psychiatry (Dnr KI 1631/2001, Dnr INT-33–00–2632; ERF 141/2001, Dnr KI 3341/2001), Stockholm.

Ekblad, S. (2003) A Swedish perspective on refugee adjustment, resettlement, acculturation and mental health. In F. Bemak, R. Chi-Ying Chung and P. B. Pedersen (eds) *Refugee mental health*, pp. 178–87. Greenwood Publishing Group Inc., Westport, CT.

Ekblad, S., Abazari, A. and Eriksson, N.-G. (1999) Migration stress-related challenges associated with perceived quality of life: qualitative analysis of Iranian refugees and Swedish patients. *Transcultural Psychiatry*, **36** (3), 329–45.

Ekblad, S., Ginsburg, B.-E., Jansson, B. and Levi, L. (1994) Psychosocial and psychiatric aspects of refugee adaptation and care in Sweden. In A. J. Marsella, T. Bornemann, S. Ekblad and J. Orley (eds) *Amidst peril and pain: the mental health and wellbeing of world's refugees*, pp. 275–93. American Psychological Association, Washington DC.

Ekblad, S., Klefbeck, E.-L., Wennström, C. and Pietkäinen, A.-L. (1997) Help for refugees. *World Health Forum*, **18**, 305–10.

Ekblad, S., Kohn, R. and Jansson, B. (1998) Psychological and clinical aspects of migration and mental health. In S. O. Okpaku (ed.) *Clinical Methods in Trans-cultural Psychiatry*, pp. 42–66. American Psychiatric Association Press, Washington, DC and London.

Ekblad, S., Manicavascar, V., Silove, D., Bäärnhielm, S., Reczycki, M., Mollica, R., Coella, M. The use of international video conferencing as a strategy for teaching medical students about transcultural psychiatry. *Transcultural Psychiatry*, (in press).

Ekblad, S., Prochazka, H. and Roth, G. (2002) Psychological impact of torture: A 3-month follow-up of mass-evacuated Kosovan adults in Sweden. Lessons learnt for prevention. *Acta Psychiatrica Scandinavica*, **106**, Suppl. 412, 30–6.

Ekblad, S. and Roth, G. (1997) Diagosing post-traumatic stress disorder in multicultural patients in a Stockholm Psychiatric Clinic. *Journal of Nervous and Mental Diseases*, **185** (2), 102–7.

Ekblad, S. and Silove, D. (1998) *Proposals for the development of mental health and psychosocial services in refugee camps August 18.* Paper from a mission for UNCHR. UNCHR, Geneva.

Ekblad, S. and Wennström, C. (1997) Relationships between traumatic life events, symptoms, and Sense of Coherence subscale meaningfulness in a group of refugee and immigrant patients referred to a Stockholm psychiatric out-patient clinic. *Scandinavian Journal of Social Welfare*, **6**, 279–85.

Essén, B., Bödker, B., Sjöberg, N. O., Langhoff-Roos, J., Greisen, G., Gudmundsson, S., *et al.* (2002) Are some perinatal deaths in immigrant groups linked to suboptimal perinatal care series. *British Journal of Obstetrics and Gynecology*, **109**, 677–82.

Essén, B., Hansson, B. S., Östergren, P.-O., Lindquist, P. G. and Gudmundsson, S. (2000) Increased perinatal morality among sub-Saharan immigrants in a city-population in Sweden. *Acta Obstetrica et Gynecologica Scandinvaica*, **79**, 737–43.

Ferrada-Noli, M. (1996) *Post-traumatic stress disorder and suicidal behaviour in immigrants to Sweden. An epidemiological, cross-cultural and psychiatric study*. Dissertation. Karolinska Institutet, Stockholm.

Ginsburg, B. E. (1994) Migration and welfare. *Scandinavian Journal of Social Welfare*, **3**, 102–8.

Hallsten, L., Bellaagh, K. and Gustafsson, K. (2002) *Burnout in Sweden – a national survey*. Arbete och Hälsa, **6**, in Swedish, with a Summary in English. National Institute for Working Life, Stockholm.

Harvey, M. R. (1996) An ecological view of psychological trauma and trauma recovery. *Journal of Traumatic Stress*, **9** (1), 3–23.

Hjelm, K. (1998) *Migration, health and diabetes mellitus. Studies comparing foreign – and Swedish-born diabetic subjects living in Sweden*. Dissertation. Department of Social sciences, Dalby/Lund.

Hjortsberg, C. and Ghatnekar, O. (2001) *Health care systems in transition: Sweden*. Available at http:/www.observatory.dk. European Observatory on Health Care Systems, Copenhagen.

Hollifield, M., Warner, T. D., Lian, N., Krakow, B., Jenkins, J., Kesler, J., *et al.* (2002) Measuring trauma and health status in refugees. *Journal of the American Medical Association*, **288** (5), 611–21.

Jaranson, J., Forbes Martin, S. and Ekblad, S. (2001) Refugee mental health. In R. W. Manderscheid and M. J. Henderson (eds) *Mental health, United States, 2000*, pp. 120–33. US Department of Health and Human Services, Substance Abuse and Mental Health Services Administration (SAMHSA), Center for Mental Health Services, Rockville, MD.

Johansson, L. M. (1997) *Migration, mental health and suicide. An epidemiological, psychiatric and cross-cultural study*. Dissertation. Karolinska Institutet, Stockholm.

Kirmayer, L. J. and Minas, H. (2000) The future of cultural psychiatry: an international perspective. *Canadian Journal of Psychiatry*, **45**, 438–46.

Kjellin, I., Brant-Segerström, G., Kjellin, L. and Sörensen, S. (1992) Flyktingkvinnors hälsa måste förbättras. *Läkartidningen*, **92** (89), 4251–5.

Kuyken, W. (1995) The World Health Organization quality of life assessment (WHOQOL): Position paper from the World Organization. *Social Science and Medicine*, **10**, 1403–9.

Lindencrona, F., Ekblad, S. and Charry, J. (2001) Kartläggning av levnadsomständigheter, behandlingskontakter och samverkansinsatser för patienter på Fittja psykiatriska öppenvårdsmottagning 1998–1999. Stressforskningsrapport nr **296**.

Lindencrona, F., Johansson Blight, K. and Ekblad, S. (2002) Teori och val av metod för att studera hälsofrämjande insatser ur ett transkulturellt perspektiv. *Nordisk Psykologi*, **54** (1), 7–26.

Livsmedelsverket (1998) Hälsoupplysning till invandrare. Livsmedelsverket. Intern promemoria daterad 1998–11–12. Livsmedelsverket.

McLeroy, K. R., Bibeau, D., Steckler, A. and Glanz, K. (1998) An ecological perspective on health promotion programs. *Health Education Quarterly,* **15** (4), 351–77.

Moberg, V. (1951) *The emigrants.* Simon and Schuster, New York.

Moberg, V. (1957) *Unto a good land.* Reinhardt, London.

Mollica, R. F., Cui, X., McInnes, K. and Massagli, M. P. (2002) Science-based policy for psychosocial interventions in refugee camps: a Cambodian example. *Journal of Nervous and Mental Disease,* **190** (3), 158–66.

Moos, R. H. (2002) The mystery of human context and coping: An unraveling of clues. *American Journal of Community Psychology,* **30** (1), 67–88.

National Board of Health and Welfare (2000) *Innehåll i och omfattning av den vård landstingen åtagit sig att ge till asylsökande m.fl. Rapport av regeringsuppdrag 2000–04–27 III:15.*

National Board of Health and Welfare (1998a) *Hur skall Sverige må bättre? – första steget mot nationella folkhälsomål. Delbetänkande från Nationella folkhälsokommittén.* Nr **43**.

National Board of Health and Welfare (1998b) *Levnadsförhållanden hos fyra invandrargrupper födda i Chile, Iran, Polen och Turkiet.* Invandrarprojektet – rapport nr **1998: 1,** Invandrares levnadsvillkor 1. Stockholm.

National Board of Health and Welfare (1997) *National public health report.* National Board of Health and Welfare, Stockholm.

Överenskommelsen om utveckling av introduktionen för flyktingar och andra invandrare (2001) (Agreement concerning development of the introduction for refugees and other immigrants). The National Labour Market Board Dnr 01–2151–21, the Swedish Integration Board Dnr INT 19–01–538, the Swedish Migration Board Dnr MV-11–2001–3005, the National Agency for Education Dnr 07–2001–734, the Swedish Association fo Local Authorities Dnr 2001/0527.

Oxenstierna, G. (1998) Invandrare, sjukvård och socialförsäkring. In S. Ekblad, G. Oxenstierna and A. Akpinar (eds) *Invandrarbakgrundens betydelse för sjukvård och socialförsäkring. En folkhälsorapport för Stockholms län 1998,* pp 23–103. Stockholm County Council and National Institute of Psychosocial Factors and Health, Stockholm.

Riksrevisionsverket (The Swedish National Audit Office) (2002) *Att etablera sig i Sverige. En granskning av introduktionsverksamheten för flyktingar och deras anhöriga.* 2002: **15.**

Roth, G. and Ekblad, S. (2002) Decreased levels of cortisol and testosterone among mass evacuated adults from Kosovo with trauma experiences and PTSD. Abstracts of 11th Congress of the Association of European Psychiatrists, Stockholm, 4–8 May. *The Journal of the Association of European Psychiatrists,* **17,** Suppl. 1, 94s.

Roth, G. and Ekblad, S. (1993) Migration and mental health: current research issues. *Nordic Journal of Psychiatry,* **3,** 185–89.

Silove, D. (1999) The psychosocial effects of torture. Mass human rights violations, and refugee trauma-toward an integrated conceptual framework. *Journal of Nervous and Mental Disease,* **187** (4), 200–7.

Silove, D. and Ekblad, S. (2002) How well do refugees adapt after resettlement in Western countries? *Acta Psychiatrica Scandinavia,* **106,** 401–2.

Silove, D., Ekblad, S. and Mollica, R. (2000) Health and human rights. The rights of the severely mentally ill in post-conflict societies. Invited Lancet commentary. *The Lancet*, 355, 1548–9.

Somerfield, M. R. and McCrae, R. R. (2000) Stress and coping research. Methodological challenges, theoretical advances, and clinical applications. *American Psychologist*, 55 (6), 620–5.

Söndergaard, H. P. and Ekblad, S. (1998) Traumatiska belastningar hos vuxna flyktingar: När ohälsan tiger still – eller pratar bruten svenska. (Abstract in English) *Läkartidningen*, 13, 1415–22.

Söndergaard, H. P., Ekblad, S. and Theorell, T. (2001) Self-rated life event patterns and their relation with health among recently resettled Iraqi and Kurdish refugees in Sweden. *The Journal of Nervous and Mental Disease*, 189, 838–45.

Söndergard, H. P. (2002) *Post-traumatic stress disorder and life events among recently resettled refugees*. Dissertation. Karolinska Institutet, Stockholm

Sundquist, J. and Johansson, S.-E. (1997) Long-term illness among indigenous and foreign-born people in Sweden. *Social Science and Medicine*, 44, 189–98.

Tärnvik, A. (2002) Tuberkulossituationen oroar. För att stå emot trycket från omvärlden krävs bättre epidemiologisk beredskap. *Läkartidningen*, 99 (23), 2616–17.

Thulesius, H. and Håkansson, A. (1999) Screening for post-traumatic stress disorder symptoms among Bosnian refugees. *Journal of Traumatic Stress*, 12 (1), 67–74.

van Willigen, L. (1992) Organization of care and rehabilitation services for victims of torture and other forms of organized violence: a review of current issues. In M. Basoglu (ed.) *Torture and its consequences. Current treatment approaches*, pp. 277–298. Cambridge University Press, Cambridge.

Wennström, C., Klefbeck, E.-L. and Ekblad, S. (2000) Samverkansmodell mellan flyktingmottagande och psykiatrin. *Socionomen*, 6, 54–56.

World Health Organization (1948) *Constitution of the World Health Organization*. World Health Organisation, Geneva.

World Health Organization (1993) *The health of Europe. Regional publications*. European Series, 49, World Health Organization, Copenhagen.

World Health Organization (2001) *World health report 2001. Mental health: new understanding, new hope*. World Health Organization, Geneva.

Chapter 11

Asylum Seekers and Refugees in the United Kingdom

Naaz Coker

The challenge

Since the 1970s, western Europe has seen growing numbers of asylum seekers and refugees, largely from countries where there is civil war, persecution or human rights abuses. In the United Kingdom (UK) the lengthy procedures for asylum determination can undermine the health and well-being of these vulnerable people. Managing their health needs is a complex process requiring a sensitive approach to identifying, assessing and responding to the particular needs of these people, many of whom are traumatized, depressed and lack resources. They need support to rebuild their lives and to regain their identity and self-esteem. The health care system has to respond to the challenge of meeting the needs of asylum seekers and refugees who are being dispersed throughout the UK.

Most refugees will have had little medical help in their own countries due to war, persecution or natural disaster. Many refugee women will need health care: some may have been subjected to rape, torture and sexual abuse, resulting in both physical and mental complications. Refugee children, too, will have complex needs. A significant number have suffered the same traumas and distress as their parents, who, due to their own frailty, are unable to provide the much needed parental support, leaving the children in a vulnerable state.

Although asylum seekers have restricted and fixed housing and cash benefits, they are entitled to National Health Service (NHS) care, both primary and secondary. Unfortunately, entitlement does not transform into ease of access; many are denied access through actual refusal or through lack of culturally sensitive services and interpreting facilities. Complaints of racial discrimination and intolerance within the system abound. Public hostility and marginalization result in this group becoming isolated and frustrated. Many, who arrive in reasonably good health, report depression and ill health some months later.

Some of the recurrent issues in delivering health services to this group include:

◆ lack of knowledge about available health services;

◆ in some cases, significant and complex health needs;

◆ uneven distribution of refugees and asylum seekers between primary care practices;

◆ diversity of culture and languages;

◆ the additional workload for refugees and asylum seekers (and health and welfare professionals) in applying for housing, legal advice and other needs;

◆ lack of knowledge of cultural and special health needs on the part of health professionals;

◆ increased time needed for consultations due to the need for interpreting;

◆ lack of additional resources for general practitioners;

◆ risk that general practitioners may lose funding if they miss immunization and cervical screening targets (the funding system requires that general practitioners meet certain performance targets to trigger payments); and

◆ the lack of effective collaboration between agencies working with asylum seekers.

In many parts of the United Kingdom those working with asylum seekers have developed innovative ways of overcoming these difficulties. The good practice examples described in more detail later in the chapter illustrate the use of imaginative ways of delivering and funding services to refugees and asylum seekers.

Who are refugees and asylum seekers?

The word refugee has a very particular meaning, set out in the 1951 United Nations Convention Relating to the Status of Refugees. At the end of the Second World War, the needs of an estimated 40 million displaced Europeans resulted in the establishment of the Office of the United Nations High Commissioner for Refugees (UNHCR). In the same year, the UN Refugee Convention was adopted, which set out the precise definition of a refugee as:

> Any person who owing to well-founded fear of being persecuted for reasons of race, religion, nationality, membership of a particular social group or political opinion, is outside the country of his/her nationality, and is unable to, or owing to such fear, is unwilling to avail himself of the protection of that country; or who, not having

a nationality and being outside the country of his former habitual residence, as a result of such events, is unable to or, owing to such fear, is unwilling to return to it.

Convention and protocol relating to the status of refugees – 1951 Geneva Convention, Article 1A

In 1967, a UN protocol extended the convention to include anybody, anywhere in the world. The United Kingdom, along with 135 other countries, is a signatory to the refugee convention and its protocol, which commits all the signatories to certain obligations including allowing any person fleeing persecution the legal right to seek asylum and protection in that country. The UNHCR also includes as refugees persons who:

- are recognized as refugees under the 1969 Organization of African Unity Convention governing The Specific Aspects Of Refugee Problems in Africa;
- are recognized by countries which apply an extended refugee definition, such as the Latin-American countries that adhere to the Cartagena Declaration;
- have been granted refugee status on humanitarian grounds;
- have been granted temporary protection.

Even now, this Convention remains the only international instrument that defines the duty of states towards those who fear persecution and that sets out minimum standards for their treatment. Yet there is growing debate amongst European Union (EU) governments on whether the spirit and wording of the convention is still valid. Some wish to review the definition. The concern is

Box 11.1 **Definitions of asylum seekers and refugees**

Asylum seekers: people who have made an application for asylum in the United Kingdom.

Exceptional leave to remain (ELR): people who, for compassionate reasons, are allowed to stay for specified period of time ranging from one to four years.

Indefinite leave to remain (ILR): people who are granted refugee status and who can apply for their dependents to join them.

People with ELR or ILR status have the same entitlements to welfare benefits, health, housing, education and employment benefits as United Kingdom citizens.

that the review is in response to the self-interests of western countries and not necessarily to the needs of the world's refugees.

Refugees are not a new phenomenon in Britain. In previous centuries there were significant movements of people for political and religious reasons. In the sixteenth century the reformation led to the influx of Calvinist exiles to the UK. The most well known influx of religious refugees came in the seventeenth century, as the French Protestants, the Huguenots, were expelled from France following the Revocation of the Edict of Nantes. In the eighteenth century, Roman Catholics and members of the aristocratic classes who were fleeing the French Revolution in 1789 also moved to Britain. In 1848, described as the year of the revolutions, the UK was seen as a bastion of tolerance for royalists, socialists and republicans from across Europe.

The twentieth century, however, has seen mass population movement worldwide; wars and armed conflicts have resulted in enforced migration of civilians from the growing areas of the world's trouble spots. Almost every part of the world has been affected, from West Africa to Indonesia, Bosnia to Afghanistan. In 1971, ten million people fled from East Pakistan (Bangladesh) into India. The 1970s also saw ideological conflicts in Indochina, the Horn of Africa, Afghanistan, Central America, Mozambique and Angola and the expulsion of South Asians from Kenya and Uganda. The 1980s and 1990s saw conflict and war in Former Yugoslavia, Bosnia and Kosovo, the Rwandan genocides, the persecution of Kurds in Iraq and Turkey, continuing conflicts in Sri Lanka, the Horn of Africa and East Timor. There has been war in Afghanistan since 1979 and many refugees have fled their homes: nearly

Box 11.2 **The century of the refugee**

A Holocaust survivor, Rabbi Hugo Gryn said just before he died in 1996 that 'future historians will call the twentieth century not only the century of the great Wars, but also the century of the refugee. Almost nobody at the end of the century is where they were at the beginning of it. It has been the century of genocide.

Speech made in Autumn 1996

The writer John Berger commented:

Wave after wave of emigrants, emigrating for either political or economic reasons but emigrating for survival. Ours is the century of enforced travel . . . the century of disappearances. The century of people helplessly seeing others, who were close to them, disappear over the horizon.

Berger 1992

2 million Afghan refugees fled to Iran and 1.2 million to Pakistan. A relatively small number have sought refuge in Europe. The situation in Afghanistan, after the removal of the Taliban, is still fragile and whilst it is considered by the European Union as a 'safe' country the circumstances for returning Afghani people are far from stable.

Refugees and internally displaced people

Today there are nearly 14 million refugees in the world. They are ordinary people who have fled from their homes because their lives are in danger. Of these, a relatively small number, about three million, have actually made it to Europe or the UK (European Council for Refugees and Exiles (ECRE) 1996). Most refugees are in the poorer countries in the developing world, particularly India and Africa, and many are living in camps where illness and death rates are extremely high. India has given sanctuary to a large number of refugees from Tibet, Burma and Sri Lanka. War in Sierra Leone and Liberia has caused nearly two million people to flee from their homes into neighbouring countries.

About 25 million people worldwide have fled from their homes, but have gone into hiding in their home country. The needs of these internally displaced people are much the same as refugees. (The main difference between displaced people and refugees is that refugees have left their own countries and crossed international borders.)

It is estimated that one person out of every 150 alive today is a refugee or a displaced person (European Council for Refugees and Exiles (ECRE) 1996). Furthermore, there is a growing body of migrants who leave their homes and countries to seek educational opportunities and economic prosperity.

In 2001, Britain had 76,000 new asylum applicants: of these 31 per cent were granted refugee status or extended leave to remain. These figures do not take into account the refusals that were overturned on appeal. In 1999, the total acceptance rate was 54 per cent. Of the 76,000 applicants, 50 per cent were from Iraq, Sri Lanka, Former Yugoslavia, Iran, Somalia and Afghanistan: all countries with continuing turmoil, conflict and serious human rights abuses. In the first quarter of 2002, the highest numbers of asylum applicants were from Iraq, Afghanistan, Zimbabwe and Somalia – all countries with well-documented instances of persecution and conflict (European Council for Refugees and Exiles (ECRE) 1996).

The distinction between refugees and immigrants

The distinction between immigrants and refugees has become blurred in the media and in the public debate, aided by government rhetoric that has been used to push an increasingly restrictive asylum determination process. As Europe tightens immigration controls, it is virtually impossible for people fleeing abuses to reach the United Kingdom legally. Those who enter Britain illegally may have no other option. As an Iraqi woman once told me, how could you ask the official who is persecuting you to give you papers to leave!

The main distinction is about choice; immigrants have a theoretical choice of staying or going back, while refugees face persecution in their home country. As discussed later, the media often portray refugees as immigrants seeking better economic conditions. Economic migrants are not bad people, however, they are human beings, mothers and fathers, brothers and sisters, who are travelling to the West because they are seeking opportunities to improve their lives and those of their families. Whilst they may not qualify as refugees under the convention criteria, they should still be treated with respect and dignity.

The legislative environment

On 29 October 2001, the British Home Secretary (Interior Minister), David Blunkett, announced proposals for a 'fundamental reform of our asylum and immigration policy'. The new proposals were outlined in the Government white paper *Secure borders, safe haven: integration with diversity in modern Britain* (Home Office 2002). This was followed by the Nationality, Immigration and Asylum Act, which came into force in January 2003.

This bill was the fourth major shake-up of the asylum system in less than ten years; each time the changes were heralded as a radical reform of the system. Whilst some measures were welcomed by refugee agencies, it was obvious that the underlying ethos of the legislation focused on the control and the removal of rejected asylum seekers rather than the provision of sanctuary and protection to refugees, which should be the primary purpose of any asylum system.

The Immigration and Asylum Act 1999

The 1999 Asylum and Immigration Act (Home Office 1999) was a complex piece of legislation whose key features impacting on asylum seekers were:

- Dispersal: all newly arrived asylum seekers would be dispersed outside London and the South East of England across the United Kingdom;

- Introduction of vouchers: asylum seekers were entitled to the equivalent of 70 per cent of income support issued as vouchers to be exchanged at designated stores for food and other items;

- No choice of accommodation: asylum seekers had to accept the accommodation offered to them or lose their benefits;

- A new system of support: the Home Office (Interior Ministry) established a new administrative unit called the National Asylum Support Service to administer and support newly arrived asylum seekers, which has been operating since April 2000.

The substantial impact of this legislation on asylum seekers was as follows:

- Poverty and isolation: Asylum seekers received £36.54 (€57.5) worth of vouchers a week, £10 (€15.7) of which was exchangeable for cash. They were not allowed to claim mainstream welfare benefits. The £36.54 amounted to 70 per cent of the standard income support given to British citizens and was 30 per cent below the national income support rate. When vouchers were exchanged the few shops taking them were not allowed to give change. Asylum seekers had to stay in emergency accommodation for up to four months prior to dispersal and the majority were put in very poor quality housing in deprived inner city areas.

- Humiliation and racist attacks: The Government justified the voucher scheme on the grounds that it would deter unfounded asylum applications. However, the use of vouchers was humiliating and stigmatizing for asylum seekers who were immediately identified as 'different' as they shopped with their 'funny money'. A young refugee girl described vouchers as 'getting a stamp saying you don't belong'. The hostile climate fuelled by negative media reporting and political rhetoric also resulted in an increase in racist attacks on asylum seekers; many continue to be subjected to violent attacks and abuse. The scheme was expensive and did not deter people from seeking asylum, as the government had hoped. The government was forced to review the voucher system as a result of pressure by the trade union movement, faith leaders, the Refugee Council, Oxfam, the King's Fund, and many other organizations and individuals: who all called for vouchers to be scrapped and replaced with a cash-based system.

- Dispersal to areas away from known communities: Previously the majority of asylum seekers settled in London where they gradually established a network of support systems. Dispersal resulted in isolation and loss of community networks leading to further exclusion and depression.

Nationality, Immigration and Asylum Act 2002

This new law came into force on 8 January 2003. Several changes were made in advance of the legislation. In February 2002, the Home Secretary announced the withdrawal of vouchers in favour of a cash based system from April 2002 accompanied by in increase in cash support in line with inflation; this still left support at 70 per cent of income support rates. The removal of vouchers represented a significant victory for the organizations and individuals who had campaigned for an end to the discriminatory system that had imposed stigma and hardship on already vulnerable people.

The key proposals in the new law are:

- Smart cards: smart cards or application registration card will be used for identification and may be used for accessing services and support.

- Dispersal: Dispersal of asylum seekers to areas outside London and the south east of England will continue with renewed emphasis on dispersing people to language clusters and areas that will best meet their needs.

- Induction centres: Asylum seekers will be referred to an induction centre located near ports of entry. These centres will undertake all the screening and identification required for the determination of asylum applications. Induction centres will also provide accommodation for those who need it. All asylum seekers will be dispersed from these induction centres.

- Accommodation centres: New accommodation centres are central to the Government's proposals. It is intended that these centres will be managed by the National Asylum Support Service and people waiting for their asylum decisions will stay in these centres. On a trial basis, the government intends to open four new centres with 750 bed spaces each; these will offer full-board accommodation with on-site access to basic health care, education for children and purposeful activity for adults.

- Reporting centres: The government proposes to establish a network of reporting centres where asylum applicants will be required to report on a regular basis.

- Detention and removal centres: The government proposes to increase the current 1900 detention places to 4000 places. These will become 'secure removal centres' intended to facilitate an increased rate of removals from the United Kingdom.

- Integration: The proposals promise improved integration procedures with support for education in language and citizenship.

- An eleventh hour amendment (section 55 of the 2002 Act) was pushed through just before the Act became law, which denied support to all asylum seekers who made their application in-country, i.e. not at the port of entry. This has resulted in some asylum seekers becoming destitute. Many of those involved have mounted legal challenges.

The refugee agencies, whilst welcoming some of the humanitarian improvements, are keen to remind the government that the purpose of the asylum system is to provide protection to refugees: thus an asylum system should ensure that the quality of decision-making is speedy, fair and treats people with dignity. The Refugee Council agrees with the need for reform, but also believes that at the heart of any credible asylum system is a fair and transparent asylum process. Asylum decisions must be legally robust and subject to proper scrutiny. Fairness demands that asylum seekers receiving support be treated with respect and also means that detention should only be used when there is sufficient evidence – which will stand up in court – that an asylum seeker has committed a crime or is likely to abscond.

As the Refugee Council said in its Parliamentary Briefing:

> Change after change generates confusion, damages the credibility of the asylum process in the eyes of the general public and, of course must be demoralising for the men and women working within the system. This time the government must listen to key stakeholders in an effort to get it right and put in place the foundation of a system that will endure.
>
> Refugee Council 2002

Box 11.3 The Refugee Council's Response to the New Immigration and Asylum Act

Welcomes:

- More positive tone and language
- The abolition of the voucher scheme and the decision to replace vouchers with cash for destitute asylum seekers
- The Government's commitment to widen access to quality legal advice for asylum seekers
- The age at which children can be registered as British citizens has reduced from ten to five years
- Confirmation that asylum seekers will no longer be detained in prisons

Opposes:

- Detention capacity being increased and the increased use of detention for families
- The proposed confidential immigration hotline
- Support levels for destitute asylum seekers remaining 30 per cent below income support levels
- The removal of asylums seekers being able to apply for support only
- The lack of access to legal advice for asylum seekers during the induction process
- Plans to widen measures regarding interviewing unaccompanied asylum-seeking children about their asylum claims

Source: Alison Fenney, Head of Policy, The Refugee Council

Media and public views of asylum seekers

Refugees and asylum seekers receive daily media attention as this remains a hotly debated issue. Unfortunately, not all coverage is balanced or truthful. Sloppy and inaccurate reporting has continued in many sections of the press with some papers suggesting that the United Kingdom is being 'swamped' by 'bogus' refugees who are 'scroungers and criminals' intent on exploiting the social welfare system and living in luxury at the taxpayer's expense. Such misleading reporting has fuelled hostility and violent racially motivated attacks on asylum seekers.

In November 2000, the Reader's Digest (Bouquet and Moller 2000) published the results of a MORI survey of 2118 adults throughout Britain on immigration and asylum issues. The poll showed that:

- 80 per cent of British adults believed that refugees came to Britain because they regard Britain as a 'soft touch';

- 66 per cent thought that 'there are too many immigrants in Britain';

- 66 per cent felt that 'too much is done to help immigrants';

- Respondents overestimated the financial aid asylum seekers receive;

- Respondents thought that 20 per cent of the population were immigrants: the real figure is 4 per cent;

- 37 per cent of the respondents felt that those settling in this country 'should not maintain the culture and lifestyle they had at home'.

Reader's Digest editor-in chief, Russell Twisk, commented that: 'This widespread resentment of immigrants and asylum seekers has worrying implications in a society that has traditionally prided itself on its racial tolerance.'

A more recent survey into public attitudes on asylum, published during Refugee Week in June 2002 (MORI Social Research Institute 2002) revealed that young people in Britain were more negative in their attitudes towards asylum seekers and refugees and were less likely to be welcoming than adults. The poll also suggested that the media had been unhelpful in providing an informative and positive view of refugees and asylum seekers. This evidence suggested that considerable work still needed to be done to raise awareness among young people about asylum and refugee issues.

Entitlements to health and welfare benefits

All asylum seekers (including those whose asylum applications have been refused and are either appealing or awaiting deportation), and people with Refugee Status or Exceptional Leave to Remain are entitled to free medical

Box 11.4 Excerpt from Statutory Instrument no. 306: The National Health Service (Charges to Overseas Visitors) Regulations 1989

Overseas visitors exempt from charges:

4. No charge shall be made in respect of any services forming part of the health service provided for an overseas visitor, being a person, or the spouse or child of a person . . . c) who has been accepted as refugee in the United Kingdom, or who has made a formal application for leave to stay as a refugee in the United Kingdom . . .'

Excerpt from Health Service Circular HSC 1999/018

Overseas visitors' eligibility to receive free primary care:

A refugee given leave to remain in the United Kingdom should be regarded as ordinarily resident. A refugee who is in the United Kingdom awaiting the result of his application to remain in this country should also be regarded as ordinarily resident because he or she is residing lawfully for a settled purpose.

treatment under the National Health Service (HSC 1999/018 & Statutory Instrument 1989 No. 306).

Primary care

All asylum seekers and refugees have the right to be permanently registered with a general practitioner and have access to all primary care services free of charge. The services provided by general practitioners are governed by a national contract as defined under the 1977 NHS Act. Every resident has a right to register with a general practitioner, but general practitioners also have the right to decide who to accept onto their patient list. However, they are expected to treat asylum seekers and people with Refugee Status or Exceptional Leave to Remain as NHS patients.

Under the Immigration and Asylum Act 1999 and the Asylum and Immigration Act 1996, most asylum seekers are not entitled to welfare benefits. However, they may qualify for:

- free NHS prescriptions;
- NHS dental treatment and checks;
- sight tests and full-value vouchers towards the cost of spectacles or contact lenses;
- travel costs to and from hospital for NHS treatment.

Asylum seekers are not, however, entitled to obtain free milk, formula milk or vitamins which can cause considerable hardship to mothers with young children. There is no requirement to show official documentation when registering with a general practitioner, however some practices are unwilling to register an asylum seeker or refugee without seeing a Home Office letter. It is important to note that the practice has no right to demand to see a passport before agreeing to register a person. If asylum seekers are unable to register with a GP, they should contact their local Primary Care Trust (the authority responsible for primary care in an area), which has the right to allocate them a general practitioner. Everyone is supposed to try to register with three practices before contacting their Trust.

Secondary care

Asylum seekers and refugees have free and full access to all NHS accident and emergency, maternity and inpatient and outpatient services. There is a registration procedure to determine free entitlement to hospital services, such as being added to a waiting list for an operation, which applies to everyone and not just refugees and asylum seekers. As refugees are in the UK for the purpose of settlement, there should be no problem in establishing free eligibility to the NHS.

Poverty and health

Poverty is a major issue facing asylum seekers in the UK. Asylum seekers were allowed to work after six months if they had not received a decision on their application, but the government withdrew this concession in July 2002, which is likely to cause additional hardship for this group who are already impoverished. Organizations working with asylum seekers remain deeply concerned at the 'unacceptable levels of poverty' experienced by these people. Oxfam and the Refugee Council (Penrose 2002) commissioned a study to explore the levels of poverty amongst asylum seekers. Their findings showed that the support given to asylum seekers fell well short of that available to Income Support (social benefits) claimants even when all benefits were taken into account. These levels of poverty undermine Government policies on social exclusion, human rights and integration.

Unaccompanied refugee children

In recent years there has been a sharp increase in the numbers of unaccompanied children seeking asylum in the United Kingdom, numbers having risen from 631 in 1996 to 5000 by April 2000, 80 per cent of whom were 16–17 years old (Audit Commission 2000). The United Nations High Commissioner for

Refugees defines unaccompanied children as 'those who are separated from both parents and are not being cared for by an adult who, by lay or custom, has the responsibility to do so' (United Nations High Commissioner for Refugees 1993). An estimated 2–3 per cent of all refugees are unaccompanied children, who have either been separated from their parents during mass population movements caused by war, or whose parents have been killed or have elected to send their children abroad to ensure their safety. Young unaccompanied asylum seekers and refugees therefore present a significant and growing challenge for policy makers and service providers.

The European Council on Refugees and Exiles maintain that young asylum seekers and refugee children should be granted the full rights of children and the full rights of refugees which are described in the *UN Convention on the rights of the child* and the UNHCR's 1994 *Guidelines on refugee children* (European Council for Refugees and Exiles (ECRE) 1996). They have the same needs for care education and support as any other child even though, in some cases, young people who have lived through conflict may have developed a high degree of maturity.

Like any other young person, the health of asylum-seeking children must be considered in a broad context. The social and economic background in which children find themselves has important implications for their health and well-being and will also influence the type of health and welfare services which they need (Hargreaves 1999). Young refugees and asylum seekers are also likely to have a range of specific needs relating to their experiences in their home countries, their circumstances of travel to this country as well as any underlying conditions for which they may not have received treatment.

Although the UK is a signatory to the *UN Convention on the rights of the child*, it reserved the right to apply this legislation in cases of immigration, a decision that has been widely challenged by both refugee organizations and children's charities. Young asylum seekers describe arrival in the United Kingdom as a traumatic process (Rutter 2001). Ports and airports are not well equipped to deal with young people who may not speak English, are unlikely to have a clear idea what will happen to them next, and who often have faced long and traumatic journeys to the UK. Local government social services in the area of the port of entry are responsible for collecting asylum seekers under the age of 18 from the port of arrival. Whilst some have put in place innovative solutions to support young arrivals, such as tapes in appropriate languages that can be played on the journey from the airport or port explaining what will happen to them next, other councils are finding it difficult to provide cover, particularly when children arrive at night. In some cases young people are left at their port of arrival until the following morning.

Age determination

Young asylum seekers may arrive in the UK with no or inadequate identification. Determining the age of an asylum seeker, and thereby determining what level of support he or she will receive, remains the responsibility of immigration officers. Home Office guidelines state that 'adjudicators tend to give the applicant the benefit of the doubt' and that there must be firm grounds for any decision to deny the age stated by the applicant. However, under the 1999 Asylum and Immigration Act, final responsibility for age determination rests with the Home Secretary.

Determining age remains an inexact science. Estimates, even those given by a paediatrician, have a margin of error of plus or minus five years. Guidelines issued jointly by the Royal College of Paediatricians and the King's Fund (Levenson and Sharma 1999) criticized the practice of using bone scans to determine age. Although this practice is now less common, some paediatricians have expressed concern that they are now not consulted in age disputes and that asylum determinations are made without reference to medical expertise.

Whilst young people generally suffer from the same conditions as adult asylum seekers, they have a number of specific needs. Young asylum seekers arriving from areas of chronic conflicts, such as Bosnia or Angola, may not be immunized. Lack of street knowledge may mean that young refugees, particularly those from rural areas, are at risk from road traffic injuries. Health promotion and surveillance services should be coordinated by geographical or practice based health visitors, liaising closely with school medical services (Levenson and Sharma 1999). Health professionals as well as young asylum seekers report a need to improve the availability of appropriate health education, particularly information on sexual health and drugs (Gosling 2000).

When such children arrive, they can apply for asylum at the port or in country. Referrals for children up to 17 years old are made to the Refugee Council, which has a panel of advisors. The advisor, who usually speaks their language then advises them through the asylum process, helping them to get access to schools, health services, etc. The social services, acting under the Children's Act, have to accommodate them in foster or children's homes and sometimes in bed and breakfast accommodation. Many of these children arrive alone and bewildered and are forced to make adult decisions before their time. Some find it very difficult to get over their distressing experiences and their experiences at school in the UK may also distress them. Many complain that because they do not speak good English, they are considered stupid and ignored, while some are bullied and accused of living on state subsidies. Because of their poor English when they first arrive, they are often put in classes with younger children, which adds to their anguish and isolation.

These children generally arrive in reasonably good health, but poor housing, poor nutrition, loneliness, uncertainties over their asylum claim and lack of emotional support have a detrimental effect on their health and well-being. In a survey carried out in south London, half the young asylum seeking children interviewed said that their health had deteriorated since arrival in the United Kingdom (Gosling 2000).

Women

Women are frequently the most seriously affected victims of exile and displacement, and women and girls make up an estimated 75 per cent of the world's refugee population. An estimated 50 per cent of women claiming asylum in Britain have been raped, according to the UNHCR London office. In exile, women are vulnerable to physical assault, domestic violence, sexual harassment and rape and their experiences and fears have tended not to be taken seriously (Wallace 1990). They need to be offered sensitive sexual health care and coun-selling, screening and health promotion advice as well as maternity care. As refugees, many have to assume responsibility as sole bread winner and head of family in households where the men may be absent or, if present, are unable to assume their responsibilities due to stress or loss of status and self-esteem.

Obstacles to accessing health services

The delivery of health services is designed for people who understand the health system, live in permanent accommodation, and who are able to com-municate their needs in English. In order for people to use health services, they need to know where those services are and how to use them. Refugees and asylum seekers often receive poor health care in the United Kingdom, despite their entitlement to free NHS treatment (Audit Commission 2000).

Refugees are expected to find their way through an unfamiliar health system. If they find a general practitioner, they may have problems commun-icating their needs without an interpreter, and some general practitioners are unwilling to use interpreting services, which are often provided by health authorities at no cost to the practice, although provision of interpreting serv-ices is often patchy. Many asylum seekers are unaware that they are entitled to register with a general practitioner, and are therefore dependent on others to advise them on how to find a general practitioner. Asylum seekers' eligibility to health services is often questioned before they can access these services.

General practitioners are often reluctant to register asylum seekers because they may think that homeless people and people placed in temporary accom-modation will soon move on. They may also think that asylum seekers and refugees make for a time-consuming workload due to their greater psychological and physical needs. Some feel that they lack the skills and support to cater for asylum seekers' and refugees' health needs.

Cultural differences may pose some problems too. Asylum seekers and refugees often find it difficult to approach strangers with their problems. They may be less prepared to discuss physical complaints or emotional problems outside their family. They may therefore only contact a health professional once the health problem has become acute. If they have experienced violence and torture they may feel very frightened and distrustful of people in an official capacity, including health workers. Confidentiality and trust are therefore critical.

Refugees and asylum seekers may fear that consultations will not be confidential. The confidential nature of the doctor-patient relationship, and the relationship with others in the primary health care team, are not always clearly explained. Trust builds up quite slowly. Many may fear that the doctor will give information about their physical or mental health to the Home Office or to other government departments, and that this will jeopardize their chances of being allowed to stay in the UK. A study in South London in 1994 found that 4 per cent of refugees believed that their general practitioner worked for the Home Office (Grant and Deane 1995).

Increased risk of hostility and discrimination is a major hurdle for refugees and asylum seekers. The negative portrayal of asylum seekers in some sections of the media and by some politicians is reflected in the attitudes of the health professionals. These create unnecessary barriers to access.

Funding health services for asylum seekers and refugees

The Primary Care Trust or the Strategic Health Authority in the area where the patient is resident is responsible for funding the medical treatment provided by a general practitioner, a hospital, or any other NHS facility. There is no special funding from the Home Office or any other statutory body for asylum seekers or refugees. However, the Department of Health has set out a model of a Local Development Scheme for general practitioners and other primary care providers, which allows access to additional funds in recognition of the increased workload (Audit Commission 2000).

Managing health needs

Asylum seekers are not a homogeneous population. Their health status varies according to the areas and countries from which they come, their experiences pre exile, the circumstances of their journeys and their experiences post exile. Many undertake arduous routes to the UK, travelling in cramped lorries or boats, having to consume rotting and contaminated food and water. Some asylum seekers come from countries where the health care system is well developed whereas others come from areas with poor health systems. Again others, the Roma gypsies of Eastern Europe being a case in point, have been excluded from accessing their country's health care system on discriminatory grounds. Their experiences in the UK post exile can further aggravate their health as they face hostility, poverty, poor housing and social isolation.

Many of the health problems experienced by refugees are not necessarily specific to them but may also be shared with deprived or excluded groups or other new entrants to the country. Whilst the health status of many refugees and asylum seekers is generally good (Mathews 2001), some experience particular health problems including tropical and infectious diseases such as malaria and hepatitis B or C. Some groups may also have a high incidence of tuberculosis or HIV/AIDS. Earlier studies have found that 'one in six refugees has a physical health problem severe enough to affect their life and two-thirds have experienced anxiety or depression' (Burnett and Peel 2001).

An area that requires particular attention is immunization. Most children and adults are incompletely immunized (Le Fevre 2000) and do not have a clear history of their vaccination. Again this varies from country to country. The World Health Organization websites give a useful country by country summary of immunization schedules.

In 1998, the then Health Education Authority in a report of the expert working group on refugee health made a series of recommendations to promote the health of refugees and asylum seekers (Health Education Authority 1998). These include:

- The provision of written information, in an appropriate language, about the structure and routes of access to NHS;
- The introduction of client-held records for newly arrived refugees;
- Encouraging general practitioners to offer permanent registration to refugees;
- Improving the quality of interpreting services;
- The establishment of multidisciplinary primary health care teams to deal with the health needs of newly arrived asylum seekers and refugees;
- The development of a guide for clinicians and health authorities on refugee health needs;
- Development of cross-cultural programmes at undergraduate and postgraduate level;
- The provision of culturally sensitive services by female health workers for refugee women's obstetric and sexual health needs;
- The development of a culturally appropriate mental health strategy for refugees based on a multi-agency approach.

Refugees and asylum seekers are not a homogeneous group: also, they and their health needs are liable to change over time depending on their context and experiences. However, any model of service provision has to ensure non-discriminatory services that promote equity of access and facilitate independence supported by well coordinated health and social care partnerships. The key areas that require to be addressed are access, communication and advocacy, needs assessment, mental health and training.

Access

The ignorance of refugees and asylum seekers about NHS structures and services and the ignorance of NHS staff about entitlements and rights of refugees and asylum seekers, coupled with the prejudices of health professionals, often create unnecessary barriers. Asylum seekers, refugees and those with Exceptional Leave to Remain have full entitlement to NHS care, both primary and secondary. Yet many experience problems in registering with a general practitioner (Fassil 2000). Refugees have often described their desperate search for general practitioners, finding some practices reluctant to register them because of high workload. Many end up in hospital emergency departments. There is also an uneven distribution of refugees between practices, with some practices taking on a much higher proportion of refugees.

Refugees should be offered permanent registration, with information about how the NHS works, which will enable ongoing care and access to health promotion and preventative services, including physiotherapy, dental and pharmaceutical services. Continuity of care is a factor particularly for sensitive consultations such as rape, torture or mental health problems.

Screening and assessment

Initial health screening should focus on communicable diseases such as tuberculosis (TB), HIV, and hepatitis B, followed by a comprehensive health assessment that should address the needs of the individual and not just see the individual as a source of contagion. Some asylum seekers are screened for TB at the port of entry to the United Kingdom but most require a further assessment. This will enable the system to provide information, advice and support to those in need, especially those who are suffering from trauma and psychological distress. Many refugees and asylum seekers will not have been immunized against the common communicable diseases and vaccination should be offered as soon as possible.

Communication and language support

The inability to speak English poses the biggest problem when working with recently arrived asylum seekers. Language and cultural barriers add to the natural reluctance to speak about their experiences (Jones and Gill 1998). Services should ensure that, wherever possible, interpreters or trained advocates are used during consultation. Out of sheer necessity, some professionals use family members as interpreters, but using family members or children can be inappropriate and may result in inaccurate interpretation or incomplete information, especially when sensitive issues need to be discussed.

Interpreters need to be trained and supervised. Establishing trust is crucial to the relationship. For the asylum seeker, it is essential that they trust and feel safe enough to disclose intimate information, especially in cases of torture or rape. In situations where interpreters are not available, then telephone interpreting can provide a limited, but useful alternative.

Mental health

Not all asylum seekers and refugees suffer from mental health problems. Many have shown incredible resourcefulness and resilience in their flight to safety. However, their experiences pre-asylum and post exile can generate mental health problems. The pre-flight experience may include oppression, imprisonment, violence, conflict and abuse. People who have been tortured or caught up in war may have seen their family members killed or tortured and their needs will relate to that loss and bereavement. In escaping persecution, they may undertake hazardous journeys across borders, suffer from hunger and exhaustion, and may experience constant fear and anxiety of being discovered or killed. The example of families attempting to enter the UK hanging on to channel tunnel trains illustrates their desperate and dangerous journey.

People who have been subjected to torture or have seen their family and friends tortured will require specialist support. It is well documented that many survivors of torture are initially reluctant to disclose their experiences until they begin to feel safe and secure and trust the professionals they encounter (Burnett and Peel 2001; Summerfield 1995). Referrals to appropriate clinical help are critical. In addition to clinical expertise, torture victims also need the social and community support from their communities in order to recover and re-experience the feelings of belonging and independence. Helen Bamber, director of the Medical Foundation for the Care of Victims of Torture, describes torture as 'the act of killing a man without his dying. The perpetrator has total power; the victim is totally helpless. Being subjected to such an experience destroys the integrity of body and mind' (Bamber 2000).

Training health care professionals

Many health professionals often do not know how best to support the needs of refugees. They feel overwhelmed by their experiences and resulting health needs; some are unable to give the time needed to manage their health needs and become frustrated by the seemingly unrealistic expectations. Some refugees become demanding and dependent on the professionals. Primary care services are crucial and yet many general practitioners are confused about the entitlements of refugees and offer only temporary registration leading to fragmented patterns of care.

All health care professionals should have access to training and ongoing support, and this training should include:

◆ knowledge of the refugee situation, where they come from and their circumstances;

◆ some knowledge of cultural differences;

◆ knowledge of the entitlements and rights of refugees;

◆ working with interpreters;

◆ knowledge of specialist services;

◆ assessment of mental health problems.

The current provision of health services

Many NHS organizations, especially in London, have made attempts to improve access to health services for refugees in their areas. However, many claim that they need additional resources to meet the needs of newly arrived asylum seekers. With the present national shortage of general practitioners, especially in urban and deprived areas, where many asylum seekers are dispersed, many lists are closed. Others blame the shortage of resources on asylum seekers.

Many trusts have set up refugee-specific initiatives in primary care (see below), however, it is important that these complement mainstream services rather than operating as a parallel health system. If services for asylum seekers are perceived to be better than those for the local community this can generate resentment and hostility. Where a separate service is established it has the advantage of being able to provide more specialized support, including dedicated language support, longer appointments and a more comprehensive assessment. Ultimately, however, the aim should be to integrate people into local health services. In some areas, such as Newham in East London, asylum seekers register initially with a designated practice specializing in their needs and, after a period of 12–18 months, are expected to register with another local practice. It has been reported that practices are keener to take on asylum seekers who have had thorough health checks and an assessment of their needs.

The government is keen to promote flexible contracts for general practitioners and encourages them to develop innovative models of care and services appropriate for local need and circumstances. The 1997 NHS (Primary Care)

Act provided the catalyst for change. The new legislation allowed new providers such as individual nurses, acute trusts and community trusts to get involved in the provision of primary medical care services (Lewis and Gillam 1999). Allowing primary care practices to opt out of the national contract and enter into local contracts opens up a host of opportunities to develop appropriate services for groups such as asylum seekers and refugees. Some of the models piloted are listed below.

Personal medical services

These have been created as pilot practices to develop new approaches to primary care. The intention is that the new pilots will be able to respond better to the needs of their local communities by offering specialist services and working with multidisciplinary teams. Many have chosen to address the specific needs of marginalized populations such as refugees, asylum seekers and the homeless (Jenkins 1999).

Salaried general practitioners

In areas with relatively high density of refugee populations, a primary care service is established specifically for this group using general practitioners paid salaries (rather than the usual model of independent contractor). For example, in east Kent, the general practitioners running such a service found that through using a positive non-judgemental approach, they found refugees willing to communicate and use their services, even without interpreters (Montgomery et al. 2000).

Local development scheme

These allow general practitioners flexibility to improve the responsiveness of general medical services to local need. The schemes allow funds to be transferred from secondary care budgets to be used for specific primary care services provided by practices working to the national contract. The additional funding is used to meet more complex needs of patients by allowing longer consultation times. This model can be used to encourage primary care teams to provide services to asylum seekers and refugees without suffering financial penalties.

Walk-in centres

These have been set up in some areas for emergency care and have the advantage of not requiring registration. Whilst they are good for emergencies, they are not a good option for long-term care.

NHS Direct

Launched in 1998, NHS Direct is a nationwide 24 hour nurse-led advice and health information service that provides a valuable access point for health advice. Interpreters are available for people who do not have a good command of the English language. The intention is that this service will encourage self-reliance and self care.

Refugee community organizations

Many of these organizations are willing and able to work with the health system in meeting the specific needs of newly arrived asylum seekers and refugees. Many communities have organized themselves to provide health advocacy services that inform refugees about health matters and refer them to appropriate health services. The Tamil Relief Centre in Edmonton, in north London, for example, employs a women and children's health worker whose role is to educate and inform both women and local health professionals. Several London health authorities and trusts have set up specialist services to meet refugees' needs. Camden and Islington Community Health Trust, for instance, has a stress trauma clinic for Bosnian refugees who have experienced atrocities in their former homes.

Conclusion

The twentieth century experience has shown that no one is safe from becoming a refugee. The UK has provided sanctuary to less than 2 per cent of the world's refugees and it is developing countries that continue to bear the greatest burden in giving sanctuary to refugees. Understanding why refugees seek exile and the importance of giving sanctuary and protection is a key moral and human rights requirement. All people fleeing persecution should be given the opportunity to reclaim a future.

The challenges of meeting the needs of refugees and asylum seekers in the UK have been reflected by changes in Government legislation. By the end of 2002 there will have been four major pieces of asylum legislation in less than a decade. A sense of panic dominates the political debate about asylum and immigration both in the UK and in other parts of Europe. In the Refugee Council's press release in June 2002, Nick Hardwick, its Chief Executive, said:

> The lack of political leadership to foster confidence in the asylum system has fuelled public insecurities about Europe's capacity to shape and manage a coherent migration and asylum policy. Unless EU governments show true commitment to fulfil our obligation to provide protection to refugees and share our global responsibility then I believe we will look back on this period of our history with shame.

Asylum seekers and refugees have particular health needs that frequently reflect the traumas they experienced in their countries of origin, the difficult journeys they may have made, and the exclusion they experience on arrival in the UK. Many of their health problems are linked to the atrocities experienced in their own countries, prior to exile, such as physical trauma and injuries through torture, mental health problems including post-traumatic stress syndrome, nutritional deficiencies and infection. In exile, they suffer from separation and loss of family and friends, community and cultural reference points. Homesickness coupled with anxiety and guilt about those they have left behind create further stresses which are compounded by lengthy asylum procedures, fear of deportation, poverty and hostility from the host society.

Health professionals will need training and support in order to meet the needs of these groups. An important component of this support includes information on the entitlements of refugees and asylum seekers to NHS services and an understanding of why people become refugees and the circumstances which they have come from. The current organizational changes within the NHS offer new opportunities for meeting the challenges in managing the health and social care needs of asylum seekers and refugees and provide lessons for those facing similar challenges in other countries.

References

Audit Commission (2000) *Another country: implementing dispersal under the Immigration and Asylum Act 1999.* Audit Commission, Oxford.

Bamber, H. (2000) *Working effectively with victims of torture in St George's House consultation report on asylum seekers in Britain – responding to the challenge.* St George's House Trust, London.

Berger, J. (1992) *Keeping a rendezvous.* Granta Books, London.

Bouquet, T. and Moller, D. (2000) *Are we a tolerant nation?* Reader's Digest, London.

Burnett, A. and Peel, M. (2001) Health needs of asylum seekers and refugees. *British Medical Journal,* **322,** 544–7.

European Council for Refugees and Exiles (ECRE) (1996) *Position on refugee children.* European Council for Refugees and Exiles. www.ecre.org

Fassil, Y. (2000) Looking after the health of refugees. *British Medical Journal,* **321,** 59.

Gosling, R. (2000) *A survey of the health needs of young asylum seekers in Lambeth, Southwark and Lewisham.* Lambeth, Southwark, Lewisham, Health Action Zone, London.

Grant, C. and Deane, J. (1995) *Stating the obvious – factors which influence uptake and provision of primary health services for refugees.* Lambeth, Southwark, Lewisham, Health Commission, London.

Hargreaves, S. (1999) *Child health in London: the health and social characteristics of London's children.* Health of Londoners' Project, London.

Health Education Authority (1998) *Promoting the health of refugees: a report of the health education authority's expert working group on refugee health.* The Inkwell Company, London.

Home Office (1999) *Immigration and asylum act 1999*. The Stationery Office, Norwich.

Home Office (2002) *Secure borders, safe haven: integration with diversity in modern Britain*. The Stationery Office, Norwich.

Jenkins, C. (1999) Personal medical services pilots – new opportunities. In R. Lewis and S. Gillam (eds) *Transforming primary care*. King's Fund, London.

Jones, D. and Gill, P. S. (1998) Refugees and primary care: tackling the inequalities. *British Medical Journal*, 317, 1444–6.

Le Fevre, P. (2000) Personal communication.

Levenson, R. and Sharma, A. (1999) *The health of refugee children: guidelines for paediatricians*. King's Fund and the Royal College of Paediatrics and Child Health, London.

Lewis, R. and Gillam, S. (1999) *Transforming primary care*. King's Fund, London.

Mathews, P. (2001) Preventative healthcare for asylum seekers. Seminar paper presented at Kings Fund. King's Fund, London.

Montgomery *et al.* (2000) Health care for asylum seekers. *British Medical Journal*, 321, 893.

MORI Social Research Institute (2002) *Attitudes towards refugees and asylum seekers: A survey of Public opinion*. www.refugeecouncil.org.uk

Penrose, J. (2002) *Poverty and asylum in the UK*. Oxfam and the Refugee Council, UK.

Refugee Council (2002) Parliamentary briefing: Nationality, Immigration and Asylum Bill 24 June.

Rutter, J. (2001) *Supporting refugee children in twenty-first century Britain*. Trentham Books, Stoke on Trent.

Summerfield, D. (1995) Addressing human response to war and atrocity. In R. Kleber, C. Figely and B. Gersons (eds) *Beyond trauma*. Plenum, New York.

United Nations High Commissioner for Refugees (1951) *Convention relating to the status of refugees*. United Nations High Commissioner for Refugees, Geneva.

United Nations High Commissioner for Refugees (1993) *Guidelines on refugee children*. United Nations High Commissioner for Refugees, Geneva.

Wallace, T. (1990) *Refugee women: their perspectives and our responses*. Oxfam, Oxford.

Chapter 12

Multicultural Health Care in Britain

Rory Williams and Seeromanie Harding

Recognition of cultural groups in Britain

It is a political question whether a modern state will recognize the existence of groups whose ancestry, religion, culture, language or customs differ. Thus an account of the extent to which health care is multicultural must begin with a brief synopsis of which groups are, or have been, recognized by the state concerned.

At the beginning of the nineteenth century, the British state's aspiration was to unify its citizens within a single culture. At that point, Britain was the 'British Isles', a union of England, Wales, Scotland and (from 1800) Ireland. As the nineteenth century wore on, however, the union began to prove fragile. The Great Famine of 1845–9 devastated Ireland and West Scotland, but while relief was organized for West Scotland on a national British basis, Ireland was left to provide its own relief (Mokyr 1983). Similarly the Irish immigration, which rose to unprecedented levels as a result, was often seen as a population of different nationality, and in this way became the first modern ethnic minority to compel recognition by the British state. Agitation for Home Rule for Ireland, followed by the 'troubles' and the creation of the Irish Free State in 1922, and later the Irish Republic, finally exploded the unitary concept of the British Isles.

The numbers of migrant Irish steadily declined, however, through the rest of the nineteenth century and into the early twentieth, to a low point in the 1930s, and no statistics were thought necessary on the second and subsequent generations of this first wave of Irish migration. Instead, concern began to shift towards the Jewish immigration from Eastern Europe, which was set in motion by economic pressures and a series of pogroms from the 1880s onwards. The British response to this movement resulted in the state's first immigration legislation, the Aliens Act of 1905. However, the partially religious character of the Jewish minority, and the fact that it derived from minorities in various Eastern European countries, meant that information even about the migrant generation was not easily captured in country of birth statistics – and religion had been excluded from the British census since the religious census of 1851.

As these two minorities passed into their second and subsequent generations, therefore, they disappeared from official view and official concern, or (in the case of the Irish) were officially deemed to be assimilated for strategic reasons (Hickman 1998).

By the end of the 1950s, however, the state had to recognize new minorities, mainly from the Caribbean, India and Pakistan. Race riots were amongst the factors that stimulated successive governments into sweeping legislation to control immigration from what became known as the New Commonwealth, beginning with the Immigration Act of 1962. The years following were the era of Powellism, when the fear was expressed, most notably through the speeches of the Conservative MP Enoch Powell, that British culture would be 'swamped' by the new arrivals. These repressive tendencies were to some extent gradually redressed by later efforts to control racial discrimination, beginning with the Race Relations Act of 1976. An assumption that ethnic minorities in Britain are always 'black' minorities grew out of the politics of this era. In 1981 an attempt to count this 'black' population through a question on ethnic group in the census, thus bringing in the second and subsequent generations, was sidelined by the declared mistrust of the groups concerned. In 1991, however, the advantages of such a question for these groups were acknowledged, and Black, Asian and Chinese minority ethnic groups became an official construct.

Reaction to the racialized dichotomy of 'black' and 'white' was a long time coming, and eventually emerged mainly from the second surge of Irish migration to England, which began after the Second World War and still continues. At an official level, little is still heard of the Jewish community as a minority presence, and much the same is true of minorities deriving from the population movements of the Second World War and earlier periods, such as the Poles and Italians. But the Irish and their advocates were able to use census data on country of birth of self and parents, collected for the first and only time in the census of 1971, to demonstrate the continuing deprivation and high mortality experienced by the Irish second generation (Harding and Balarajan 1996; Raftery et al. 1990). The Department of Health began to recognize the Irish as a minority of concern, and campaigns were then fought both in England and Scotland to ensure that they were recognized in the census of 2001.

In preparations for this same census of 2001, religious minorities also began to be recognized. In England, recognition was confined to the religions of New Commonwealth minorities; but in Scotland, following claims of continuing disadvantage among the Catholic minority (mainly Irish in the West of

Scotland) and of prejudice against them, a breakdown of Christian denominations was also introduced for the first time in 150 years (Walls 2001).

In Britain ethnic and religious minorities have emerged and submerged again, for reasons that are part of British political history, and there is no time at which more than a few potential minority candidates have been recognized. At present, recognition of minorities is more extensive than it has ever been, and coincides with devolution of aspects of government to Scotland and Wales, which has reversed three centuries of policy towards Scotland and more centuries still of policy towards Wales. Whether this movement will continue, or recede with another swing of the pendulum, remains to be seen.

Disease patterns among minority ethnic groups

Mortality and morbidity patterns of the largest minority ethnic groups currently recognized in the United Kingdom, mainly the Irish, South Asians and Caribbeans, are well documented. The most comprehensive of these descriptions is undoubtedly the decennial volume (Marmot et al. 1984), based on data from the 1971 census and mortality data around that census. This exercise was repeated using data from and around the subsequent decennial censuses (Balarajan and Bulusu 1990; Harding and Maxwell 1998). A major limitation of these data is that they refer only to migrant populations. Minority ethnic groups born in the UK cannot be identified in these data, as although ethnic origin has been collected in the last two censuses, it is not collected at death registration. National morbidity data relating to ethnicity are sparse and come mainly from The Fourth National Survey (Nazroo 1997). It is fairly simple to describe the morbidity and mortality patterns of these minority groups, but less so to discuss the causes of the differences in morbidity and mortality between these groups and the host population.

Disease profiles

Table 12.1 shows mortality for selected causes of death for migrant Scots, Irish, Indians, Pakistanis, Bangladeshis, Sri Lankans, Caribbeans, other Africans and East Africans, aged 20–69. The denominators were from the 1991 Census and the numerators from death registrations for the years 1989–93. Mortality varies among these groups. An often overlooked point, however, is that the main causes of death among these groups, for example coronary heart disease (CHD), strokes, diabetes, lung and breast cancers, are similar to that of the whole nation. For some groups these causes are associated with lower mortality relative to that for England and Wales (for example lung cancer

Table 12.1 Number of deaths, age-standardized rates~, for persons aged 20–69 years by sex, country of birth and selected causes, 1988–1992

	Males		Females	
	Deaths	**Rate**	**Deaths**	**Rate**
All causes (ICD 001–999)				
England and Wales	483363	607.47	300744	352.60
Scotland	12785	786.21	7562	469.38
All Ireland	17015	860.26	9298	423.07
India	5796	631.00	3216	366.60
Pakistan	2077	576.24	814	299.13
Bangladesh	1055	718.36	182	258.22
Caribbean Commonwealth	4012	528.03	2401	338.51
East Africa	1395	546.31	679	291.82
Other Commonwealth Africa	671	618.49	331	356.53
Malignant neoplasm of stomach (ICD 151)				
England and Wales	10538	13.18	4126	4.78
Scotland	246	14.85	107	6.75
All Ireland	362	17.63	161	7.27
India	59	6.32	19	2.16
Pakistan	15	4.37	8	2.10
Bangladesh	11	7.44	0	0.00
Caribbean Commonwealth	117	14.29	46	6.31
East Africa	12	5.33	6	1.30
Other Commonwealth Africa	7	6.36	6	4.53
Malignant neoplasm of colon (ICD 153)				
England and Wales	10777	13.60	9154	10.79
Scotland	282	16.98	229	14.40
All Ireland	380	18.48	307	13.81
India	58	6.23	56	6.30
Pakistan	14	3.93	8	1.91
Bangladesh	9	7.49	4	2.65
Caribbean Commonwealth	56	6.92	50	7.43
East Africa	17	6.52	6	4.60

Table 12.1 (Continued)

	Males		Females	
	Deaths	**Rate**	**Deaths**	**Rate**
Other Commonwealth Africa	9	7.77	4	4.95
Malignant neoplasm of trachea, bronchus and lung (ICD 162)				
England and Wales	52292	65.18	24166	27.99
Scotland	1632	99.43	761	46.45
All Ireland	2061	98.88	912	39.97
India	273	29.74	84	9.58
Pakistan	68	20.48	16	6.69
Bangladesh	76	55.12	9	15.87
Caribbean Commonwealth	269	32.74	67	9.28
East Africa	40	24.91	12	7.75
Other Commonwealth Africa	33	44.87	7	13.51
Malignant neoplasm of female breast (ICD 174)				
England and Wales			34432	43.28
Scotland			744	49.20
All Ireland			854	41.49
India			258	28.73
Pakistan			59	18.51
Bangladesh			6	6.43
Caribbean Commonwealth			257	34.23
East Africa			74	27.95
Other Commonwealth Africa			43	40.03
Malignant neoplasm of cervix uteri (ICD 180)				
England and Wales			5553	6.93
Scotland			152	10.41
All Ireland			180	9.12
India			67	7.83
Pakistan			6	1.41
Bangladesh			4	5.21
Caribbean Commonwealth			49	6.99

Table 12.1 (Continued)

	Males		Females	
	Deaths	**Rate**	**Deaths**	**Rate**
East Africa			12	5.17
Other Commonwealth Africa			5	5.03
Malignant neoplasm of prostate (ICD 185)				
England and Wales	8040	9.56		
Scotland	174	9.99		
All Ireland	234	10.55		
India	59	6.44		
Pakistan	6	2.12		
Bangladesh	3	1.35		
Caribbean Commonwealth	125	15.43		
East Africa	9	6.59		
Other Commonwealth Africa	12	19.41		
Diabetes mellitus (ICD 250)				
England and Wales	5226	6.55	4126	4.74
Scotland	105	6.43	68	4.14
All Ireland	111	5.27	79	3.44
India	185	19.99	144	16.57
Pakistan	93	28.32	45	21.94
Bangladesh	65	42.65	3	5.56
Caribbean Commonwealth	192	23.32	186	27.45
East Africa	34	17.60	14	9.84
Other Commonwealth Africa	18	20.30	5	6.00
Hypertensive disease (ICD 401–405)				
England and Wales	2748	3.44	1750	1.99
Scotland	54	3.31	38	2.22
All Ireland	106	5.10	49	2.02
India	52	5.60	30	3.46
Pakistan	13	3.73	10	4.67
Bangladesh	3	1.82	1	0.85

Table 12.1 (Continued)

	Males		Females	
	Deaths	**Rate**	**Deaths**	**Rate**
Caribbean Commonwealth	106	12.69	87	12.19
East Africa	10	5.36	4	1.56
Other Commonwealth Africa	20	21.62	11	14.73
Ischaemic heart disease (ICD 410–414)				
England and Wales	157336	198.71	55982	62.34
Scotland	3695	225.97	1306	77.47
All Ireland	5097	248.28	1730	73.72
India	2538	272.72	856	98.33
Pakistan	995	282.02	151	64.83
Bangladesh	427	291.53	27	49.24
Caribbean Commonwealth	819	100.01	307	43.72
East Africa	444	218.55	89	63.74
Other Commonwealth Africa	103	108.98	16	43.00
Cerebrovascular disease (ICD 430–438)				
England and Wales	27029	33.39	22065	25.05
Scotland	682	40.89	526	30.75
All Ireland	969	46.76	706	31.02
India	409	44.62	300	34.14
Pakistan	172	49.30	90	34.31
Bangladesh	122	88.46	22	32.13
Caribbean Commonwealth	477	59.80	282	40.04
East Africa	71	33.05	51	25.80
Other Commonwealth Africa	79	89.70	30	31.58
Bronchitis, chronic and unspecified, emphysema and asthma (ICD 490–493)				
England and Wales	8395	10.29	5645	6.53
Scotland	230	14.05	167	10.36
All Ireland	360	17.23	179	7.75
India	92	10.29	47	5.37
Pakistan	27	6.80	21	8.70

Table 12.1 (Continued)

	Males		Females	
	Deaths	**Rate**	**Deaths**	**Rate**
Bangladesh	19	16.24	4	2.98
Caribbean Commonwealth	53	6.97	28	3.60
East Africa	23	10.43	16	6.48
Other Commonwealth Africa	6	9.47	2	1.79
Chronic liver disease and cirrhosis (ICD 571)				
England and Wales	6213	8.25	4308	5.37
Scotland	331	21.04	208	14.21
All Ireland	389	21.06	261	13.12
India	205	21.51	31	3.45
Pakistan	34	9.53	9	2.77
Bangladesh	33	15.97	4	4.96
Caribbean Commonwealth	66	8.71	30	4.26
East Africa	71	21.51	4	1.43
Other Commonwealth Africa	6	4.25	5	5.99
Suicide & self-inflicted injury (ICD E950–E959)				
England and Wales	12553	16.05	3607	4.53
Scotland	312	20.44	86	5.92
All Ireland	280	19.02	95	5.18
India	140	18.14	60	6.68
Pakistan	31	5.98	10	1.75
Bangladesh	10	7.33	3	1.17
Caribbean Commonwealth	65	12.55	19	3.01
East Africa	69	14.60	30	7.25
Other Commonwealth Africa	21	8.71	7	5.18

~ Death rates directly standardized using age distribution of the European population.

among Indians), but all cancers account for about 40 per cent of all deaths within each group. This has major significance in terms of the planning and provision of health care. For example, low lung cancer death rates could lead to complacency among health care providers in terms of preventative care.

The pattern of cardiovascular (CVD) mortality differs between south Asians and black Caribbeans. A striking feature of south Asian mortality, whether Pakistani, Indian or Bangladeshi, is excess cardiovascular mortality including both coronary heart disease and stroke mortality, relative to the national average (Balarajan and Bulusu 1990; Marmot *et al.* 1984). Excess hypertensive, diabetes and end-stage renal failure mortality is also known (Cruickshank *et al.* 1991a; Raleigh 1997; Roderick *et al.* 1999). A paradoxical feature in the mortality (and prevalence) patterns of people of West African heritage is that mortality (and prevalence) from hypertension and diabetes is very high (Chaturvedi *et al.* 1993; Cruickshank *et al.* 2001a; Riste *et al.* 2001), as is the burden of these diseases in terms of stroke and end-stage renal failure, but mortality from CHD is low relative to the national average for England and Wales.

The Irish and Scots, on the other hand, have excess mortality from a range of causes – cardiovascular disease, various cancers, respiratory disease and accidents. The incidence of cancers, including lung, laryngeal and oesophageal cancers among the Irish and lung among the Scots, is also high in these populations (Harding and Rosato 1999). The Irish are the only group for which we have some knowledge of the health and mortality of their children (UK-born Irish with Irish-born parentage). Raised mortality has persisted in the second (parents born in Ireland) and third generations (grandparents born in Ireland but parents born in the UK) (Abbotts *et al.* 1998; Harding and Balarajan 2001; Harding and Balarajan 1996) as well as raised cancer incidence (Harding 1998) in spite of intergenerational improvements in socio-economic position (Harding and Balarajan 2001).

Other health concerns do not account for a large number of deaths but can, nevertheless, result in significant morbidity. Poor mental health in Black Caribbeans, and excess schizophrenia and psychotic conditions in particular, are well known regardless of whether they were born in the Caribbean or in the UK (Arai and Harding 2002; Bhugra *et al.* 1997; Harrison *et al.* 1997; Sharpley *et al.* 2001). High suicide death rates among South Asian women (Raleigh 1996) point to poor mental health in this population, but psychiatric morbidity rates appear to be low suggesting lack of sensitivity in the instruments used to measure such disorders. Sexual health among Black Caribbeans is also of concern. Rates of sexually transmitted diseases, such as gonorrhoeal, chlamydial and herpes simplex virus (HSV-2) infections are high in Black Caribbeans, some 10 times higher than for whites (Low *et al.* 2001). Age of coitarche (first sexual intercourse), a factor strongly associated with infections in Black Caribbean men, is lower. There is also a high prevalence of some autoimmune conditions, such as systemic lupus erythematosus, the cause of which is unknown (Johnson *et al.* 1995; Molokhia *et al.* 2001). The prevalence of human T-cell lymphoma/leukaemia virus type 1 is also high, transmitted both perinatally and sexually and leads uncommonly to two separate conditions – tropical spastic paraparesis and adult T-cell leukaemia/ lymphoma, (Cruickshank *et al.* 1991b; Hale *et al.* 1997; Nightingale *et al.* 1993). Haemoglobinopathies, attributed to genetic factors, such as sickle cell disease and thalassaemia, in people of West African and Middle Eastern ancestry are also well known but, as with auto-immune conditions, account for a small number of deaths.

Possible explanations for ethnic differences in outcomes

The cause of the specific excess chronic disease mortality in these groups is the focus of much research attempting to quantify the contribution from social and biological or genetic factors. Most agree that environmental and modifiable risk factors relating to social disadvantage, diet and lifestyle play an important role in understanding the specific patterns of chronic disease mortality and morbidity among ethnic groups. Social and economic disadvantage, as measured by labour market participation rates, occupational class and standard of living items, is greater among Pakistanis, Bangladeshis, Caribbeans and Irish than among the whole population in England and Wales (National Institute for Ethnic Studies in Health and Social Studies 1997; Berthoud 1999; Nazroo 1997).

The contribution of socio-economic disadvantage to ethnic differentials in health status has been under scrutiny since the 1970s. In the 1970s, occupational class was not consistently related to the mortality of South Asian or Caribbean migrants. Later work in the 1990s, however, showed an emergence of the conventional class morbidity and mortality gradients (Harding and Maxwell 1998; Nazroo 1997). Adjustment for differences in class distributions attenuated the specific patterns of excess mortality in the different groups, but did not remove the excess. For example, excess (relative to the national average) stroke mortality among migrant Caribbeans, in 1990–92, reduced from 69 to 46 per cent after adjustment for occupational class differences (Harding and Maxwell 1998). Among migrant Pakistanis, excess CHD reduced from 93 to 78 per cent after adjustment for class differences (Harding 2000). For the Irish, occupational class was a strong predictor of mortality differences within this group in the 1970s and 1990s and relative class differences appeared to widen. As with Caribbeans and South Asians, adjustment for class did not remove the excess mortality for these groups either. Interpreting class differentials in minority groups is problematic and a key issue relates to methods of measurement, including the residual excess mortality observed after adjustments for measurements such as occupational class. The limitations of uni-dimensional indicators (for example occupational class or access to cars) (Harding and Balarajan 2001; Nazroo 1997) the heterogeneity within classes (for example in each class Black Caribbeans earn less than their white counterparts (Nazroo 1997), the cultural sensitivity of certain measures (for example high house ownership among Indians is well known but so is overcrowding), the impact of persisting disadvantage (Harding and Balarajan 2001), social mobility, including significant upward mobility (Harding 2003), and the disruption of class chances after migration (Williams *et al.* 1998), are all implicated to some degree. A failure to appreciate these issues could lead to mistaken conclusions about the contribution of deprivation to ethnic differences in health.

Metabolic profiles differ among these groups. Cardiovascular disease in South Asians is associated with unfavourable lipid profiles – high low-density lipoproteins (LDL), low high-density lipoproteins (HDL) and high triglycerides (McKeigue *et al.* 1991). In contrast, Black Caribbeans and black Africans have low LDL, high HDL and low triglycerides and low plasma fibrinogen (Cappuccio *et al.* 1997; Whitty *et al.* 1999). Very little is known about metabolic risk factors for the Irish. There are differences in body size; the prevalence of obesity is greater for South Asians and Black Caribbeans (particularly women) compared with same aged white men and women (Cappuccio *et al.* 1997) reflecting differences in energy intake and energy expenditure/ physical exercise. Differences in nutritional intake and energy balance at different phases of the lifespan are thought to be a major contributor to differences in diabetes rates based on proportions of known 'cases' and also on the impact of small shifts in blood sugar distributions used to define type 2 diabetes (Cruickshank *et al.* 1991a; Landman and Cruickshank 2001). The prevalence of smoking, a major risk factor for CVD, is lower among Indians and Pakistanis, higher among Bangladeshis and Irish people, and the same among Black Caribbeans compared with whites (Department of Health and National Institute for Ethnic Studies in Health and Social Policy 2000). Alcohol consumption has a complicated relationship with vascular outcomes, being protective if consumption is mild to moderate but harmful if excessive. With the exception of the Irish, alcohol consumption is lower in these groups compared with whites. Another behavioural factor that would influence health outcomes concerns health care, access, use and quality of health care, and the empirical evidence is discussed below.

Growth *in utero* and in childhood has been consistently related to chronic diseases in later life (Barker 1998) and there is a growing support for the use of this approach to understand ethnic differences in chronic disease patterns. Caribbean and South Asian babies are lighter than those born to UK-born mothers (Office for National Statistics 2000). The importance of early growth was demonstrated in a study of Jamaican school children aged 15 years, in which blood pressure and the propensity of diabetes by the level of glycosylated haemoglobin was inversely related to birth weight and crown to heel length (Forrester *et al.* 1996). The findings of the migration studies, however, argue against an interpretation based on genomic variation. In a study of genetically similar populations of West African descent in rural and urban Cameroon, the Caribbean and in the UK, there were clear differences in blood pressure, fasting glucose levels and body mass index (BMI) between these sites, with those in rural Cameroon at the lower end and those in Manchester at the higher end; (Cruickshank *et al.* 2001a,b; Mbanya *et al.* 1999). There were also differences in dietary intake and exercise with Black Caribbeans in Manchester having higher energy foods and more sedentary life style than people in rural Cameroon (Mennen *et al.* 2000, 2001). These findings would support a model of non-genetic intergenerational transfer of risk that leads to differences in vascular and other organ development. (Cruickshank *et al.* 2001a,b). Clearly growth is important, but it is not yet understood how this interacts with later growth and risk factors acquired only in adulthood to produce different outcomes in ethnic groups.

There are no known studies in which risk factors or health status were measured before and after migration. There are a few studies of migrants in their new environments compared with that of those left behind. For example, in a study of the Luo people in Kenya (Poulter *et al.* 1985), blood pressure was higher in those who had moved from rural to urban areas compared with that of those who had been left behind. This shift was thought to be linked to higher salt intake. In the Tokalau island study (Finau *et al.* 1982) those who had settled in New Zealand after evacuation from the island following a hurricane had higher blood pressure and more diabetes than those who had not moved. These findings would add further support for an environmental role in the aetiology of these diseases.

Many polymorphic genetic variants have now been found both within and between different ethnic groups. Many studies in the 1990s attempted to link disease outcomes to variants in these 'candidate genes' including for hypertension, diabetes and coronary heart disease, in mental health for schizophrenia and depression, in bone disease for osteoporosis and for many other chronic diseases. An interesting and popular concept has been that based on the thrifty genotype hypothesis. Neel (1962) proposed that individuals with a gene or genes that increased the ability to conserve and store food energy in times of plenty would survive recurrent periods of near famine better than those without such a gene. However, when food supplies became more universally plentiful so that obesity becomes frequent, those with such genes would develop diabetes more frequently than those without the gene(s). As yet, no such gene or genes have been isolated and an alternative concept, much more amenable to social and other environmental pressures, is that of the thrifty phenotype (Hales and Barker 1992), which emerged from Barker's hypothesis of intrauterine origins of adult disease. Here, developing foetuses of poorly nourished mothers or those with poor placental nutrient supplies during pregnancy adapt by growth restraints in less vital organs than the brain. Specific organ development, such as the islet cells of the pancreas which make insulin, may be permanently impaired. After birth and during later growth, particularly if obesity occurs, vascular beds and other organ function are still constrained which leads to maladaptive changes leading to disease (e.g. hypertension, poor or inadequate insulin secretion leading to diabetes, or poor bone mass). Both these versions of the nature–nurture debate are under intensive biomedical investigation, but the thrifty phenotype hypothesis and its variants offer a powerful pathway for intergenerational, non-genetic transmission of disease risk to occur.

In summary, there is a large body of evidence about the patterns of diseases among ethnic groups but less is known about the cause of the specific patterns. The shift in research focus towards social and biological conditions in early life, childhood and over the life course is promising. An important gap in knowledge concerns the health of UK-born minority groups. The conventional wisdom from epidemiological studies (Haenszel and Kurihara 1968; Syme et al. 1975), is that we should see a shift in disease patterns towards that of the host population. The evidence on lifestyle patterns such as smoking, (National Institute for Ethnic Studies in Health and Social Policy 1997; Nazroo 1997) and dietary patterns (Sharma et al. 1999), though incomplete, suggests that this may be the case for Black Caribbeans and South Asians. The Irish, however, appear to be a counter example to the convergence hypothesis, in that the death rates of those born in England and Wales do not appear to be converging towards that of the national population.

Access: use or quality of health care?

Ethnic differences in mortality could reflect differences in survival, in morbidity or both. Studies in the United States have shown potential barriers at various stages of the pathways to quality care, which could contribute to the high cardiovascular related mortality of African Americans through differential survival. In the UK, our knowledge about the health of minority ethnic populations has grown in recent years, but knowledge about access to health and other care in minority groups is less developed, and what there is suffers from methodological limitations, making interpretation difficult. A consideration of the health needs of minority groups did not begin until the late 1970s, (McFarland *et al.* 1987; McNaught 1985, 1988). Much of this research examines access and utilization issues and patient/provider interactions, such as health seeking behaviour, frequency of use, satisfaction and cultural appropriateness of services. There are few studies that examine the *quality of medical management*, that is, type of treatment at the primary and secondary level including referral patterns to specialist care.

There are consistent themes regarding perceived barriers to access and health seeking behaviour that are noteworthy, despite methodological problems concerning the inability to adjust for need/level of morbidity or differences in socio-economic circumstances. South Asians appear to use primary health services more than whites (Chaturvedi *et al.* 1997) but they appear to report higher dissatisfaction in relation to lack of access to female doctors, language barriers or in relation to white ethnicity staff in primary care reception areas (Campbell *et al.* 2001). Linguistic difficulties appear to be less for younger South Asians but the elderly continue to use relatives as interpreters, reflecting some level of unmet need (Ebden *et al.* 1988; Free *et al.* 1999). Link workers are used to address difficulties with communication in some areas and are thought to be successful. For example, in the Hackney Multi-ethnic Women's Health Project, this advocacy approach was thought to result in a reduction in caesarian rates, rates of induction and changes in length of antenatal stay (Ahmad 1993).

Black Caribbeans use the services less than expected, report high levels of mistrust for doctors (particularly Black Caribbean men), and often seek private health care (Donovan 1996; Scott 1998). There is high usage of natural remedies, such as bush teas, evening primrose oil and laxatives, and non-compliance with prescribed medication may be related to the poor management of conditions such as hypertension, diabetes and sickle cell disease (Ahmad 2000; Cappuccio *et al.* 1997; Scott 1998; Shaw *et al.* 1999). Adherence to prescribed drugs among Black Caribbeans is influenced by traditional beliefs concerning long-term harmful effects of drugs and religious beliefs, but also by lack of communication between Black Caribbeans and their GPs. Scott (1998) argues that most practitioners are concerned with clinical features of conditions rather than with the health beliefs and practices of this group.

Cultural and education issues are also implicated for Asian asthmatic patients. They have an increased risk of admission to hospitals with poor self management associated with passive control and lack of understanding of the role of drugs in the management of asthma (Griffiths *et al.* 2001; Moudgil and Honeybourne 1998). The evidence on high usage of home remedies is consistent but generally their health impact has not been assessed (Chen 1999).

Studies focusing on specific conditions have provided some information about differences in referral patterns and in severity of disease at presentation. Black Caribbeans with schizophrenia are more likely than whites to be admitted to services via a police station with little involvement from a General Practitioner (GP), and more frequently under a section of the Mental Health Act (Davies *et al.* 1996; McGovern and Cope 1991; Singh *et al.* 1998; Thomas *et al.* 1993). The reasons for higher compulsory admission rates in this group are not clear. Prejudicial stereotyping by the police and mental health practitioners (Lewis *et al.* 1990), an increase in severity of illness because of delay in seeking treatment, poor compliance with medicines, and social isolation have been considered likely factors (Davies *et al.* 1996). Differential routes of referral to mental health services also apply to black children with psychosomatic and medical illness, Black children being more likely than White children to be referred by education services and mixed race children by social services (Daryanani *et al.* 2001).

Other work suggests that there may be inequity at the referral level from GPs (Cooper *et al.* 1998; Smaje and Le Grand 1997). For example, there is high use of primary care services but low use of secondary care services by minority children and young people. Whites are more likely than Indians to attend hospital diabetes clinics and also GP clinics, which is at odds with the higher rates of diabetes and diabetic mortality in Indians (Goyder and Botha 2000). Asians are more likely to receive renal replacement therapy because of end stage renal failure associated with diabetes (Roderick *et al.* 1996, 1999). This could reflect poor control of diabetes and associated high blood pressure, but whether this is due to health seeking behaviour at the individual level or organizational issues of poor access to specialist care remain unclear. Retinopathy can result from diabetes and late presentation at services is a significant risk factor for blindness. Black Caribbean patients are over four times more likely (South Asians, 22 per cent) to present with advanced loss of vision than whites after adjusting for referral source (Fraser *et al.* 1999). South Asians also have a greater risk of coronary disease than whites but appear to wait twice as long for coronary angiography (Shaukat *et al.* 1993), although referral bias was not thought to be major problem. Diagnosis of heart attacks in South Asians might be missed since they are less likely to present with classic symptoms

(Lear *et al.* 1994). A recent study of invasive management of coronary disease, however, found no differences in clinical presentation, previous investigations and interventions between South Asians and whites who had coronary angioplasty and coronary artery bypass grafting but South Asians were more likely to be younger, male and non-obese (Feder *et al.* 2002). Whites were more likely to be given a follow-up appointment after leaving the GP surgery and also to be referred for home visiting than Caribbeans and Irish (Gillam *et al.* 1989).

Ethnic minorities tend to live in poor urban areas and often face the prospect of seeking care in facilities with fewer resources. Structural and organizational issues could limit access to quality care. For example, the uptake of cervical screening in deprived areas (and where there are large proportions of minority ethnic populations) is low (Majeed *et al.* 1994). GPs are unevenly distributed across England and some areas do not have enough GPs for the needs of their population (Benzeval and Judge 1996). We know that higher levels of satisfaction are reported if the ethnic origin of the patient is concordant with that of the provider of services, but little is known about whether or not this means that they receive a high quality of care. An earlier study noted that the GPs of Asian mothers were less likely to be qualified obstetricians (as they were not on the Royal College of Obstetricians and Gynaecologist obstetric list) than the GPs of white mothers, which has been associated with poorer perinatal outcomes (Clarke and Clayton 1983). Some suggest that discrimination in the health care setting might also compromise the quality of care, (Ahmad and Atkin 2000; Anionwu and Atkin 2001; McNaught 1988; Webb 2000). This is particularly relevant to haemoglobinopathies, such as sickle cell anaemia, which could be seen as a 'black disease', with health professionals attributing illnesses to some aspect of culture (Maxwell *et al.* 1999).

In summary, the empirical evidence on access to health care among minorities is patchy but there is sufficient basis to be concerned about the cultural appropriateness of health care provision, whether or not there is equitable access to quality care, and whether or not these issues impact on health outcomes.

How effective and efficient are health services to ethnic minorities in Britain?

There are serious problems in addressing this question. At the broadest level, something might have been gleaned from progress against the ten-year targets set by the United Kingdom Government in *The health of the nation* (Department of Health 1992) but no specific targets were set for ethnic minorities. More informative have been analyses of change in mortality among ethnic groups around the decennial census for England and Wales, where analyses were more extensive on the 1979–83 data compared with the previous decade (Balarajan and Bulusu 1990). At this time, the greatest improvements in all-cause mortality were observed for African and Caribbean groups, who on the whole had had the highest mortality in 1970–72, and the smallest improvements were observed among Scots and Irish, who were not far behind in 1970–72 and had the highest mortality by 1979–83. Groups from the Indian subcontinent were intermediate in mortality at both census points and in their improvement in between. These were surprising results in terms of the common assumption at the time that Black and Asian groups were faring worst in the British environment, but whether the causes lay in the social environment or in aspects of health care could not be ascertained.

In order to be more specific about the effectiveness of health services, intervention studies among ethnic minority populations are needed, but the Independent Inquiry into Inequalities in Health found a dearth of these (Acheson 1998). Research in this area has continued to be concerned with the logically prior task of identifying what factors are responsible for health variations among ethnic minorities, and has barely begun to try to control and influence these factors. Nevertheless, some records of past interventions have been made and some suggestions for the future noted, for instance in the area of diet and nutrition (Bush *et al.* 1997).

A serious obstacle to effectiveness, however, is the existence of the 'inverse care law' – that those who have the greatest needs receive the least and poorest services. Originally coined to reflect the fact that the poor often received the worst services in Britain, the term has also been applied to the situation of ethnic minorities, many of whose members are relatively poor and live in areas with a historically poor supply of services. These minorities also have additional needs, such as for interpreters, and encounter services that are less able to provide a high quality of care; for example, as we noted in the last section, general practices with less experience of obstetric training.

The plight of such areas is not generally counteracted by separate services provided for or run by particular racial, cultural or religious groups. There are exceptions in particular contexts, such as day centres for the elderly – an age group where adaptation to multicultural norms is likely to be slowest – but the overall thrust of the NHS and social services is firmly towards a single public service that is responsive to the whole range of groups. In so far as counteracting strategies have been undertaken, these have usually been in the form of campaigns for greater access to mainstream services, for example, by sufferers from sickle cell or thalassaemia, children with rickets, mothers and babies etc.

The efficiency of services to ethnic minorities is still harder to assess, but the tiny proportion of the national budget allotted to their needs makes any assessment somewhat superfluous.

The nature of health claims by racial, cultural or religious groups on the British state

From the British state's perspective, the health claims of racial, cultural or religious groups were initially seen in terms of threats that they were thought to pose to the established home population. This was true of the Irish and Jewish immigrations; and similarly, the health education literature designed for New Commonwealth migrants showed a marked tendency at first to focus on infections, and otherwise, in terms reminiscent of Powellite fears, on family planning and contraception (Bhopal and Donaldson 1988).

From the minority perspective, on the other hand, health claims have been based on concepts of citizenship. Such claims were not easy to make when health care was private or depended on voluntary or charitable institutions. However, in 1948 the National Health Service (NHS) instituted an explicit commitment to universal health care. At the same time this move gave unprecedented power to the medical profession. While private medicine continued to coexist with the NHS, affording choice to a small stratum who could pay, models of care within the NHS were increasingly conceived as population-wide medicine, to be varied only according to scientific considerations. Variations in care, where they were not historical hangovers, thus became increasingly dependent on variations in medical research interests and on theories of aetiology or treatment. From the 1960s to the 1980s increasing evidence emerged in Britain and in Western countries generally of variations in medical practice (tonsillectomy, prostatectomy or hysterectomy being obvious examples), which were hard to account for on grounds of morbidity, with the implication – documented in some cases – that variations in clinical judgement were the principal cause (Andersen and Mooney 1990; Bloor 1976). There was nothing multicultural in such thinking, and the claim of citizenship in the early decades of the NHS was simply to equality on the terms of the dominant culture, in this case the dominant medical culture.

At the same time, ethnic minorities were occasionally seen to have a special claim to the interest of the medical profession because differences in morbidity and mortality amongst them were suggestive of aetiological hypotheses. A number of these considerations were put forward in the first government study of immigrant mortality in 1984 (Marmot *et al.* 1984), and formed the principal basis of the argument throughout, suggesting 'the potential link between way of life and way of death' (Marmot *et al.* 1984 p. 3). In accordance with this perspective, ethnic minorities had a special place in the first British government health plan (Department of Health 1992), and for each disease group ethnic minorities appeared as a subheading under the general rubric of 'social variations' in the disease pattern. This was under the long Conservative administration of Mrs Thatcher.

An additional argument of the 1984 report on immigrant mortality, however, was its claim to 'point to particular health problems of immigrants that merit attention by the health services' (Marmot *et al.* 1984). This argument was to evolve rapidly. The phraseology was a standard part of the discourse of discerning needs in the NHS at the time; but from the point of view of the ethnic minorities, the criticism of this type of approach was that it fixed on minorities as bearers of health 'problems', rather than of good health. At the same time, the critics linked this with the aetiological interest in ways of life, and argued that the focus on health problems rather than successes led to a selective emphasis on negative aspects of ways of life. This conjunction came to be identified as 'culture blaming' (Sheldon and Parker 1992). These critics argued that material disadvantage, deriving from factors such as discrimination in the labour and housing markets, were a more fundamental determinant of health problems in ethnic minorities than culture, and as we have noted, these material influences are now an increasingly obvious factor in ethnic minority health.

The formulation of health claims on the state by ethnic minorities have thus become an aspect of claims on the basis of inequalities generally, and this approach was ratified at governmental level when the new Labour administration accepted the language of inequalities and set up an Independent Inquiry into Inequalities in Health. This report included summaries of the latest research on ethnic minorities (Acheson 1998), and was followed by a new health plan in which inequalities were cited as a major source of ill health (Department of Health 1998).

At the same time, claims on the state formulated in the language of inequalities have also been increasingly accepted in health care as well as in public and preventive health. An amendment introduced into the Race Relations Act in 2000 placed a statutory duty on public authorities, including the NHS, '(a) to eliminate unlawful racial discrimination; and (b) to promote equality of opportunity and good relations between persons of different racial groups' in carrying out their functions.

Moreover the positive duty of public bodies expressed under (b) above is in fact capable of extension in a multicultural direction. While the language here was still based on a Black/White racial dichotomy, it has not been interpreted so narrowly in some areas of the NHS. This broader basis for claims on the state has also been reinforced in some associated policy statements that verge on a multicultural approach. The notion of a 'culturally competent' service is gaining ground: one that shows respect for the diverse beliefs and consequent needs of clients. Another development of the inequalities approach, which has a multicultural potential, is the policy of 'mainstreaming'. As one formulation puts it, this 'entails rethinking mainstream provision to accommodate gender, race, disability and other dimensions of discrimination and disadvantage, including sexuality and religion' (Scottish Executive 2000).

Whether these developments can be made to work in practice has yet to be seen; and they will in any case have to prevail against a reaction towards reasserting a single culture, precipitated by the attack on the World Trade Center in New York. In the aftermath of the attack, the British Home Secretary emphasized the importance of all British residents speaking English and assenting to agreed civic values. This is a somewhat empty manifesto, considering the rapidity with which English has been adopted to the best of their ability by ethnic minorities in Britain.

At the same time, proponents of the dominant culture continue to make universal moral claims that impinge on ethnic and religious differences, and which in some cases make use of health grounds. For example, attacks on arranged marriage sometimes cite the mental health or suicide risk of the wives, despite its defenders pointing to the great variation in forms of arranged marriage. Universal claims are also made in counter-attacks by minority groups, which again involve health issues. Catholics feel particularly strongly about what they see as forms of murder in practices surrounding abortion, some types of contraception, and termination of life. Other issues of a similar kind still slumber because as yet they are poorly articulated. The practice of cousin marriage among Muslims has been connected with genetic risks; but too often the only remedy which genetic counselling can offer is abortion, about which Muslims too have considerable reservations.

These are radical disagreements and it is difficult to see how multicultural approaches can grapple honestly with them, when such approaches mainly consist in vague slogans of respect and goodwill, or invoke naive secular utilitarianism, or attempt to reduce as much morality as possible to private choice. What is left when these approaches are removed?

Looking to the future

In the year 2000, the Runnymede Trust published a report that went beyond any previous description of what a future Britain could look like as a multicultural society (Runnymede Trust 2000). Having identified five models of how the state relates to ethnic diversity, the report focuses on three that it regards as historical options for Britain. In the nationalist model, the state promotes a single national culture; in the liberal model, there is a single political culture in the public sphere and diversity in private life; but the report throws all its weight into a further model, the plural model, where there is both unity and diversity in public life, and Britain is envisaged as a 'community of communities' as well as a community of individuals, reflecting the importance to individuals of their cultural and religious heritage. These communities should be recognized as equal but different – both aspects are essential – while at the same time undergoing a process of growth and transition facilitated by public dialogue. Amongst the health issues that such a dialogue could tackle are the disagreements connected with the family or the sanctity of life, which we mentioned earlier as particularly intractable within the present national culture.

As the most demanding and self-aware treatment of multiculturalism to have emerged from a British public body, this programme provides a template against which we can compare the prospects for multiculturalism in health care. The strategy proposed for change, bearing on health care as on other social institutions, begins by noting that policies for reducing social exclusion cannot be restricted to attacks on poverty, because causes of poverty, where race or culture are involved, are particular both to certain areas and to the added experience of racism and discrimination. The report notes a sea change in the Labour government dating from late 1999 and early 2000, when the limits to an anti-poverty strategy were realized, and marks the Race Relations Amendment Act 2000 as the centrepiece of a number of new measures, significant because, as we have already noted, it laid positive duties on public authorities to promote equality of opportunity and good relations between persons of different racial groups. But in the report's thinking this is only a beginning, and it looks to a number of further developments, the following being perhaps the most important in the present context:

- There is still a failure to move beyond the terminology of race, and we need to recognize the variety of racisms, which focus with equal ease on differences of culture and religion.

- Processes of inequality are essentially similar across a number of dimensions, race, culture, religion, gender, age, sexuality and so on, and should be brought together under a single Equality Act and a single Equality Commission.

- In addition to coercive measures, public authorities and other organizations should be encouraged to regulate themselves through equality audits and to have bodies that can help and advise them.

◆ It follows from these developments at the level of law that there is a corresponding emphasis on organizational change in such bodies as the health
service. This focuses on procedures for self-review, and on what we referred
to earlier as 'mainstreaming', that is, the practice of reviewing all proposed
policy aimed at the general population in order to estimate and adjust for
its impact on different racial, cultural and religious groups.

Some of these proposed developments are, the report notes, already evolving
in Scotland (Runnymede Trust 2000), which to that extent is emerging as a
test bed for the approach. The Scottish Executive has an Equality Strategy
coordinated by an Equality Unit, and the Parliament has an Equal Opportunities
Committee that scrutinizes proposed legislation using an explicit mainstreaming approach. Scotland may therefore provide advance indications of
problems that the approach will have to surmount.

One notable problem is indeed the failure to move beyond the terminology
of race. Scotland's demographic composition is very different from that of
England. The population that originated in the New Commonwealth is much
smaller in Scotland, and that which originated in Ireland much larger. Among
the Irish, disadvantage is faced primarily by people of Catholic background
(about 18 per cent of the Scottish population) (Williams and Walls 2000). It is
therefore significant that, while religion is mentioned in the Scotland Act
among a number of possible bases for discrimination that need scrutiny, the
Equality Strategy has focused first on the very small and new proportion of
the population where the issue appears as one of race, and has postponed to
an indefinite future the consideration of the large and historically long-rooted
population where the issue appears as one of religion. Such a sequence can be
justified on practical grounds; but until the problem that is numerically the
biggest and historically the oldest is faced and tackled, there will always be a
suspicion that the new approach can be reduced to official window dressing
and parliamentary moralizing of a kind attractive to a devolved administration that has not yet got its feet wet.

It is also important, therefore, to look hard at the nuts and bolts of such a
multicultural approach in a specific institutional setting like health care. Within
the arena of a single health service, the present approach stresses the importance of knowledge of differences between groups and thus the reduction of
inequalities. This emphasis creates a major requirement for good public health
data on often small population groups, which to some extent fits the increasing
trend to large public data sets made possible by electronic advances. But as we
noted earlier, we are already better informed on ethnic differences than we are
on what we can do about them, and thus there is a risk that the explosion of
data analysis will not be matched by well-constructed intervention studies.

A further emphasis of the new multicultural approach is on the link between racism and poverty in the causation of ill health. In the 1980s, the poverty hypothesis did not fare well with the evidence on British ethnic groups then available. Nor did the racism hypothesis fare much better; for example, although work in the US suggested an effect on blood pressure in Black Americans, other groups such as South Asians in Britain who could be presumed to have had similar experiences of racism did not show similar health patterns. However, research in the 1990s changed the picture (Williams and Harding 2001). Socio-economic effects reappeared, and prima facie effects of racism, possibly diversified by predisposing biological factors, began to accumulate. The Runnymede Trust report, which calls for funding to be directed towards collecting such evidence, may well catch this new wind in health research.

The emphasis on mainstreaming also makes increasingly good sense in health care. A recent provision for health authorities to formulate Health Improvement Plans for the reduction of inequalities means that there is now a vehicle ready for this kind of policy appraisal, which explicitly assesses impact on cultural and religious groups. Health authorities 'will identify local health and health care needs, and promote action to achieve demonstrable health improvements and reductions in health inequality'; and in addition a Health Improvement Programme Performance Scheme 'will recognize health communities making progress from a low base, tackling entrenched problems of ill-health, deprivation and poor or fragmented services' (Department of Health 1998).

As a final note of caution, however, we would point out that the blueprints outlined in the Runnymede Trust report are concerned with the health care of cultural and religious groups, not individuals. The report and its multicultural philosophy are chiefly concerned with the politics, identities and claims of groups, although individuals stand, of course, to benefit from any improvement in the health care of their group as a whole. But there are other sides to cultural and religious identity that have irreducibly individual aspects in practice. Redress in cases of perceived discrimination is individual by virtue of the application of case law to particular circumstances, and the same applies to difficulties in the encounter between doctor and patient. One of the few individual remedies discussed in the Runnymede Trust report is provision for telephone interpreting services. But a more urgent issue is the development of health advocacy, which is an important omission from the report's philosophy. Health advocacy can assist the doctor up to a point, but there are occasions when it should question or even oppose the doctor's decision – a result that may be unwelcome to all but the best doctors. There may also be occasions when well-meaning health advocacy could actually obstruct the interests of the patient. There is much to be argued out and clarified in areas that affect individual patients, and it would be a pity if the advance of multicultural group politics should diminish the interest in matters so critical to individual welfare.

References

Abbotts, J., Williams, R. and Davey Smith, G. (1998) Mortality in men of patrilineal Irish decent in Britain. *Public Health*, **112** (4), 229–32.

Acheson, S. D. (1998) *Independent inquiry into inequalities in health.* HMSO, London.

Ahmad, W. I. U. (1993) '*Race*' *and health in contemporary Britain.* Open University Press, Buckingham.

Ahmad, W. I. U. (2000) *Ethnicity, disability and chronic illness.* Buckingham, Open University Press.

Ahmad, W. and Atkin, K. (2000) Primary care and haemoglobin disorders: a study of families and professionals. *Critical Public Health*, **10** (1), 41–53.

Andersen, T. F. and Mooney, G. (eds) (1990) *The challenges of medical practice variations.* Macmillan, London.

Anionwu, E. N. and Atkin, K. (2001) *The politics of sickle cell thalassaemia.* Open University Press, Buckingham.

Arai, L. and Harding, S. (2002) *United Kingdom-born black Caribbeans: generational changes in health and well-being.* Occasional Paper No. 6, Medical Research Council, Glasgow.

Balarajan, R. and Bulusu, L. (1990) Mortality among immigrants in England and Wales, 1978–1983. In M. Britton (ed.) *Mortality and geography: a review of the mid-1980s.* OPCS Series DS No. 9 HMSO, London.

Barker, D. J. P. (1998) *Mothers, babies and health in later life*, second edition. Churchill Livingstone, Edinburgh.

Benzeval, M. and Judge, K. (1996) Access to health care in England: continuing inequalities in the distribution of GPs. *Journal of Public Health Medicine*, **18** (1), 33–40.

Berthoud, R. (1999) *Young Caribbean men and the labour market: a comparison with other ethnic groups.* York Publishing Services for the Joseph Rowntree Foundation, York.

Bhopal, R. S. and Donaldson, L. J. (1988) Health education for ethnic minorities – current provision and future directions. *Health Education Journal*, **47**, 137–40.

Bhugra, D., Leff, J., Mallett, R., Der, G., Corridan, B. and Rudge, S. (1997) Incidence and outcome of schizophrenia in whites, African-Caribbeans and Asians in London. *Psychological Medicine*, **27**, 791–8.

Bloor, M. (1976) Bishop Berkeley and the adeno-tonsillectomy enigma: an exploration of variation in the social construction of medical disposals. *Sociology*, **10**, 43–61.

Bush, H., Williams, R., Sharma, S. and Cruickshank, K. (1997) *Opportunities for and barriers to good nutritional health in minority ethnic groups.* Health Education Authority, London.

Campbell, J. L., Ramsay, J. and Green, J. (2001) Age, gender, socioeconomic and ethnic differences in patients' assessments of primary care. *Quality in Health Care*, **10**, 90–5.

Cappuccio, F. P., Cook, D. G., Atkinson, R. W. and Strazullo, P. (1997) Prevalence, detection and management of cardiovascular risk factors in different ethnic groups in south London. *Heart*, **78**, 555–63.

Chaturvedi, N., McKeigue, P. M. and Marmot, M. G. (1993) Resting and ambulatory blood pressure differences in Afro-Caribbeans and Europeans. *Hypertension*, **22** (1), 90–6.

Chaturvedi, N., Rai, H. and Ben-Shlomo, Y. (1997) Lay diagnosis and health care seeking behaviour for chest pain in South Asians and Europeans. *Lancet*, **350**, 1578–83.

Chen, M. S. J. (1999) Informal care and the empowerment of minority communities: comparisons between the USA and the United Kingdom. *Ethnicity and Health*, **4** (3), 139–51.

Clarke, M. and Clayton, D. G. (1983) Quality of obstetric care provided for Asian immigrants in Leicestershire. *British Medical Journal*, **286**, 621–3.

Cooper, H., Smaje, C. and Arber, S. (1998) Use of health services by children and young people according to ethnicity and social class: secondary analysis of a national survey. *British Medical Journal*, **317**, 1047–51.

Cruickshank, J. K., Burnett, M., MacDuff, J. and Drubra, U. (1991a) Ethnic differences in fasting plasma C-peptide and insulin in relation to glucose tolerance and blood pressure. *Lancet*, **338**, 842–7.

Cruickshank, J. K., Mbanya, J. C., Wilks, R., Balkau, B., Forrester, T., Anderson, S. G., *et al.* (2001a) Hypertension in four African-origin populations: current 'Rule of Halves', quality of blood pressure control and attributable risk (fraction) for cardiovascular disease. *Journal of Hypertension*, **19**, 41–6.

Cruickshank, J. K., Mbanya, J. C., Wilks, R., Balkau, B., McFarlane-Anderson, N. and Forrester, T. (2001b) Sick genes, sick individuals or sick populations with chronic disease? The emergence of diabetes and high blood pressure in African-origin populations. *International Journal of Epidemiology*, **30**, 111–17.

Cruickshank, J. K., Richardson, J. H., Morgan, O., Porter, J., Klenerman, P., Knight, J., *et al.* (1991b) Migrant study of HTLV-1 infection in British and Jamaican relatives of tropical spastic paraperesis patients in Britain: lack of evidence for prolonged sero-negative incubation. *British Medical Journal*, **300**, 300–304.

Daryanani, R., Hinley, P., Evans, C., Fahy, P. and Turk, J. (2001) Ethnicity and use of a child and adolescent mental health service. *Child Psychology and Psychiatry Review* **6**, **3**, 127–32.

Davies, S., Thornicroft, G., Leese, M., Higgingbotham, A. and Phelan, A. (1996) Ethnic differences in risk of compulsory psychiatric admission among representative cases of psychosis in London. *British Medical Journal*, **312**, 533–7.

Department of Health (1992) *The health of the nation: a strategy for health in England*. HMSO, London.

Department of Health (1998) *Saving lives: our healthier nation*. HMSO, London.

Department of Health and National Institute for Ethnic Studies in Health and Social Policy (2000) *Ethnic Differences in Drinking and smoking. An analysis of data from the General Household survey for 1984–1994*.

Donovan, J. (1996) *We don't buy sickness, it just comes. Health, illness and health care in the lives of black people in London*. Gower, Aldershot.

Ebden, P., Carey, O. J., Bhatt, A. and Harrison, B. (1988) The bilingual consultation. *The Lancet*, **1**, 347.

Feder, G., Crook, A. M., Magee, P., Banerjee, S., Timmis, A. D. and Hemmingway, H. (2002) Ethnic differences in invasive management of coronary disease: prospective cohort study of patients undergoing angiography. *British Medical Journal*, **324**, 511–16.

Finau, S. A., Prior, A. I. and Evans, J. G. (1982) Ageing in the South Pacific. Physical changes with urbanization. *Social Science and Medicine*, **16**, 1539–49.

Forrester, T., Wilks, R. J., Bennett, F. I., Simeon, D., Osmond, C., Allen, M., *et al*. (1996) Fetal growth and cardiovascular risk factors in Jamaican schoolchildren. *British Medical Journal*, **312**, 156–60.

Fraser, S., Bunce, C. and Wormald, R. (1999) Retrospective analysis of risk factors for late presentation of chronic glaucoma. *British Journal of Opthamology*, **83**, 24–8.

Free, C., White, P., Shipman, C. and Dale, J. (1999) Access to and use of out-of-hours services by members of Vietnamese community groups in South London: a focus group study. *Family Practice*, **16** (4), 369–74.

Gillam, S. J., Jarman, B., White, P. and Law, R. (1989) Ethnic differences in consultation rates in urban general practice. *British Medical Journal*, **299**, 953–7.

Goyder, E. C. and Botha, J. L. (2000) Inequalities in access to diabetes care; evidence from a historical cohort study. *Quality in Health Care*, **9**, 85–9.

Griffiths, C., Kaur, G., Gantley, M., Feder, G., Hillier, S., Goddard, J., *et al*. (2001) Influences on hospital admission for asthma in South Asian and white adults: qualitative interview study. *British Journal of Opthamology*, **323**, 962–6.

Haenszel, H. and Kurihara, M. (1968) Studies of Japanese migrants. Mortality from cancer and other diseases among Japanese in the United States. *Journal of the National Cancer Institute*, **40**, 43–68.

Hale, A., Leung, T., Sivasubramaniam, S., Kenny, J. and Sutherland, S. (1997) Prevalence of anitibodies to HTLV in antenatal clinic attenders in south and east London. *Journal of Medical Virology*, **53**, 326–9.

Hales, C. N. and Barker, D. J. P. (1992) Type 2 (non-insulin dependent) diabetes mellitus: the thrifty phenotype hypothesis. *Diabetologia*, **35**, 595–601.

Harding, S. (2000) Examining the contribution of social class to high cardiovascular mortality among Indian, Pakistani and Bangladeshi male migrants living in England and Wales. *Health Statistics Quarterly*, 26–8.

Harding, S. (1998) The incidence of cancers among second generation Irish living in England and Wales. *British Journal of Cancer*, **78**, 958–61.

Harding, S. (2003) Longitudinal study of the relationship between social mobility and morbidity among South Asians and West Indians living in England and Wales. *Social Science & Medicine*, **56**, 355–361

Harding, S. and Balarajan, R. (2001) Longitudinal study of socio-economic differences in mortality among south Asians and West Indian migrants. *Ethnicity and Health*, **6** (2), 121–8.

Harding, S. and Balarajan, R. (1996) Patterns of mortality in second generation Irish living in England and Wales: longitudinal study. *British Medical Journal*, **312**, 1389–92.

Harding, S. and Maxwell, R. (1998) Differences in mortality of migrants. In Drever and M. Whitehead (eds) *Health inequalities: decennial supplement*. ONS series DS no. 15, The Stationery Office, London.

Harding, S. and Rosato, M. (1999) Incidence of cancers in migrant groups living in England and Wales. *Ethnicity and Health*, **4** (1/2), 83–92.

Harrison, G., Glazebrook, G., Brewin, J., Cantwell, R., Dalkin, T., Fox, R., *et al.* (1997) Increased incidence of psychotic disorders in migrants from the Caribbean to the United Kingdom. *Psychological Medicine*, **27** (4), 799–806.

Hickman, M. J. (1998) Reconstructing deconstructing 'race': British political discourses about the Irish in Britain. *Ethnic and Racial Studies*, **21** (2), 288–307.

Johnson, A. E., Gordon, C., Palmer, R. G. and Bacon, P. A. (1995) The prevalence and incidence of systemic lupus erythematosus in Birmingham, England. *Arthritis and Rheumatism*, **38** (4), 551–8.

Landman, J. and Cruickshank, J. K. (2001) A review of ethnicity, health and nutrition-related diseases among former migrants in the United Kingdom. *Public Health Nutrition*, **4**, 647–57.

Lear, J. T., Lawrence, I. G., Pohl, J. E. and Burden, A. C. (1994) Myocardial infarction and thrombolysis: a comparision of the Indian and European populations on a coronary care unit. *Journal of the Royal College of Physicians London*, **28**, 143–47.

Lewis, G., Croft-Jeffreys, C. and David, A. (1990) Are British psychiatrists racist? *British Journal of Psychiatry*, **157**, 410–15.

Low, N., Sterne, J. A. C. and Barlow, D. (2001) Inequalities in rates of gonorrhoea and chlamydia between Black ethnic groups in south east London: a cross sectional study. *Sexually Transmitted Infection*, **77**, 15–20.

Majeed, F. A., Cook, D. G., Anderson, H. R., Hilton, S., Bunn, S. and Stones, C. (1994) Using patient and general practice characteristics to explain variations in cervical smear uptake rates. *British Medical Journal*, **308**, 1272–6.

Marmot, M. G., Adelstein, A. and Bulusu, L. (1984) *Immigrant mortality in England and Wales 1970–1978*. OPCS studies on population and medical subjects: no 47. HMSO, London.

Maxwell, K., Streetly, A. and Bevan, D. (1999) Experiences of hospital care and treatment seeking for pain from sickle cell disease: qualitative study. *British Medical Journal*, **318**, 1585–90.

Mbanya, J. C., Cruickshank, J. K., Forrester, T., Balkau, B., Ngogang, J. Y., Riste, L., *et al.* (1999) Standardised comparison of glucose tolerance in West African origin-populations of rural and urban Cameroon, Jamaica and Caribbean migrants to Britain. *Diabetes Care*, **22**, 434–40.

McFarland, E., Dalton, M. and Walsh, D. (1987) Personal welfare services and ethnic minorities. Scottish. *Scottish Ethnic Minorities Research Unit Research Paper No. 4.*

McGovern, D. and Cope, R. (1991) Second generation Afro-Caribbeans and young White with a first admission diagnosis of schizophrenia. *Social Psychiatry and Psychiatric Epidemiology*, **26**, 95–9.

McKeigue, P. M., Shah, B. and Marmot, M. G. (1991) Relation of central obesity and insulin resistance with high diabetes prevalence and cardiovascular risk in South Asians. *Lancet*, **337**, 382–6.

McNaught, A. (1985) *Race and health care in the United Kingdom*. Health Education Council, London.

McNaught, A. (1988) *Race and health policy*. Routledge, London.

Mennen, L., Jackson, M. and Sharma, S. (2001) Habitual diet in four populations of African origin: nutrient intakes in rural and urban Cameroon, Jamaica and Caribbean migrants in Britain. *Public Health Nutrition*, **4**, 765–72.

Mennen, L. I., Jackson, M., Cade, J., Mbanya, J. C., Lafay, L., Sharma, S., *et al.* (2000) Under-reporting of energy intake in four populations of African origin. *International Journal of Obesity*, **24**, 882–7.

Mokyr, J. (1983) *Why Ireland starved: a quantitative and analytical history of the Irish economy 1800–1850*. Allen and Unwin, London.

Molokhia, M., McKeigue, P. M., Cuadrado, M. and Hughes, G. (2001) Systemic lupus erythematosus in migrants from west Africa compared with Afro-Caribbean people in the United Kingdom. *Lancet*, **357**, 1414–5.

Moudgil, H. and Honeybourne, D. (1998) Differences in asthma management between White European and Indian subcontinent ethnic groups living in socioeconomically deprived areas in the Birmingham (IK) conurbation. *Thorax*, **53**, 490–4.

National Institute for Ethnic Studies in Health and Social Policy (1997) *Ethnic Diversity in England and Wales. An analysis by health Authorities based on the 1991 Census (London).*

Nazroo, J. Y. (1997) *The health of Britain's minorities.* Policy Studies Institute, London.

Neel, J. V. (1962) Diabetes mellitus: a thrifty genotype rendered detrimental by progress? *American Journal of Human Genetics*, **14**, 353–62.

Nightingale, S., Orton, D., Ratcliffe, D., Skidmore, S., Toswill, J. and Desselberger, U. (1993) Antenatal survey for the seroprevalence of HTLV-1 infections in the West Midlands, England. *Epidemiology and Infection*, **110**, 379–87.

Office for National Statistics (2000) *Mortality statistics, childhood, infant and perinatal.* HMSO, London.

Poulter, N., Khaw, K.T., Hopwood, B.E., *et al.* (1985) Determinants of blood pressure changes due to urbanisation: a longitudinal study. *Journal of Hypertension*, **3**, S375–S377.

Raftery, J., Jones, D. R. and Rosato, M. (1990) The mortality of first and second generation Irish immigrants in the United Kingdom. *Social Science and Medicine*, **24** (3), 91–4.

Raleigh, V. S. (1997) Diabetes and hypertension in Britain's ethnic minorities: implications for the future of renal services. *British Medical Journal*, **314**, 209–13.

Raleigh, V. S. (1996) Suicide patterns and trends in people of Indian subcontinent and Caribbean origin in England and Wales. *Ethnicity and Health*, **1** (1), 55–63.

Riste, L. K., Khan, F. and Cruickshank, J. K. (2001) High prevalence of Type 2 diabetes in all ethnic groups, including Europeans, in inner city Britain: relative poverty, inactivity, history of twenty-first century Europe? *Diabetes Care*, **24**, 1377–83.

Roderick, P., Clements, S., Stone, N., Martin, D. and Diamond, I. (1999) What determines geographical variation in rates of acceptance onto renal replacement therapy in England? *Journal of Health Services Research and Policy*, **4** (3), 139–46.

Roderick, P., Raleigh, V. S., Hallam, L. and Mallick, N. (1996) The need and demand for renal replacement therapy in ethnic minorities in England. *Journal of Epidemiology and Community Health*, **50** (3), 334–9.

Runnymede Trust (2000) *The future of multi-ethnic Britain: the Parekh report.* Profile Books, London.

Scott, P. (1998) Lay beliefs and the management of diseases amongst West Indians with diabetes. *Health and Social Care in the Community*, **6** (6), 407–19.

Scottish Executive (2000) *Towards an equality strategy.* Scottish Executive, Edinburgh.

Sharma, S., Cade, J., Riste, L. and Cruickshank, K. (1999) Nutrient intake trends among African-Caribbeans in Britain: a migrant population and its second generation. *Public Health Nutrition*, **2** (4), 469–76.

Sharpley, M., Hutchinson, G., Murray, R. M. and McKenzie, K. (2001) Understanding the excess of psychosis among the African-Caribbean population in England. *British Journal of Psychiatry*, **178** Suppl. 40, 60–8.

Shaukat, N., de Bono, D. P. and Cruickshank, J. K. (1993) Clinical features, risk factors, and referral delay in British patients of Indian and European origin with angina matched for age and extent of coronary atheroma. *British Medical Journal*, **307**, 717–18.

Shaw, C. M., Creed, F., Tomenson, B., Riste, L. and Cruickshank, J. K. (1999) Prevalence of anxiety and depressive illness and help seeking behaviour in African Caribbeans and White Europeans: two phase general population survey. *British Medical Journal*, **318**, 302–5.

Sheldon, T. and Parker, H. (1992) The use of 'ethnicity' and 'race' in health research: a cautionary note. In W. I. U. Ahmad (ed.) *The politics of 'race' and health*. University of Bradford, Bradford.

Singh, S. P., Croudace, T., Beck, A. and Harrison, G. (1998) Perceived ethnicity and the risk of compulsory admission. *Social Psychiatry and Psychiatric Epidemiology*, **33**, 39–44.

Smaje, C. and Le Grand, J. (1997) Ethnicity, equity and the use of health services in the British NHS. *Social Science and Medicine*, **45** (3), 485–96.

Syme, S. L., Marmot, M. G., Kagan, A., Kato, H. and Rhoads, G. (1975) Epidemiologic studies of coronary heart disease and stroke in Japanese men living in Japan, Hawaii and California: introduction. *American Journal of Epidemiology*, **102** (6), 477–80.

Thomas, C. S., Stone, K., Osborn, M., Thomas, C. S. and Fisher, M. (1993) Psychiatric morbidity and compulsory admission among United Kingdom-born Europeans, Afro-Caribbeans and Asians in Central Manchester. *British Journal of Psychiatry*, **163**, 91–9.

Walls, P. (2001) Religion, ethnicity and nation in the Census: some thoughts on the inclusion of Irish ethnicity and Catholic religion. *Radical Statistics*, **78**, 48–61.

Webb, E. (2000) Health care for ethnic minorities. *Current Pediatrics*, **10**, 184–90.

Whitty, C. J. M., Brunner, E. J., Shipley, M. J., Hemmingway, H. and Marmot, M. G. (1999) Differences in biological risk factors for cardiovascular disease between three ethnic groups in the Whitehall II study. *Atherosclerosis*, **142**, 279–86.

Williams, R. and Harding, S. (2001) *South Asian heart disease: the contribution of poverty, stress and racism. South Asian Health Foundation meeting on South Asian heart disease.* London.

Williams, R. and Walls, P. (2000) Going but not gone: Catholic disadvantage in Scotland. In T. M. Devine (ed.) *Scotland's shame? Bigotry and sectarianism in modern Scotland.* Mainstream, Edinburgh.

Williams, R., Wright, W. and Hunt, K. (1998) Social class and health: the puzzling counter-example of British south Asians. *Social Science and Medicine*, **47**, 1277–88.

Chapter 13

Roma Health

Problems and Perception

Martin Kovats

A question of identities

At first sight the concept of 'Roma health' appears straightforward, encompassing the health status and needs of Roma people. However, it is by no means clear who is covered by the label 'Roma', neither are there comprehensive data about the health status of such people, even within individual countries, let alone on a Europe-wide or global basis. For these reasons, this chapter begins by examining the concept of 'Roma' before discussing the health data related to these populations in the Czech Republic, Slovakia, Hungary and Bulgaria.

The available data indicate that the health of Roma minorities is substantially worse than that of the national average. This is a result of both poorer living conditions and limited access to health care information and services. However, addressing these problems requires that one takes account not only of objective disadvantages but also the (related) cultural context, notably the low social status of Roma populations. Strategies designed explicitly to address Roma needs run the risk of further isolating already marginalized individuals and communities. Consequently, targeted interventions must take account of the broader economic, social, political and cultural context and be guided by the principles of equal opportunities.

'Roma' is a collective name derived from the Romani language. However, it is not a label that most of those to whom it is applied would necessarily accept for themselves. This chapter employs the term 'Roma/Gypsies' when referring to all members of the supposed European diaspora, limiting Roma to the populations in eastern Europe. These necessarily arbitrary designations should not be taken as reflecting the preferred identity of individuals and communities themselves. In fact there are many different group names used by Roma/Gypsy communities, as shown by the work of the anthropologists Marushiakova and Popov who identify over 150, not necessarily exclusive, group names in the

Balkans alone (Marushiakova and Popov 2002). The increasingly widespread application of the term 'Roma' is best seen as a politically driven replacement for the generic term 'Gypsy'.[1]

Communities range from small, family-based (often) itinerant groups such as UK Travellers, through to large, settled, urban populations such the 70,000 strong Roma town of Shutko in Macedonia. Living conditions vary enormously from mobile homes and semi-permanent traveller sites, through to isolated rural slums, villages, suburbs or urban ghettoes. Some Roma/Gypsies are wealthy, others economically independent or employed, yet many are very poor and dependent on welfare benefits or the black/grey economy for survival.

There is also considerable linguistic and cultural diversity amongst Roma/Gypsies. Most speak the language of the country in which they live, though not necessarily as their mother tongue. The Romani language itself consists of dozens of dialects, which 'are not mutually comprehensible except at very basic levels such as words relating to food or family' (Kenrick 2002) and is spoken by only a minority of Roma/Gypsies, most of whom live in the Balkans. Culture is a more controversial subject, not least because it has often been claimed that Roma/Gypsies have no culture, or only a 'culture of poverty'. Yet anthropologists have demonstrated that communities can have very sophistic-ated codes of behaviour, perceptions of the world and means of cultural expression. However, this does not mean that all communities are the same or share the same values, though there is a very widespread conceptual distinction between Roma and non-Roma (*gadje*). Prejudice and marginalization are not the sole explanation for this dichotomy, which can have profound implications for health care provision.

There is a marked distinction within Europe between the far larger popula-tions of the east and those in western countries. Even within these regions and in individual countries there is considerable diversity between the Roma/Gypsies of neighbouring states. The situation is further complicated by the movement across state borders, whether as seasonal migrants, long term workers or asylum seekers. Finally, account also needs to be taken of the very different economic, social and cultural conditions in the countries in which Roma/Gypsies live, ranging from wealthy western nations with stable

---

[1] In April 2002 the Parliament of the Council of Europe adopted a report that identified Roma minorities in almost every European country. *Legal Situation of the Roma in Europe*, Parliamentary Assembly of the Council of Europe, Doc. 9397, 19 April 2002 or a detailed discussion of the political meaning of 'Roma' at the European level see M, Kovats, 'The Emergence of European Roma Policy' in W. Guy op. cit., pp. 93–116.

democracies and some degree of multiculturalism, through to poorer states going through a difficult process of transition and even countries that have been devastated by war in recent years.

Historically, limited interaction with and knowledge about these communities led to the generation of stereotypes, sometimes romantic but usually hostile. For example, prior to the twentieth century, Gypsies were often considered 'children of nature' who enjoyed rude health and could live to fantastic ages of well over one hundred. More sophisticated research has since demonstrated the tragic inaccuracy of such a view. If a discourse of Roma health is to develop it must take account of the observation of the Commission on Security and Cooperation in Europe's High Commissioner on National Minorities that Roma/Gypsies 'comprise an extremely heterogeneous set of communities that are perhaps best understood in their own specific circumstances'.[2]

A Roma race?

The idea that Roma constitute a single and distinct people of common origin has long dominated public understanding of these communities. This is not particularly surprising given the close association between Gypsies and nomads who, by definition, come from 'somewhere else'. The connection between nomads and Roma/Gypsies is largely historical though some communities, mainly in western Europe, still pursue an itinerant lifestyle (even if only for part of the year). Most Roma communities in eastern Europe have been settled since at least the nineteenth century. From the late Middle Ages the most widespread belief was that these people came from Egypt, from which the word Gypsy is derived, yet other labels such as 'Tartar' or 'Bohemian' were also occasionally applied. Though the Egyptian connection also has a long tradition throughout Europe, in eastern and central European Roma have historically been known by variations on the word Tsigan, Cigány, Zigeuner etc, the etymology of which is unclear, and which have conventionally been translated into English as Gypsy.

At the end of the eighteenth century the first scholarly work to be published on 'the Gypsies' identified India as their original homeland, based on the large number of Indic words in the Romani vocabulary. From the mid nineteenth century scholarship was dominated by the Romantic spirit of Gypsy Lorism

---

[2] Statement of the HCNM on his study of the Roma in the CSCE Region, Office of the High Commissioner on National Minorities, September 1993 p. 3.

dedicated, in the words of one of its leading lights, to 'cultivate the race as some care for flowers, without feeling impelled to turn nursery gardeners or scientific botanists' (Sampson 1907). In general, public knowledge about Roma/Gypsies has been conditioned less by understanding their reality than by what they are supposed to symbolize. Closer relations between Roma/Gypsies and mainstream institutions and, in particular, the recent emergence of formal interest representation have created an unprecedented opportunity to overcome stereotypes and generalizations.

Due to the conspicuous differences between Roma/Gypsy communities, the aspiration to define these people as distinct (political) community requires the claim that in the distant past they were united. The idea of a Roma race has been challenged by anthropologists, historians and sociologists. Judith Okely has argued that 'Gypsiologists make the same mistakes as the nineteenth century anthropologists in the general study of languages and racial distribution' (Okely 1983) and suggests an indigenous origin for some west European Gypsy communities. Wim Willems and others have pointed to the arbitrary application of Gypsy identity to itinerant communities (Willems and Lucassen 1998), an approach developed by Ladányi and Szelényi in respect of contemporary debates over the size of the (largely) settled Roma populations in eastern Europe (Ladányi and Szelényi 2000). It is ironic that just when social scientists are starting to provide the basis for a more sophisticated understanding of the relationship between Roma/Gypsy communities, identities and wider society, political developments are resurrecting the idea of the Roma race. For example, the Chair of the Council of Europe's Specialist Group on Roma/Gypsies (inaccurately) asserts that 'the people known . . . as Gypsies . . . came from northern India seven centuries ago in a long march that took them from the Middle East to Egypt and from Turkey to Andalusia' (European Committee on Migration 1995).

Genetic research

The question of whether or to what extent Roma/Gypsies represent a distinctive biological population is not just of cultural or political interest but has implications for health services. However, work in this field needs to be sensitive to the persistence of anti-Roma prejudices based on the perception that Roma are alien to the majority nations amongst whom they live. This problem has already been identified within the Roma health literature by McKee and Hajioff who note that the 'concentration on communicable diseases also resonates, uncomfortably, with the Social Darwinist agenda' (Hajioff and McKee 2000).

The first extensive research into Roma/Gypsy ancestry was carried out by the Research Institute for Racial Hygiene and Population Biology in Nazi Germany.

Using genealogical data rather than biological material, over 20,000 racial diagnoses were carried out, 90 per cent resulting in a categorization of 'mixed blood' (Willems 1997). Gypsy biology attracted the interest of Dr Josef Mengele who, in 1944 was proposed for a medal 'in recognition of his work on the racial origins of the Gypsies' (Lewy 2000 pp. 158–62). More recently, the Hungarian socio-biologist Tamás Bereczkei has argued that genetic difference partly explained what he claimed were the r-selected reproductive strategies of Roma in Hungary, concluding that ' "humanist" oriented politicians may increase problems in the coexistence of the two ethnic groups [Roma and Magyar] because they are convinced that political and legal equality is based on biological identity' (Bereczkei 1993). Given this intellectual environment, the Deputy Director General of the Korányi Tuberculosis and Pulmonary Institute in Hungary, Dr Dezső Kozma, insists that 'we would rather talk about family genetics . . . than the genetics of Roma as an ethnic group' (Puporka and Zádori 1998 p. 35).

Roma/Gypsies were not included in Cavalli-Sforza's comprehensive analysis of global genetic diversity, as it was assumed they represented non-aboriginal populations (Cavalli-Sforza 1994). In their review of the published literature, Kalydjieva, Gresham and Calafell (2001) note that 'post-war genetic research has been preoccupied with the Indian origins of the Roma' with most studies remaining 'in the realm of scientific exploration, away from the health needs of Roma'. Their reanalysis of the data indicates that 'most Roma are genetically closer to Indians than to European populations'. This is not surprising given the close correlation between the appearance of Gypsy identity/ communities in south-east Europe and the repopulation of the region by people from the Middle East and beyond during the expansion of the Ottoman Empire. The authors also note that 'more importantly, the analysis highlights the internal diversity of the Roma, who appear to be genetically far more heterogeneous that autochthonous European populations' with a proportion of variance between Roma/Gypsies almost twice that of between all Roma/ Gypsies and all non-Roma/Gypsy Europeans (Kalydjieva et al. 2001).

In 2001 Kalydjieva and others published the findings of their study of Y-chromosome and mtDNA markers in 14 different communities, 12 from Bulgaria and one each from Lithuania and Spain (275 individuals). A total of 13 paternal and 25 maternal lineages were found in more than one Roma group. The most common male lineage was found in 80 individuals and in all 14 groups in a haplogroup previously identified at low frequencies in India and Central Asia. The other lineages, variously distributed, represented haplogroups commonly or solely found either in Asia, the Middle East, as well as Europe (Gresham 2001).

Hereditary disorders

The extent to which different Roma individuals/communities share some particular genetic heritage has implications for the diagnosis and treatment of hereditary disorders. In their review of the literature Kalaydjieva, Gresham and Calafell identify nine Mendelian disorders caused by 'private' Roma mutations, as well as a number of conditions that are also present in the wider society such as cystic fibrosis and phenylketonuria (Kalaydjieva *et al.* 2001). In the countries covered by this chapter, the most detailed study of hereditary disorders affecting Roma has been conducted in Bulgaria as part of project that also includes a number of western countries. The distribution of conditions can vary greatly within the country, even if they have also been identified amongst Roma abroad. Hereditary motor and sensory neuropathy, Lom type has been found in over 40 different locations in Bulgaria affecting a number of different linguistic communities, yet the Rousse type appears confined to a small local region and one particular, endogamous Roma community. Congenital myasthenic syndrome, type Ia appears only amongst speakers of the Yerli dialect of Romani, whilst primary epilepsy is found only amongst those using the Wallachian dialect and spinal muscular atrophy, type 1 only amongst Turkish-speaking Roma communities (Turnev *et al.* 2002).

The extent to which prevalence of congenital disorders reflects a higher incidence of consanguinity within some Roma communities is highly controversial. In the absence of more extensive data together with stereotyped perception of Roma people, it is not surprising that a number of studies have assumed such diseases arise as a result of inbreeding amongst closed communities. The greater awareness by health professionals of the need to address the needs of Roma minorities should improve understanding of the distribution of inherited disorders. However, the utility of the recommendation that 'future studies of the epidemiology of single gene disorders should take social organisation and cultural anthropology into consideration' depends on an accurate understanding of the specific history of particular communities (Kalaydjieva *et al.* 2001).

Roma in the Czech Republic, Slovakia, Hungary and Bulgaria

The primary responsibility for the provision of health care services to Roma/ Gypsy minorities lies with the public health authorities of the countries in which these populations live. Therefore, analysis of the health circumstances and needs must be rooted in awareness of the situation of Roma communities within each state. The following discussion focuses on four countries: the Czech

Republic, Slovakia, Hungary and Bulgaria. These countries are selected not because they offer some ideal model of Roma and their circumstances, but simply because in recent years reports have been produced summarizing what is known about the health-related issues affecting their Roma minorities. Generally, the literature falls into broad categories of communicable and non-communicable diseases, reproductive health and economic and cultural factors affecting access to health care services. However, it should be recognized that the picture presented is far from comprehensive.

How many Roma?

The question of how many Roma people there are, either on a global basis or within individual countries, illustrates the conceptual problems involved in defining any Roma-specific social policy. The most commonly cited figures are those published in 1995 by the London-based Minority Rights Group. Though accepted by the European Commission, these data are not based on systematic research but can most charitably be described as the guesstimates of individual experts. As Table 13.1 indicates, these figures stand in stark contrast to those produced by census returns where categories of Roma identity and/or Romani language have been included.

This discrepancy is usually attributed to the unwillingness of many Roma people to identify themselves as such due to fear of discrimination. Though anti-Roma prejudice is clearly an important factor, the argument fails to recognize that many Roma people feel part of their country's national community (Marushiakova and Popov 2002). Given considerable cultural, social and economic diversity between Roma communities and in their relations with other population groups, it is not surprising that many people may not wish to associate themselves with other Roma. In general, self-ascription

Table 13.1 Roma population estimates

Country	Total population (2001) (1)	No. of Roma census (1990–92)	No. of Roma national estimates 1989–97	No. of Roma Minority Rights Group (6)
Czech Republic	10,264,212	32,903	200,000 (2)	250–300,000
Slovakia	5,414,937	83,988	253,943 (3)	480–520,000
Hungary	10,106,017	142,683	482,000 (4)	550–600,000
Bulgaria	7,707,495	313,396	553,436 (5)	700–800,000

Sources: adapted from 1-CIA (2001), 2-Guy (2001 p. 316), 3-Vašecka (1999 p. 5), 4-Havas et al. (1995 p. 67), 5-Marushiakova and Popov (2000 p. 16), 6-Minority Rights Group (1995, p. 7).

produces low figures, indicating that many people do not see Roma as their primary identity, at least within the public sphere.

During the 1990s, in policy oriented research, Roma people were identified by others, either researchers or on the basis of data held by public authorities, using different methods that produced different population estimates. The Hungarian sociologists János Ladányi and Iván Szelényi have argued that there is no way of objectively identifying who is Roma and that such population estimates express the preconceptions of those making the identification. For example, the surveys of the Central Statistical Office in Hungary are based on whether the research interviewer believes the subject exhibits a 'Gypsy lifestyle', a 'semi-Gypsy lifestyle' or a 'non-Gypsy lifestyle'. However, as they point out, regardless of what the individual might consider him or herself, such surveys are not without value as 'those whom their environment consider to be Gypsies will be treated as Gypsies' (Ladányi and Szelény 2000).

Countries

Given these caveats, the following discussion reflects the contemporary public discourse about the Roma minorities in the Czech Republic, Slovakia, Hungary and Bulgaria. However, before examining the health-related literature itself it is important to provide further context by considering the differences between these states in respect of the size, circumstances and history of their Roma populations.

The Czech Republic and Slovakia

The creation of Czech and Slovak nation-states in 1993 and the process of economic transition have had a dramatic effect on the situation of Roma minorities in both countries. Historically the Czech lands always had far fewer Roma than Slovakia. From 1938 the area came under Nazi occupation resulting in the extermination of almost all its 6,000 Roma, whilst most survived the war in the nominally independent Slovakia. As a result, the Czech Roma are made up of (the descendants of) post-war migrants from rural Slovakia to industrial regions. Roma became the largest minority in the new Czech state and with Roma unemployment running at over 70 per cent, Czech society has encouraged their emigration either by 'returning' to Slovakia or as asylum seekers further afield. The Czech Republic has the unique distinction of an almost entirely urbanized Roma population. However, this has not prevented social exclusion illustrated, in 2002, when the government acknowledged the existence of almost two dozen Roma ghettos.

The Roma minority in Slovakia is more economically, socially and culturally diverse. Many still live in rural areas, where they have been particularly hard hit by economic decline with almost 100 per cent unemployment in some settlements. Though a larger minority, both in absolute and relative terms, they are of less political significance for the state and society due to the presence of a substantial Magyar minority. In both countries the poor relations between Roma and the state represent a legacy of communist assimilation policies, which effectively perpetuated long-standing prejudices of Roma inferiority, whilst their material improvements have been largely undone. In both countries a large proportion of Roma children are now directed into dead-end remedial education[4] so it is not surprising that governments of both states have been at the forefront of defining the Roma as a European rather than a national issue.

Hungary

The long and complex history of Roma in Hungary reached its nadir in the first half of the twentieth century when decades of poverty and social exclusion resulted in deportations and mass murder during the Second World War. Today, the minority is conventionally divided into three linguistic groups. Approximately 80 per cent are native Hungarian speakers (Romungro) and the rest speak either an archaic form of Romanian (Beash) or a Wallachian dialect of Romani as their mother-tongue. Since the end of the Second World War Roma numbers have risen approximately fivefold and now account for 5 per cent of the country's 10 million population.

Post-war integration policies led to greater urbanization, though today 60 per cent still live in the countryside where residential segregation appears to be strengthening. The majority of Roma live in the poorest regions in the north and east of the country which, together with low levels of education, has contributed to dramatic unemployment and impoverishment in the post-communist period. The 1990s were characterized by Hungary's enthusiastic embrace of minority right and the state's willingness to develop specific Roma policies. Given that over the decade the percentage of the Roma population amongst the country's poorest 20 per cent rose from 70 to 85 per cent, such policies appear to have been ineffective (Kádet 2002). However, the establishment of over 700 Roma minority self-governments along with hundreds of other Roma NGOs mean that unprecedented opportunities have been created for Roma people to participate in public debate about themselves, including the development and implementation of policies.

---

[4] For a broad overview of the educational disadvantages faced by Roma minorities in eastern Europe, see *Denied a Future*, Save the Children Foundation (UK): London, 2001.

Bulgaria

The Roma minority in Bulgaria is characterized both by its internal diversity, as well as social, economic and cultural distinction from wider Bulgarian society. The anthropologists Elena Marushiakova and Vesilin Popov note that 'for a better understanding of the present day situation of the Gypsy minority in Bulgaria we have to consider the fundamental ethnic and social parameters that affect them, to take into account their specific ethnic and cultural features' (Marushiakova and Popov 2002). Group boundaries are very important, though they change over time as does the relationship between groups.

Bulgaria has a high proportion of native Romani speakers, though of many different dialects. The biggest group, the Yerli, is also divided into Christian and Muslim communities. There are many speakers of different Wallachian dialects of Romani representing different periods of migration into the country from what is now Romania, and these groups are also distinguished by 'traditional' professions, even if these may no longer now be practised. Some groups such as the Agyupti keep their distance from other Roma and prefer to identify as Turks or Pomaks, whilst other communities prefer a Bulgarian identity.

A legacy of long Ottoman rule is marked residential segregation, notably in urban/suburban mahallas, though many Roma also live in rural areas. Segregation in education also has a relatively long tradition back into the communist era. In the post-communist period almost all Roma have become unemployed, though many get by in the black or grey economies. Lack of state attention has led to a burgeoning growth in NGO activities in the country, though the extent to which the initiatives have been beneficial to Roma populations has been called into question (Popov unpublished).

Health data

Hajioff and McKee (2000) note that health literature about Roma is very limited in both content and scale. In the post-communist period contradictory tendencies have emerged. On the one hand, for data protection and human rights reasons states have stopped or even prohibited the publication of statistics based on ethnicity. Koupilová *et al.* have suggested that fear of further stigmatizing Roma minorities may also have inhibited some researchers (Koupilová *et al.* 2001). At the same time the redefinition of Roma as subject of social policy has led to the commissioning of broad sociological surveys as well as a growing number of local studies. Notably, more recent literature reflects the growing awareness of the importance of 'culture', in the sense both of how Roma people's values and perceptions, as well as stereotypes and prejudice, effect health care provision.

Communicable disease

The perception of Roma as a source of contagion has a very long tradition – stretching back at least into the nineteenth century – which is not confined to eastern Europe. Illustrative were the forced bathings, disinfection and even hair cropping of Roma communities widely practised in Hungary from the 1940s. Though these practices may initially have had some personal or public health justification in settlements with very poor sanitary conditions, the arbitrary and superficial enforcement of such procedures meant that they appear primarily designed to intimidate and stigmatize Roma communities (Bernath 2002). Forced bathings were eventually stopped in the 1980s, though the discrimination that they represented has proved more persistent. In 1997 a headmaster in the town of Tiszavasvári ruled that the school's Roma children must hold a separate graduation ceremony as they represented a threat of louse infection to non-Roma pupils.

Despite the unprecedented improvement in material conditions in the decades following the Second World War, Roma remained grossly over-represented amongst those living in the smallest and worst quality accommodation. For most, conditions have deteriorated during the post-communist period due to mass impoverishment and the decline in public services. In Hungary in the early 1990s over 60,000 Roma lived in more or less isolated rural settlements, the infrastructure in which has been described as 'disastrous... often with access to water supply over five hundred meters away and no sewage system. In a number of cases no electric power is supplied and gas supply is tantamount to a luxury service' (Puporka and Zádori 1998). Similar conditions are even more prevalent in Bulgaria and Slovakia. Even in urban areas impoverishment means many cannot pay bills and risk losing their gas, electricity, water supply or even becoming homeless. Poverty also leads to overcrowding. In Hungary 40 per cent live in homes with less than 10 square metres of space per person, whilst in Bulgaria this rises to 74 per cent. As Pál Banlaky observes 'even in the warmest of family environments [such scarcity of space] is unacceptable and unhealthy, both in physical and mental terms' (Puporka and Zádori 1998).

The spread of tuberculosis represents a growing threat to the health of poorer people in the region. Local studies in Roma communities in Bulgaria have identified between 0.6 and 1.8 per cent to be infected and in the cities of Sofia and Sliven Roma account for 30 and 60 per cent respectively of all patients with tuberculosis (Turnev et al. 2002). Tuberculosis is also thought to be more prevalent amongst Roma in Hungary and there was micro-epidemic in the Czech Republic in the 1990s, however no recent research has been carried out in either country to quantify the problem, nor the extent to which Roma people participate in screening programmes (London School of Hygiene and Tropical Medicine 2000).

During the 1990s there were outbreaks of Hepatitis A amongst Roma communities in Brno and Protejov in the Czech Republic (London School of Hygiene and Tropical Medicine 2000) and these are occasionally reported in Hungary. In the latter, compulsory screening of pregnant women for Hepatitis B has shown almost all infections to be amongst Roma (Puporka and Zádori 1998). In Bulgaria 'viral hepatitis is also a serious problem in Roma neighbourhoods and ghettos . . . The incidence of Hepatitis A and B is high among Roma' (Turnev *et al.* 2002).

The extent to which Roma participate vaccination programmes against diseases such as measles has yet to be thoroughly investigated in any of the four countries under discussion. One of the last outbreaks of polio in Europe affected three Roma children in Bulgaria, according to a report in The *Guardian* on 22 June 2002 (Anon 2002). In 1994 a polio outbreak in Sliven left almost all ninety of its young Roma victims permanently disabled (Turnev *et al.* 2002). Skin diseases and waterborne infections such as dysentery and *Shigella Enteritis* have been reported amongst Roma communities in the region. Despite the relative wealth of Roma-specific data on communicable diseases, the picture is far from comprehensive. It is likely that many of these problems will persist and even increase unless substantial steps are taken to improve the living conditions of many Roma people, as 'the lack of basic sanitary conditions is one of the main reasons for the higher incidence of infectious diseases among Roma compared with the rest of the population' (Turnev *et al.* 2002).

Non-communicable diseases

Though illnesses such as cardiovascular and lung diseases probably make a significant contribution to the notably lower life expectancy of Roma minorities, specific research in these areas has been extremely limited. Mortality data has not been coded for Roma ethnicity, however it is widely accepted in both Hungary and Bulgaria that the life expectancy of Roma people is at least ten years lower than the national averages. In 1989 a study based on comparing census data concluded that in Czechoslovakia the life expectancies of Roma men and women were, respectively, 12.1 and 14.4 years lower than for the country's population as a whole.

County studies in Hungary in the late 1970s found heart disease, cerebrovascular disease and illness of the respiratory and digestive systems to be the most common cause of death amongst Roma. A local study in the late 1980s found asthma to be the most common illness of men and cardiovascular and kidney

diseases amongst women. In 1998 research in a rural Roma settlement identified coronary disease to be most common amongst men and respiratory and
kidney diseases amongst women (Puporka and Zádori 1998). In 1989 a Slovak
study found cardiovascular diseases to be the primary cause of morbidity and
mortality in one Roma settlement (London School of Hygiene and Tropical
Medicine 2000).

The reasons for the high rates of chronic diseases among Roma remain
inadequately understood. Poverty is likely to be a major factor, in part mediated through so-called lifestyle factors. Roma are believed to have high rates of
smoking and to start smoking at an earlier age. Malnutrition, both in the sense
of a lack of food and eating the wrong kinds of food, also contributes to
poorer health. In the Roma settlement of Kiskundorozsma (Hungary) in 1998
almost the entire adult population was unemployed with both adults and children showing signs of under-nourishment, whilst in the former industrial city
of Miskolc 'for the majority of Roma procuring their daily meal is a serious
struggle'. It has also been argued that in some cultures obesity is considered a
sign of wealth (Puporka and Zádori 1998). Research in the Czech Republic
indicated that the diet of Roma children included a high proportion of fats
and sugars and around only half the amount of fresh fruit, vegetables and milk
than that of their non-Roma counterparts (Koupilová *et al.* 2001).

There appear very few health awareness programmes targeted at Roma
communities that include information about healthy diets, risk factors and the
importance of regular exercise. It is widely believed that many Roma see
health care professionals less frequently than other citizens, often waiting until
symptoms become unbearable. Researchers carrying out fieldwork in Roma
settlements in Bulgaria identified a number of conditions that had not been
previously diagnosed. As discussed below, the rising cost of health services and
medicines mean that some Roma people probably do not receive treatment in
time so their conditions deteriorate. In all the countries covered, Roma are
over-represented amongst the disabled, though it is unlikely that official
figures fully reflect the extent of chronic incapacity.

Reproductive and sexual health

There is much more information about the reproductive health of Roma. In
large part this stems from long standing concerns of state authorities regarding the size of their Roma minority, particularly within the context of stagnat-
ing and even falling national populations. Following the same methodology,
surveys in 1971 and 1993/4 showed the number of Roma in Hungary to
have risen almost 50 per cent from 320,000 to just under half a million. Since
the mid-1980s Hungary's total population has steadily declined leading to the

projection that by 2015 three-quarters of a million Roma will account for 8 per cent of all citizens (Havas *et al.* 1995). However, it is questionable whether such a prediction will be realized. Research in 1993 showed that family size deceased markedly amongst urban Roma (Banlaky 1993). The transition to a market economy has had a mixed effect with many Roma moving to urban areas to seek work, whilst others return to the cheaper countryside in the wake of industrial decline. A study in an isolated rural settlement in 1998 also showed that even in such an environment the birth rate had fallen sharply in recent years due to poverty, with only 6.5 per cent of the community five years old or younger compared to up to 30 per cent in the mid-1980s (Puporka and Zádori 1998).

A national picture is harder to obtain for the Czech Republic and Slovakia, as published figures are based on census data. In 1997 the Czech Government's landmark report outlining its future Roma policy gave only a vague estimate of the number of Roma and noted only that 'their birth-rate is higher than that of the non-Romani population'. The greater absolute and relative numbers of Roma in Slovakia is a far more sensitive political issue, illustrated in 2000 by the claim of the nationalist politician Robert Fico that by 2010 Roma would account for half the population of East Slovakia (Guy 2001). Despite observing that 'Roma families still tend to have four or more children' recent research carried out for the Open Society Institute in Bulgaria, also noted that 'all data are relative, different sources provide disparate information, no one seems ready to stand by any conclusive figures . . . under these conditions it is very difficult to differentiate the indictors reflecting the reproductive health status of Roma' (Turnev *et al.* 2002).

Given low life expectancy, the rise in Roma numbers over the last fifty years in eastern Europe reflects a significant decline in high rates of child mortality. In Hungary in 1970 infant mortality among Roma was 115 per 1,000 live births, a figure that had fallen to 22 in 1990, still higher than the national average of 16. Data from Czechoslovakia in the 1980s also indicated high rates of infant mortality (Czech land 23.9, Slovakia 34.8 compared to 12.1 and 14.6 respectively for non-Roma) (London School of Hygiene and Tropical Medicine 2000). A significant contributory factor seems to be the greater number of low birth weight babies born to Roma women. This in turn is felt to reflect the poorer general health of the women whose own weight is lower than the national average for pregnant mothers (Puporka and Zádori 1998).

To a certain degree, the relatively higher fertility of Roma women reflects the family orientation of communities (frequently noted in the anthropological literature) that have traditionally enjoyed little economic security and have had to rely upon close social contacts rather than more distant institutions for economic and social support. This indicates not only cultural diversity within east European societies but also that social exclusion has obstructed processes of social integration.

Some Roma communities are clearly more conservative than others. Maria Neményi's research among women of different Roma groups in Hungary found that almost two-thirds of Romanians speaking Beash had never used contraception compared with 38 per cent of those from Budapest (Nemenyi 1998). Young marriage is also common in some communities because of the 'tradition that the bride should be chaste' (Open Society Foundation 2001). In 1997 a local survey in Bulgaria estimated that half of pregnancies in the 13–16 age group were Roma (Hajioff and McKee 2000). For many Roma people life-long relationships are the norm and a review of Czechoslovak medical records (1953–79) showed a very low rate of cervical cancer amongst Roma women (London School of Hygiene and Tropical Medicine 2000). However, in the 1990s it was estimated that many of the prostitutes in the Czech Republic's were Roma and similar high-risk behaviour has also been noted in Hungary and Bulgaria. No research appears to have been conducted into the sexual health of Roma men.

Access to health services

Problems identified affecting the access of Roma people to health care services can be divided into material and cultural. Residents of isolated rural settlements often face a journey of several kilometres to see a doctor, thus incurring both additional physical effort and financial costs. Poor road conditions also obstruct the access of emergency vehicles. Patients requiring specialist examination or treatment are further disadvantaged as

> the road from the primary health care unit in the village to the regional hospital in the small town, to the district hospital in the bigger town to the university hospital in the city, where treatment has to be conducted, turns out to be too long for Roma and is an insurmountable obstacle to receiving specialised medical care.
>
> Turnev *et al.* 2002

Such fundamental problems appear to be increasing due to both the process of resettlement occurring throughout the region and a general decline in national health services. Puporka and Zádori note that 'it is undeniable that the health care system is ailing in Hungary, but in our experience certain groups in society, including Roma . . . feel this pain more acutely' (Puporka and Zádori 1998). Research amongst the 11,000 Roma of a sub-urban settlement in Bulgaria found that 85 per cent viewed recent health service reforms as 'negative'.

Former universal provision has been replaced by compulsory insurance systems. Due to high rates of unemployment, many Roma have their contributions paid by the state, however failure to register with the authorities and confusion over the need for health insurance mean that Roma people are probably over represented amongst those without entitlements (Zoon 2001). Even when insured, patients often have to make some financial contribution. In Bulgaria it has been noted that

> many families are forced to make the difficult choice between buying food or paying for medicines. . . many Roma often choose not to see their general practitioner because they know that they would be unable to fulfil his or her prescription. . . thus they resort to self-treatment which is seldom appropriate.
>
> Turnev *et al.* 2002

Across the region it is increasingly common for hospital patients to pay gratuities to staff or to contribute to the cost of their care (Balabanova and McKee 2002).

Health provision has received little attention in the Roma policies developed by governments in the region in recent years. The focus on Roma representation, cultural recognition and education may all contribute to improving health care in the longer term, though the efficacy of these policies is unclear while they lack significant financial backing. Consequently Roma-related health initiatives have remained the preserve of NGOs, the limited resources of which mean they are usually confined to the collection and dissemination of information.

Two cases illustrate the dilemma of Roma-specific health initiatives. In the former industrial town of Ózd (northern Hungary) the Roma minority self-government launched health education, vaccination and contraception programmes but costs proved prohibitive because, according to the programmes director, the multiple disadvantages faced by the Roma population means that 'we can't request the unpaid participation of the professionals involved in associated programmes . . . because this work is far more tiring than usual information giving' (Anon 1997).

In other words, additional resources (unforthcoming) were required to provide equal opportunity for the Roma population. However, the district of Krasna Poliana in Sofia had one health care facility and the authorities decided to build an extra one in the Roma mahalla of Fakulteta. As Ina Zoon notes:

> This met with the approval of the non-Roma from Krasna Poliana who no longer need to wait in line and to share 'their' clinic with Roma. For Roma, however, the 'branch' is only a source of never-ending problems . . . On any given day, the clinic has

no more than one doctor and one nurse. The place is continually overcrowded . . . In urgent cases, doctors, even when actually present, cannot provide much assistance because they lack equipment for emergencies and have little or no medication.

Zoon 2001

The story illustrates the likelihood that separating Roma is likely to lead to lower quality provision, a phenomenon that is particularly noticeable in respect of education.

The roots of this dilemma lie in the need to address objective disadvantages with limited means against a background of profound and widespread negative attitudes towards Roma people. It is far too simplistic to see prejudice as a resulting from 'ignorance of Roma culture'. It is a very complex phenomenon relating not only to ideas of national/ethnic belonging, but also to class antagonisms and contempt for poor people. The post-communist period has allowed for an unprecedented level of debate about racism, yet impoverishment and growing inequality have also made problems appear so intractable that there is inevitably a tendency to seek explanations in cultural difference. Hostile attitudes and discriminatory behaviour not only impede access to health care service by denying people the care to which they are entitled as citizens, but can also undermine the confidence of Roma people to seek advice and treatment and increases fear and suspicion of representatives of mainstream authorities.

Organizations such as the Open Society Institute and the European Roma Rights Centre have publicized numerous instances of discrimination against Roma in relation to health, ranging form patronizing behaviour through to denial of treatment and the segregation of Roma patients. Research in two Roma settlements found that most people disliked or were disappointed with their GP (Turnev et al. 2002). Problems might arise from a wide variety of reasons such as patients not following a doctor's orders that clash with cultural traditions, or from the many family visitors a Roma patient might receive whilst in hospital. Researchers report that some doctors find Roma aggressive, itself an indication that the individuals may feel that they are not being treated fairly. Maria Neményi's research amongst Roma mothers and health care workers in Hungary provides an important insight into the problems of communication, observing that the 'two sides' had radically divergent perceptions of the same events. However, she also noted that 'neither on one side or the other can we talk about homogenous groups' and that the health care workers with the closest relationship with their Roma clients were more likely to consider each as individuals and to have a less distorted attitude and to use more appropriate language and behaviour towards them (Nemenyi 1998).

Conclusion

The limited data available demonstrates that the health of Roma people in eastern Europe is consistently worse than the national average of the countries in which they live. There is clearly an urgent need to improve not only understanding of this phenomenon, but also to develop practical interventions which can ensure that Roma individuals and communities receive the information and care appropriate to their needs. How this can be achieved is a far more difficult question. To be effective, any discourse of Roma health has to take into account not only the extensive cultural and social diversity of different Roma communities and their different health care needs and perceptions, but also the broader economic and political contexts that determine their circumstances, as well as the effect of the low social status of Roma populations within wider society.

Within the field of health care some Roma-specific areas can be identified, such as research into the needs of specific populations, targeted health information and the development of more effective methods of delivering health services, including improved communication between Roma patients and practitioners. However, without addressing problems such as high unemployment, poverty, poor housing and environment, low education and weak interest representation such initiatives cannot make a significant impact on the health status of Roma people.

Growing inequality throughout eastern Europe indicates that states are not prepared to allocate sufficient resources towards the less economically productive of their citizens (amongst whom Roma are substantially over-represented) who are either ignored or for whom responsibility is devolved to non-state actors. There is a danger that a discourse of Roma health may develop that cherry-picks certain high profile initiatives whilst neglecting to address the far more costly factors behind Roma health disadvantage. Thus the appearance is given that action is being taken whilst the fundamental problems remain or even worsen. Rather than being a means for overcoming the disadvantages of Roma people, such an approach to Roma health would facilitate the perpetuation of inequality and social exclusion. Roma people are integral to the societies in which they live. It is unrealistic to think that the health of Roma people can be significantly improved without improvements in the health services and circumstances of their home societies as whole. Therefore, the discourse of 'Roma health' must be incorporated into national health care systems and be guided by the principles of equal opportunity for all citizens, rather than being taken out of context and defined through the narrow prism of ethnicity.

References

Anon (1997) Nem nő nagyra a cigányság korfája, *Népszabadság* 8 July 1997.

Anon (2002) Polio is eradicated from Europe, The *Guardian*, 22 June 2002.

Balabanova, D. and McKee, M. (2002) Understanding informal payments for health care: the example of Bulgaria. *Health Policy*, 62, 243–73.

Banlaky, P. (1993) *Cigánycsaládok Vizsgálata*, pp. 21–2. Budapest, Ministry of Welfare.

Bereczkei, T. (1993) Selected reproductive strategies among Hungarian gypsies: a preliminary analysis. *Ethology and Sociobiology*, 14, 71–88.

Bernath, G. (2002) *Forced bathings in Romani settlements*. Roma Press Centre Books, Budapest.

Cavalli-Sforza, L. (1994) *The history and geography of human genes*. Princeton University Press, Princeton, NJ.

CIA (2001) *World Fact Book*. Available at http://www.cia.gov/cia/publications/factbook.

European Committee on Migration (1995) *The situation of gypsies (Roma and Sinti) in Europe*. Council of Europe., Strasbourg.

Gresham, D. (2001) Origins and divergence of the Roma (gypsies). *American Journal of Human Genetics*, 69, 1314-31.

Guy, W. (2001) The Czech lands and Slovakia: another false dawn? In W. Guy (ed.) *Between past and future – the Roma of Central and Eastern Europe*. University of Hertfordshire Press, Hatfield.

Hajioff, S. and McKee, M. (2000) The health of the Roma people: a review of the published literature. *Journal of Epidemiology and Community Health*, 54(11), 864–9.

Havas, G., Kertesi, G. and Kemeny, I. (1995) The statistics of deprivation. *Hungarian Quarterly*, 36, Summer, 67–80.

Kádet, E. (2002) Röppalyán. Emelkedik, avagy süllzed a romák rakétája? *Beszélő*, March, 93–9.

Kalaydjieva, L., Gresham, D. and Calafell, F. (2001) Genetic studies of the Roma (Gypsies): a review. *BMC Medical Genetics*, 2, 5.

Kenrick, D. (2002) Inflections in Flux. *Transitions Online*, April, 2.

Koupilová, I., Epstein, H., Holcik, J., Hajihoff, S. and McKee, M. (2001) Health needs of the Roma population in the Czech and Slovak Republics. *Social Science and Medicine*, 53, 1191–204.

Ladányi, J. and Szelényi, I. Ki a Cigány? (2000) In Á. Horváth, E. Landau and J. Szalai (eds) *Cigánynak Születni*. Új Mandátum, Budapest.

Lewy, G. (2000) *The Nazi persecution of the gypsies*. Oxford University Press, Oxford.

London School of Hygiene and Tropical Medicine (2000) *Health needs of the Roma population in the Czech and Slovak Republics*. London School of Hygiene and Tropical Medicine (LSHTM), London.

Marushiakova, E. and Popov, V. (2000) *Gypsies/Roma in times past and present*. Litavra Publishing, Sofia.

Marushiakova, E. and Popov, V. (2002) Historical and ethnographic background: gypsies, roma and Sinti. In W. Guy (ed.) *Between past and future – the Roma of Central and Eastern Europe*. University of Hertfordshire Press, Hatfield.

Minority Rights Group (1995) *Roma/Gypsies: a European minority*. Minority Rights Group, London.

Nemenyi, M. (1998) Két Külön világ – Cigány anyák és a magyar egészségügy, *Beszélő*, 2, 53–64.

Okely, J. (1983) *The traveller – gypsies*. Cambridge University Press, Cambridge.

Open Society Foundation (2001) *Education and health problems confronting Roma women*. OSI, Sofia.

Popov, V. (unpublished) *The Roma – a nation without a state? Historical background and contemporary tendencies*.

Puporka, L. and Zádori, Z. (1998) *The health status of Romas in Hungary*. Roma Press Centre, Budapest.

Sampson, J. (1907) Gypsy language and origin. *Journal of the Gypsy Lore Society Second Series*, 1, 4–22.

Turnev, I., Kamenov, O., Popov, M., Makaveeva, L. and Alexandrova, V. (2002) *Common health problems among Roma – nature, consequences and possible solutions*. Open Society Foundation, Sofia.

Vašecka, M. (1999) *The Roma*. Institute for Public Affairs: Bratislava.

Willems, W. (1997) *In search of the true gypsy*. Frank Cass, London.

Willems, W. and Lucassen, L. (1998) The Church of Knowledge: representation of gypsies in encyclopaedias. In W. Willems, L., Lucassen and A. Cottar (eds) *Gypsies and other itinerant groups*. Macmillan Press, London.

Zoon, I. (2001) On the margins – Roma and public services in Romania, Bulgaria and Macedonia. New York, Open Society Institute 92.

Chapter 14

'On Our Terms'

The politics of Aboriginal health in Australia

Robert Griew, Beverly Sibthorpe,
Ian Anderson, Sandra Eades and Ted Wilkes

> We will welcome government cooperation and
> collaboration, but your history and our history
> demand that such takes place on our terms.
> Victorian Aboriginal Health Service, quoted in
> *National Aboriginal Health Strategy* 1989 p. xiv

We start with three assertions. Access to effective health care is a right. Diversity among populations is a fact. Therefore, to be effective in meeting citizen's rights, health care systems must embrace diversity.

In Australia, the health care system's greatest challenge is to address the significantly poorer health status of its indigenous people, who make up only around 2.6 per cent of the population. Life expectancy for Aboriginal and Torres Strait Islander people is nearly twenty years less than for non-Aboriginal Australians and mortality rates from cardiovascular, endocrine and respiratory conditions and poisoning and injury are all measured at rates several times greater (Australian Bureau of Statistics 2001). Aboriginal health status is also significantly worse than that of the indigenous populations of the other settler colonial nations with which Australia shares a similar past – New Zealand, Canada and the United States (Kunitz 1994).

So this chapter concerns indigenous claims against the Australian state for decent health care in the context of an enormous burden of disease, disability and premature death. However, the claims are complex and contested even among those who make them. Further, embracing diversity is not a one-way process – it is not something that the system 'does to' its diverse communities. Nor does it occur in a vacuum. It is part of a larger political process, involving contest and negotiation. This chapter is about this political process.

There are two groups of indigenous people in Australia, Aboriginal people and Torres Strait Islanders. The three indigenous authors of this chapter are Aboriginal people, as are most of the political activists driving the movement and organizations described in this chapter. Torres Strait Islanders have their own aspirations and structures in health. This chapter is, therefore, about Aboriginal health politics.

Our analysis focuses on the period since the development, by a joint community and government steering committee, of the National Aboriginal Health Strategy in 1989. This Strategy is generally viewed as the seminal document that articulates Aboriginal aspirations in health, and Aboriginal health political processes to the present day have in many ways revolved around ebbs and flows in the relationships of government and Aboriginal organizations around its implementation.

Theoretical framework

In order to analyse the politics of this period we have drawn on the Advocacy Coalition Framework developed by Sabatier and Jenkins-Smith (1993). This provides a theoretical framework for analysing policy development and decision-making in the politics of Aboriginal health in Australia. They insist that we look outside the traditional political science models of the machinery of government and lobby groups in a number of respects. Analysis needs to encapsulate the full range of stakeholders in any given public policy domain, including, in a federal system, stakeholders at provincial as well as central government levels. Change needs to be measured and analysed over longer time frames (ten years at least) and to take more account of ideas and knowledge in adjoining policy domains.

Sabatier and Jenkins-Smith argue that within any public policy domain, coalitions or policy 'subsystems' develop. The analytical tools offered by the framework are aimed at understanding the internal and external factors that cause these coalitions or subsystems to evolve over time.

According to Sabatier and Jenkins-Smith, policy coalitions develop and are maintained around shared core beliefs, even though their members may have different vested interests, articulated as competing claims. Coherence and stability are maintained by prioritizing these core beliefs and policy propositions over second order ones, which are not agreed. We return later in the chapter to critique this emphasis on belief structures, rather than interests, in understanding the system dynamics that operate within coalitions.

The parties that make up the Aboriginal health policy coalition are defined by history and include:

- the leadership of the Aboriginal health movement;
- a number of senior media players;
- leaders in health professional groups;
- senior public servants (many being Aboriginal and Torres Strait Islander people);
- Aboriginal health researchers (increasingly including Aboriginal and Torres Strait Islander people);
- senior politicians and Ministers; and
- Aboriginal and Torres Strait Islander leaders outside the health sector.

Three questions about this coalition arise from the Sabatier and Jenkins-Smith framework. They are:

(1) What are its key policy components?

(2) Given apparent consensus around these components, what is the nature of continuing conflict between Aboriginal and non-Aboriginal members of the coalition?

(3) Where are the dynamics within the coalition likely to take it over the next ten years?

Historical context

In order to address these questions it is first necessary to examine the historical context.

Australia is a colonial society, first settled by Europeans in 1788, in which no treaty, compact or deed of settlement was ever made between its indigenous inhabitants and the settler peoples. Australia is also a federal system and only in 1967 was the Australian Constitution amended by referendum to allow the national (Commonwealth) government for the first time to make laws for Aboriginal people (previously a State prerogative). Although not technically correct, many, in both the Aboriginal and non-Aboriginal communities in Australia, refer to this as the granting of citizenship rights to Aboriginal people (Attwood and Markus 1998).

The 1967 referendum was significant both in terms of the powerful popular movement that campaigned for the 'Yes' vote and the 90.7 per cent 'Yes' vote achieved – by far the highest endorsement of any Australian referendum. A number of other legislative and policy changes were made around this time. In 1959, the Commonwealth *Social Services Consolidation Act* gave the first clear legislative signal of the dismantling of the previous exclusion of Aboriginal people from social security entitlements. In 1962, the *Electoral Franchise Act* extended the vote to all Aboriginal people for the first time (Chesterman and Galligan 1997). Serially, State liquor licensing laws were becoming less discriminatory. The systematic removal of Aboriginal children, and the oppressive State laws regulating movement of people and life on Aboriginal reserves, were also coming to an end.

The Aboriginal medical service

The 1967 referendum was also important for radicalizing a generation of Aboriginal leaders, the attention of whom then turned to building new movements. Independent Aboriginal medical and legal services were established in Redfern (a poor, Sydney inner-city area with Aboriginal residents from across the country) in 1972. In its first years, the Aboriginal Medical Service was run largely on voluntary labour, with support from a few radical doctors, the local Catholic Church and the building unions. Throughout the 1970s and 1980s, other Aboriginal Medical Services were established successively in the capital cities of each of Australia's States and Territories and then through regional and finally many remote areas. These provided an alternative to existing inadequate means for Aboriginal people to access health care. These services, in common with other Aboriginal social movements of this time, embraced the politics of self-determination or self-management, an increasingly central (albeit contested) construct in Aboriginal Affairs that emerged in the post referendum era (Anderson 1994; Burgman 1993; Kunitz 1994).

Poor mainstream engagement in Aboriginal health was partly due to the fact that the health professions engaged late in all aspects of social or public medicine, including being in outright opposition to successive public health insurance systems, up to and including the current Medicare system (Mackay 1989). Involvement in Aboriginal health issues fell to a small number of individual doctors, for example through the National Trachoma and Eye Health Program that travelled around rural and remote areas in the 1970s and highlighted the appalling lack of primary health care services in Aboriginal Australia.

The first public funding for Aboriginal Medical Services came in grants from the Commonwealth Department of Aboriginal Affairs, established in 1972. Since then, Commonwealth funding has been switched around between national bodies. In 1973, the Department of Health also became involved in Aboriginal health, but in 1984, funding was consolidated in the Department of Aboriginal Affairs. In 1989 the Department of Aboriginal Affairs was reconstituted with the passage of legislation creating the Aboriginal and Torres Strait Islander Commission, an innovative elected commission set up to run special indigenous programs on a directly accountable basis (Anderson and Sanders 1996). Funding for the Aboriginal Medical Services was transferred to this new body.

As the number of Aboriginal Medical Services grew, so too did their political organization. The national representative body, the National Aboriginal and Islander Health Organisation, which later became the National Aboriginal Community Controlled Health Organisation (NACCHO), was established in 1974 (Saggers and Gray 1991). During the latter half of the decade, this national body and its member organizations established a claim to the legitimacy of Aboriginal community control of primary health care services. During the same period, the World Health Organization developed a vision for primary health care based on a radical engagement of primary health care with environmental and social change, not just to provide care to the sick, but to improve health at a population level (World Health Organization 1978). This model was immediately recognizable to Aboriginal activists, based as it was in the same politics and understanding of health issues.

National Aboriginal Health Strategy

The most important illustration of the impact of the Aboriginal Medical Services sector was the development of the 1989 National Aboriginal Health Strategy by representatives of Commonwealth and State governments, the National Aboriginal and Islander Health Organisation and the Department of Aboriginal Affairs (Commonwealth Department of Health and Aged Care 1989). This Strategy does not read like a government document (for which it is often criticized in unguarded moments by non-Aboriginal health bureaucrats.) It sets out key principles and a large number of often quite detailed claims and budget allocations, ranging from development of strategies to tackle specific health conditions to new primary health care and environmental health infrastructure. An overview of this Strategy is given here and its key policy components are discussed later in this chapter.

Constructed around a number of key themes, the Strategy was explicitly based on the World Health Organization model of primary health care with an emphasis on the introduction of

(1) . . . fundamental change on a preventive health-care basis to effect lasting improvements in Aboriginal health, as well as

(2) . . . alleviating the acute, existing health problems in the short term, (but) without adopting a panaceic approach that might make the application of (objective) (1) more difficult in the longer term (p. vii).

The Strategy starts with a holistic definition of health, 'Not just the physical well-being of the individual but the social, emotional and cultural well-being of the whole community' (p. x). Consistent with this is an emphasis on inter-sectoral action, such as housing and legal rights. The first task of new Aboriginal health forums in each State would be 'to finalize arrangements for ongoing mechanisms to promote intersectoral collaboration' (p. xxiii).

According to the Strategy, Aboriginal people had to be more closely involved in all aspects of the health system. In particular, the claim of the Aboriginal Medical Services for the legitimacy of Aboriginal control of primary health care was reinforced. Its recommendations supported the 'strong argument for the adoption of community controlled Aboriginal Health Services as the most appropriate service type, and for the transfer of primary level health services (from State Health Department control) to community control' (p. xxiv).

There was also a strong case made for action to improve the Aboriginal health workforce. This included both Aboriginal health workers (as primary health care workers who 'have become an integral part of the clinical staff of Aboriginal Health Services') and 'supporting Aboriginal people in courses which will qualify them for careers as health professionals' (p. xxviii). Conscious of 'the growing concern on the part of governments. . . with the effectiveness of special programs for Aboriginal people' (p. xi), the Strategy also included a whole chapter on accountability mechanisms to provide a 'closer nexus between services and needs' (p. 218).

The Strategy also included 80 pages relating to specific health challenges, from diabetes mellitus to alcohol and other drug related issues, but argued that these had to be dealt with through an 'integrated coordinated health policy' (p. 128). And it recommended an all party multi-jurisdictional Council of Aboriginal Health, a large increase in investment in environmental health and housing, and increased funding for community controlled 'Aboriginal Health Services'.

The process involved in the development of the Strategy (including community level consultation around the country) produced a real sense of ownership by Aboriginal people, and it remains to Aboriginal participants in the policy process the touchstone statement of principles from which legit-imate action can be designed. Although those involved at the time recall significant negotiation and contest on the part of the States, especially regarding their financial obligations, all Australian health ministers, as well as the National Aboriginal and Islander Health Organisation, endorsed the Strategy (Commonwealth Department of Health and Human Services 1994). It is unclear in the record how much ownership, if any, State govern-ments felt for the Strategy, but it is unusual for a strategy developed with such a strong community engagement to be endorsed by governments (Anderson 1997).

Aboriginal and Torres Strait Islander Commission

Taking up National Aboriginal Health Strategy recommendations, the Commonwealth government committed substantial amounts of funding, especially to an ambitious environmental health and housing plan. This funding flowed through the Aboriginal and Torres Strait Islander Commission, no longer a Commonwealth Government department, but a democratically elected representative structure with regional, State and a national council, each with administrative responsibilities. This proved an unhappy arrangement for many Aboriginal Medical Services, as local politics played out through the elected regional councils undermining the security of funding needed to run increasingly complex primary health care services. In 1993, the ex-head of the Commonwealth Health department was commissioned to review the Council of Aboriginal Health (that was established under the Strategy) and in 1994, a committee chaired by a senior elected executive from the National Aboriginal Community Controlled Health Organisation, evaluated the Strategy. While this committee noted that some progress had been made, the report's introduction, which was added later, presented a much harsher view, arguing that while the Strategy was the right policy, it had never been properly implemented (Codd 1993). The Aboriginal and Torres Strait Islander Commission's administrative capacity was criticized, as was the commitment of State and Territory governments.

The report fuelled intra-governmental political moves within the Commonwealth Labor government, and in 1995 that government transferred responsibility for funding Aboriginal health services away from the Aboriginal and Torres Strait Islander Commission to the Commonwealth Health Department, where it has remained ever since. The Commission, however, was to remain involved, with its continuing roles codified in a Memorandum of Understanding between itself and the Health Department. It retained an involvement in 'health hardware' including housing, water, sewerage etc. and was also to continue to be involved as an elected community representational voice on policy, and as an 'upstream' watchdog of progress.

Commonwealth and State health departments

The Commonwealth Health Department had prepared the way for the transfer of health responsibility over a couple of years prior to 1995, by establishing a national Office of Aboriginal and Torres Strait Islander Health Services. This Office would be responsible for the Aboriginal Medical Services funding program and Aboriginal-specific substance abuse services, but would equally importantly, at least in the eyes of Departmental officials, take responsibility for substantially increasing the Department's commitment across all its programs to improving Aboriginal health outcomes.

The Aboriginal Medical Services and the National Aboriginal Community Controlled Health Organisation sought the 1995 transfer back to Health. They wanted access to larger funding sources and to the greater power of a large mainstream Commonwealth Department. They were also wooed by two successive federal Labor Health Ministers and a number of senior bureaucrats who assured them that they understood the principles underpinning the National Aboriginal Health Strategy and would stand up to State governments on issues of funding and community control.

State Health Department Aboriginal health branches and the Australian Medical Association also supported the move. The consensus was that governments needed to give higher priority to Aboriginal health and to deliver on the promises made. The Australian Health Ministers Advisory Council endorsed a group of the Heads of Aboriginal Health Units to meet and establish a senior national network, largely comprised of Aboriginal people working within the government health system. This group was itself, at stages, a significant counterpoint to the Aboriginal community controlled health sector.

The Commonwealth also negotiated unorthodox funding arrangements with the State health authorities, such as allowing Medicare (the Commonwealth insurance system for private medical costs) to be billed by the States for provision of public medical officers to remote Aboriginal communities. A subsequent period of sustained funding growth followed, nearly doubling funds in five years to the Commonwealth Aboriginal health program from $116 million in 1996–97 to $203.2 million in 2001–02 (Australian Institute of Health and Welfare 2001; Treasurer 2002).

State governments in parallel also developed their own Aboriginal health plans. The Australian Health Ministers Council endorsed a set of Aboriginal health performance indicators and targets, and within eighteen months of the transfer, six of eight jurisdictions signed Commonwealth–State Framework Agreements to guide joint action on Aboriginal and Torres Strait Islander health. An influential report mapped Commonwealth and State expenditures on Aboriginal health (Commonwealth Department of Health and Aged Care 1989), and the first two-yearly report on Aboriginal health and welfare statistics by the Australian Bureau of Statistics also attracted considerable attention (Australian Bureau of Statistics 1997, 1999, 2001).

Human rights reports

Also during this time, parliamentary and human rights watchdogs continued to prompt government, sometimes more vigorously than the governments intended. The Royal Commission into Aboriginal Deaths in Custody (Johnston 1991) made recommendations across governments to reduce the rate of Aboriginal and Torres Strait Islander incarceration. The Deaths in Custody report endorsed the National Aboriginal Health Strategy (Recommendation 264) and about a third of its other recommendations referred to health issues. The Human Rights and Equal Opportunity Commission (1997) documented the 'stolen generation' of Aboriginal children who were removed from their parents by government and church authorities during the first half of the twentieth century. The latter became a significant national political issue in its own right when the conservative Commonwealth government refused both the apology and the reparations it recommended. Also, the Australian Parliament produced a report called *Health is Life* (House of Representatives Standing Committee on Community Affairs 2000) and the powerful Commonwealth Grants Commission (Commonwealth Grants Commission 2001) reported on the distribution of funds for programs that affect Aboriginal and Torres Strait Islander people. These last two reports repeated much that had been said in previous reports, although the Grants Commission report, in particular, produced much debate within the conservative Commonwealth Government, with central agencies arguing that it showed that Aboriginal specific funding had failed and in urban areas was not really needed.

National Aboriginal Community Controlled Health Organisation

Despite a high degree of apparent consensus on key aspects of policy, such as the principles underpinning the National Aboriginal Health Strategy, the last years of the decade also were characterized by conflict. As it took up its new role, the Commonwealth Health Department came into conflict with the National Aboriginal Community Controlled Health Organisation and a number of its State affiliates. In 1997, an Aboriginal Medical Service in Queensland was defunded by the Commonwealth Minister for Health following a Department commissioned review into its functioning. Then in 2000, at its annual general meeting, the National Aboriginal Community Controlled Health Organisation decided to withdraw from participation in the National Aboriginal and Torres Strait Islander Health Council that advised the Commonwealth Health Minister.

While the trigger for the 2000 withdrawal was the drafting by the Council of a new national Aboriginal and Torres Strait Islander health framework, the National Aboriginal Community Controlled Health Organisation also cited a retreat from agreed principles and processes by both the Minister and his

Department. Issues of contention cut across National Aboriginal Health Strategy principles, including an allegedly unequal burden of accountability, support by government for new, non-community controlled models of primary health care and inaction on the intersectoral agenda, especially the response to the 'stolen generations' report. Senior Health Departmental officials were accused of behaving like the 'mission managers' of old. In response, the Minister instigated a review of government funding for Aboriginal health representative structures. Eventually the National Aboriginal Community Controlled Health Organisation rejoined the Council, but not before a damaging period of open conflict and fracturing of a number of key relationships between Aboriginal activists and government officials.

Against this background, the remainder of this chapter is concerned with our three questions of the Aboriginal health policy coalition, namely its key policy components; the nature of conflict within it; and its likely future.

Key policy components

Our analysis reveals five key policy propositions around which there is *some degree* of consensus within the Aboriginal health policy coalition. The first is:

- an emphasis on primary care as the sector where Aboriginal claims in health were first established and institutionally reside, and also because the National Aboriginal Health Strategy tied the coalition to that term, as spelt out by the WHO in the 1978 Alma Ata Declaration (World Health Organization 1978).

Nested under this are the other four key policy propositions that are:

- the notion of holism as a defining concept in both health and health care and intersectoral action;
- the value of Aboriginal and Torres Strait Islander community control and/or participation;
- the Aboriginalization of the health workforce; and
- the need for fairness and balance in accountability for both government and non-government providers.

An emphasis on primary health care

There is broad agreement within the policy coalition about the need for an emphasis on primary health care. The National Aboriginal Health Strategy is a primary health care policy agenda and the main focus of the Office of Aboriginal and Torres Strait Islander Health is primary health care. However, in a health system long dominated by hospitals and primary *medical* care, delivery of primary health care was always going to be a struggle.

The service elements through which primary care is delivered to Aboriginal and Torres Strait Islander people are a complex matrix of private general medical practitioners (subsidized through the Medicare Benefits Schedule), Commonwealth and/or State funded health, and community care services (Office of Aboriginal and Torres Strait Islander Health 2001). It also includes over 100 Aboriginal Medical Services, now distributed across urban, regional and remote settings and funded in several ways: a block grant base fund, billing under Medicare for individual patient consultations, and tied health program grants (e.g. for diabetes or sexual health programs). This allows a more comprehensive approach to primary health care than the Medicare billing base of private general practice.

General medical practice reform was a central plank of the Commonwealth Labor administration of health in the early 1990s, and the process was continued by the subsequent conservative government. However, this was a primary *medical* care agenda 'with general practice at its heart' and much narrower than the aspirations of the National Aboriginal Health Strategy and its supporters. The new policy disposition played out predominantly as support for a more population-health focus in Divisions of General Practice. These regional, voluntary coalitions of GPs were established in the early 1990s and receive Commonwealth funding to 'improve the health outcomes for patients by encouraging general practitioners to work together and link with other health professionals to upgrade the quality of health service delivery at the local level' (Department of Health and Ageing 2002).

One of the central points of difference in the Aboriginal arena was comprehensiveness, many elements of which lie outside the purview of general medical practice. The Office of Aboriginal and Torres Strait Islander Health recently articulated comprehensiveness in the Aboriginal primary health care setting as including all of the following elements:

- Clinical care covering treatment of acute illness, emergency care, and the management of chronic conditions;
- Population health programs (e.g. immunization, ante-natal care, screening);
- Facilitation of access to secondary and tertiary care; and
- Client/community assistance and advocacy on health related matters within the health and non-health sectors (Office of Aboriginal and Torres Strait Islander Health 2001).

Mobilising all the disparate elements of the health system to achieve a comprehensive service, especially given the limited workforce on which both Aboriginal and non-Aboriginal services can draw, is a very difficult task (Office of Aboriginal and Torres Strait Islander Health 2000). The most significant achievement in the period since 1995 has been increased funding for

Aboriginal Medical Services, including access to Medicare funding. As well, Commonwealth Health supported managed care pooled funding models, several of which targeted Aboriginal communities (Anderson 2002a).

However, by the end of the decade, the leadership of the Aboriginal Medical Services was far from sanguine about the extent to which progress had been made on a primary health care agenda. From their perspective, funds were too often tied to general medical practice or to very specific vertical programs, not to a comprehensive model of primary health care (National Aboriginal Community Controlled Health Organisation 2000). Some saw nothing but danger in the new, pooled funding arrangements, especially the erosion of their public health, political and preventative emphasis.

As new funds were poured into Divisions of General Practice, some Aboriginal organizations pursued direct relationships with Divisions in order to influence primary care infrastructures. Others withdrew in frustration at the amount of funds they saw being given on lesser pretext to organizations with a lesser vision of primary health care and lower standards of accountability. From their perspective, while the Office of Aboriginal and Torres Strait Islander Health within Commonwealth Health had issued guidelines on the meaning of primary health care, which corresponded largely to the view of the Aboriginal Medical Services, in practice Commonwealth Health was directing resources to a narrower view of primary medical care.

More recently, some disquiet has been expressed within the policy coalition about the almost exclusive focus on primary health care. A small number of coalition members are now seeking greater emphasis in Aboriginal health on secondary and tertiary care and especially on the role of specialist medical leadership (Anderson 2002a, 2002c; Cunningham 2002). None of these argue that Aboriginal Medical Services or primary health care have failed or are not important. They do, however, point to the need to pay more attention to secondary and tertiary care.

Holism

Holism is generally accepted as a defining concept in Aboriginal and Torres Strait Islander health, invoked in relation to both health and health care. In relation to health, it pertains not only to the whole person (physical, mental, emotional, spiritual and social) but to the whole community. In relation to health care, it pertains to providing care to the whole person (not just 'body parts') and to the contribution that housing, education, employment, and justice etc. make to Aboriginal individual and community health and well-being.

While governments signed off to the principle of holism when they agreed to the National Aboriginal Health Strategy and at the time of the transfer in 1995, many subsequent initiatives injected funds into vertical programs. These included, for example, the National Indigenous Australians Sexual Health Strategy in 1997 and the National Eye Health Review in 1998, both of which have community support, but nonetheless signify a government commitment to 'body part' programs. In addition, intersectoral initiatives have not attracted the same level of support as in the original Strategy response (which was dominated by big housing and environmental health programs), although some housing for health campaigns have continued to be funded.

The Aboriginal health movement is not alone in criticizing the conservative Commonwealth Government for de-emphasising 'whole of government' health initiatives. For example, the HIV community sector is concerned about the lack of progress on law reform agendas. Within Aboriginal health, there has been progress in improving housing through a national health hardware initiative, but little action in linking primary health care to other initiatives.

The debate around horizontal versus vertical programs, however, has become confused. There is room for dedicated health programs within the primary health care context, as the National Aboriginal Health Strategy made clear in 80 pages of proposals for integrated programs to address a host of specific health problems. Within the policy coalition, the critique of the narrowing of an intersectoral agenda goes further than attacking government conservatism on social issues and land rights, but also opposes targeted programs within primary health care, where they see a proliferation of 'body parts' programs. However, the Commonwealth Health Department (and some in the Aboriginal Medical Services) want to target certain areas, and want more accountability on the part of services for running a range of vertical programs (such as maternal and infant health programs).

Aboriginal and Torres Strait Islander control and/or participation

There is also widespread though hard won *general* support within the policy coalition for the participation of Aboriginal people and organizations in primary health care, along the lines of the World Health Organization *Alma Ata Declaration* (World Health Organization 1978), the *Ottawa Charter* (World Health Organization 1986) and the *Jakarta Declaration* (World Health Organization 2001). Advocates of Aboriginal community controlled health services want community *control* of service delivery – the single most important principle around which the modern Aboriginal health movement was built.

For this reason, it remains an important issue of contention between governments and Aboriginal health organizations and activists (Anderson 2002b).

A general commitment to community participation and empowerment is widely shared by governments, and the politics of self-determination have dominated Aboriginal Affairs in Australia since the 1970s. However, Aboriginal controlled health organizations believed, when governments signed the 1989 National Aboriginal Health Strategy, that they were signing off not to a general notion of participation or self-determination, but to Aboriginal community *control* of primary health care, exercised through elected Aboriginal boards of *independent* and *local* primary health care services. Despite the strategy being fairly explicit on this point, governments have preferred more general formulations of the principle.

State governments in the north of the country have traditionally run primary health care services in remote communities. These governments have begun to accept more community participation, even including a move to some form of community control. But previously they had resisted models advocated by urban Aboriginal leaders because, they claimed, these were not relevant to the more traditional communities in remote areas. The legacy of antagonism between State governments and Aboriginal activists will take a while to overcome, even though both sides have made a positive decision to change the patterns of the past (Aboriginal Medical Services Alliance of the NT 2001). Support for formal Aboriginal governance of independent health services has remained a lightning rod for this legacy and absorbs large amounts of community leadership capacity.

On the other hand, a substantial proportion of Aboriginal people cannot access an Aboriginal community controlled health service, either because of distance or the lack of such a service in their region. While growth in the number of Aboriginal Medical Services is one answer to this problem, the reality is that many communities have no chance of access in the foreseeable future, largely because of diseconomies resulting from the small and dispersed nature of the Aboriginal population in remote areas. Further, some communities seek alternative forms of health care delivery, such as maintaining government provided health clinics or accessing local town or city general practitioners. Thus a singular model of stand-alone community controlled health services will not meet the needs of all Aboriginal people now, or in the future.

Aboriginalization of the health workforce

Aboriginalization of the health workforce is one of the most difficult areas of policy discussion within the coalition. Training of Aboriginal and Torres Strait Islander people to work in health services commenced in Australia long after indigenous participation in training began in New Zealand and North America. For example, the first indigenous medical graduates in North America and New Zealand were in 1889 and 1899 respectively, whereas the first Aboriginal medical practitioners did not graduate until the 1980s.

Australia developed the model of the Aboriginal health worker in the Northern Territory, based on a hospital assistants' course that started in the mid-1960s. Aboriginal health workers are meant to receive a year of training and then practice at the front line in Aboriginal primary health care settings, being seen as a kind of primary care 'barefoot doctor' by some advocates of the model.

There are now two courses in Queensland universities that cater for Aboriginal health worker training at a higher level. Mostly, however, health workers are trained in vocational, not tertiary settings. Numbers of Aboriginal people enrolled in vocational courses have climbed sharply since the mid-1990s, while those enrolled in tertiary level courses has remained stagnant, and in the case of nursing students, actually fallen (Schwab and Anderson 1998). A robust discussion is emerging about the future of Aboriginal health workers and the competencies that should be expected of them. Now that they are paid wages comparable to Nursing Assistants, value for money questions arise about the relative contributions of these workers compared to those with mainstream health training (Office of Aboriginal and Torres Strait Islander Health 2001).

Despite support for more Aboriginal medical graduates, there is some ambivalence about the role of Aboriginal doctors and nurses. Professional associations for Aboriginal doctors and nurses have been established and graduates work in community controlled services, State government and private practice. They are not always well received within community controlled organizations, however, being sometimes seen as 'tall poppies' or a threat to management. Governments have supported curriculum initiatives for medical training, but have generally failed to support initiatives to boost Aboriginal nursing numbers, or to promote more Aboriginal workers in public health, dentistry, allied health, nursing or health management (Anderson 2002a; Office of Aboriginal and Torres Strait Islander Health 2001).

The need for fairness and balance in accountability

There is acceptance within the policy coalition of the notion of accountability, as illustrated in the National Aboriginal Health Strategy. However, its shape or form continues to be the subject of dispute. Despite the limited monitoring of infrastructure, processes and outputs of mainstream primary health care in Australia, Aboriginal primary health care, in contrast, has been subjected to considerable scrutiny.

When the Aboriginal Medical Services funding program transferred to the Health Department in 1995, the imposition of some standard form of account-ability was inevitable. The previous administration under the Aboriginal and Torres Strait Islander Commission, conscious (and possibly resentful) that health was such a big component of their funding pool, considered an account-ability system based on individual services improving health outcomes for their communities. This was resisted by Aboriginal Medical Services on the basis that improvements in health status require strategies outside the health domain and sustained over a long time (Anderson and Brady 1995). Under Health, a system of Service Activity Reporting for Commonwealth funded services was estab-lished. Jointly endorsed after extended disputation, these data are now jointly collected and analysed by the Office of Aboriginal and Torres Strait Islander Health and the National Aboriginal Community Controlled Health Organisation. Some services are also beginning to undergo accreditation, simi-lar to that established in private general practice.

The current argument is less about the amount of accountability – too much or too little – than about the purposes for which performance informa-tion is gathered, and the lack of perceived reciprocity in the accountability of governments to community organizations. Some argue that service account-ability is still process and financially driven and the nature and quality of programming is largely unknown. Aboriginal Medical Services also point out that they are much more accountable than State services, or the general Medicare Benefits Scheme that funds patient consultations with private general practitioners. They strongly criticize the Commonwealth Health Department for not holding the States more accountable.

While recognizing the need for accountability, *all* Aboriginal service sectors resent being held more accountable than mainstream services. Aboriginal activists also fear the day that accountability turns from a reasonable relationship of reciprocity to a hostile relation that will seek again to hold services accountable for impossible outcomes that would never be applied to non-Aboriginal services. This fear is not unfounded, since in the face of the continuing poor health status of Aboriginal people, Government central agencies frequently ask how continued investment in Aboriginal primary health care can be justified. In fact, prior to the transfer of the Aboriginal health program to Commonwealth Health, the Aboriginal and Torres Strait Islander Commission had precipitated a significant controversy by asking an Aboriginal Medical Service (in Walgett, NSW) to endorse performance targets on which their funding would depend. These included targets such as reducing the incidence of non-insulin dependent diabetes mellitus by 20 per cent within two years, a target unachievable by a single health service working alone, and probably unachievable in any circumstances (Anderson and Brady 1995). In contrast, the mainstream health system is so far seldom assessed in terms of health gain. Aboriginal activists are well aware of these Government discussions and, in health as in other areas, take a sceptical view of government accountability as a result. Aboriginal health bureaucrats are forced on the defensive, caught between their defence of health service funding as providing basic equity, their advocacy of a primary health care solution in the long run, and their own accountability agendas to pursue quality and effectiveness. Accountability is not the only issue that is compromised by this dynamic.

Conflict and consensus within the coalition

From this brief discussion of the coalition's key policy components, elements both of underlying agreement and conflict emerge. Occasionally, the conflict has reached substantial levels, for example in late 2000 when the National Aboriginal Community Controlled Health Organisation 'walked out' of the National Aboriginal and Torres Strait Islander Health Council. They cited some of the concerns discussed above, but the trigger was the Council's attempt to rewrite the National Aboriginal Health Strategy, seen as losing both the principles and the community engagement.

We can identify four overarching causes for conflict in the Aboriginal health policy system, as follows.

First, there has been a general decline in political consensus about Aboriginal affairs since the election of the conservative Coalition Government in Canberra in 1996. The first term of the new government was characterized by outright conflict with Aboriginal organizations. The Government made substantial funding cuts to the Aboriginal and Torres Strait Islander Commission, refused to make a formal apology for past wrongs, especially the removal of children, when recommended by the Human Rights and Equal Opportunities Commission (even when every State parliament did so), and rejected any discussion of a treaty. Senior Ministers also criticized the High Court for its decisions in the Mabo and Wik land rights decisions, which rejected the historic fiction that Australia had been no man's land – *terra nullius* – when settled by English colonizers in the 18th century.

Despite this inauspicious background, the new Health Minister, Dr Michael Wooldridge, who stayed in the job for five years, had a strong personal commitment to Aboriginal people and was widely respected within the Aboriginal community. His good relationship with the leaders of the National Aboriginal Community Controlled Health Organisation probably limited conflict within the Aboriginal health coalition for several years. However, preserving this good relationship (by both sides) in such a hostile environment also meant that some issues were allowed to fester rather than being brought out into the open and dealt with.

Second, other parts of the Commonwealth bureaucracy have argued explicitly against elements of the underlying health policy consensus, including the role of primary health care and any notion of community control of services. The relevance of Aboriginal-specific services for urban Aboriginal populations also has been contested, most clearly in public pronouncements from the Commonwealth Minister for Aboriginal Affairs regarding the Commonwealth Grants Commission report. Paradoxically these criticisms may have suppressed debate within the policy coalition, in the face of a shared sense of threat.

Third, not all underlying beliefs are shared by all. These include the 'compensation' argument, embraced by many Aboriginal activists, but inevitably at odds with government precepts of needs-based policy. Another contested belief is the meaning of community participation. White administrators complain that Aboriginal communities (and some service organizations) see community development as more important than the quality and sustainability of the services they deliver. Aboriginal activists reply that community development is an internationally recognized path to health gain, often invoking past experiences of being patronized by non-Aboriginal sympathizers. Bureaucrats are concerned about the vulnerability of the program as a whole, if timeframes are not met and they cannot demonstrate improved health outcomes.

Finally, there remain unresolved differences in the meaning given to some key policy components. For example, non-Aboriginal coalition members often decry the lack of a government-style strategy in the National Aboriginal Health Strategy. Aboriginal members argue that the Strategy principles would solve the current problems if only governments would implement them.

Similarly, the rationale for the transfer of Aboriginal health from the Aboriginal and Torres Strait Islander Commission to Commonwealth Health in 1995 (which was strongly supported by nearly all members of the Aboriginal health policy coalition) clearly had different meanings to the parties concerned. As noted earlier, the Health Department had two objectives at the time of the transfer, first, supporting Aboriginal community control of health services, and second, improving access and effectiveness for Aboriginal people across the health system. The latter objective included a component of mainstreaming, that is, making mainstream services more accessible to and effective for Aboriginal and Torres Strait Islander people. While everyone endorsed improved access, especially to hospitals, the priority given to access to private

General Practice and the use of the language of mainstreaming are all points of tension.

Aboriginal players expected that an alignment with a powerful Commonwealth Department would allow them to really 'take the States on'. But the intricacies of Commonwealth–State relations across a portfolio as complicated as Health were never going to allow the Commonwealth to play the kind of advocacy role expected of them by community organizations. Similarly, it was not realistic of the Health Department to expect the radicals of the Aboriginal health sector to suddenly embrace mainstreaming.

Likely future path

Two issues are key to predicting the future of Aboriginal health politics. The first issue concerns the role of conflict within the system. Within the Advocacy Coalition Framework, conflict among coalition members is seen as normal, not pathological. From this it flows that lack of conflict may pose as great a danger to the coalition as conflict. Although there is consensus on some basic policy components, we would argue that some unresolved issues should to be exposed to open debate and argument in order for the players in the coalition to move forward. These central issues include:

- The centrality of primary health care compared to more emphasis on secondary and tertiary health care;
- The lack of progress in collaboration between the Aboriginal health system and other sectors, such as education, justice, planning, local government, public works, welfare and community services;
- The nature of Aboriginal community control of service delivery including the centrality of the Aboriginal Medical Services model as opposed to alternative new models (such as regionalized services);
- The future of Aboriginal people in the health workforce – specifically support for a full range of Aboriginal and Torres Strait Islander health professionals;
- The extent of accountability that can reasonably be expected of health programs; and
- The best strategies for producing change in State government services within a federal system of government.

The second issue concerns the role of shared core beliefs in binding a policy coalition or subsystem as proposed by Sabatier and Jenkins-Smith (1993). Examination of Aboriginal health policy has shown that within the coalition there are fundamental differences in core beliefs.

We would argue that it is instead shared interests that bind the coalition. These include:

- Resistance to populist notions that there is a simple solution to the complex problems in Aboriginal health;
- Fighting off attacks against policy and funding, such as misinterpretations by central agencies of demographic and epidemiological data in the Grants Commission 2001 report; and
- A shared interest in defending hard won policy structures and processes.

The problem is that when only basic interests, generated for the most part by a sense of external threat, bind the members of a coalition together, addressing difficult issues arising from the lack of shared core beliefs will be difficult. Thus it appears that some core precepts from the National Aboriginal Health Strategy (at least from an Aboriginal perspective) are not widely shared, but fear of the consequences of unpacking those disagreements may be enough to stifle important debate by either government or non-government parties.

On the other hand, sustained resistance on the part of Aboriginal leaders to notions like mainstreaming helps maintain a focus upon core Aboriginal claims. It is not yet clear if the emergence of a greater number of younger Aboriginal people with technical training of various kinds will lead to a more accommodating politics with government. There is little sign of that at present, with very similar politics apparent on the part of the younger leaders emerging within the health movement.

The key questions, therefore, are what are the dynamics of change within the coalition and how will these shape future policies? Factors we have identified include the following:

- Senior Aboriginal personnel within the coalition are changing. Although their leadership has been extraordinarily stable for a long period, change is now inevitable as the current leaders retire to less punishing roles and are themselves affected by the illness and disability burden they have fought so long to lift.
- Although the new generation of leaders has adopted largely the same politics, they are also the product of more formal education and bring a technical as well as political perspective to their new leadership roles.
- Some of the underlying debates are driven from outside the coalition, for example by changes in the wider health system, such as the availability of or restrictions on funding.

- There is an important role for new knowledge and technology in the Aboriginal health coalition. For example, new vaccine technologies may make it harder to resist targeted child health programs.
- There will continue to be powerful pressure for evaluation. For example, the Aboriginal Health Performance Indicators and Targets adopted by Australian Health Ministers in 1997 will lead to questions of responsibility if progress is inadequate.

Conclusion

This chapter has considered nearly a decade and a half of political process in historical context and has examined the political advocacy coalition that has been created. We have argued that although a broad policy consensus has been reached, it is underpinned by conflict and dispute among the members of the coalition. Rather than being bound by common beliefs alone – often the main reason for dispute – we argue that common interests bind the players together. Our analysis points to important changes in the politics of Aboriginal health over the next decade as contested beliefs are argued out, and as the Australian health system incrementally improves its response to Australia's Indigenous peoples.

We have also examined the role of conflict within Aboriginal health politics and have argued that there are constructive as well as dysfunctional aspects. Such conflict helps maintain key Aboriginal claims in the face of government inertia and the impatience of technocrats, and will also, depending on how the dynamics of change unfold, ensure that some of the key issues are argued out over the next years.

Non-Aboriginal members of the coalition often experience such conflict as highly dysfunctional to progress. Our advice for them is that they should not be put off but engage in debate, trusting that constructive answers will be found, even though at times differences appear to defy resolution. One of the key barriers to overcome, however, is the view held by many Aboriginal players that all argument on these key issues is just cover for simplistic attacks from both within and outside government.

References

Aboriginal Medical Services Alliance of the NT (2001) Presentation to 2001 Public Health Association annual conference. Sydney.

Anderson, I. (1994) Power of health – on the politics of self-determining Aboriginal health. *Arena Magazine*, **11**, June–July, 32–36.

Anderson, I. (1997) *The national Aboriginal health strategy.* In H. Gardiner (ed.) *Health policy in Australia.* Oxford University Press, Melbourne.

Anderson, I. (2002a) *National strategy in Aboriginal and Torres Strait Islander health: a framework for health gain?* Discussion Paper No 6. VicHealth Koori Health Research and Community Development Unit, Melbourne.

Anderson, I. and Brady, M. (1995) *Performance indicators for Aboriginal health services.* Discussion Paper 81. Centre for Aboriginal Economic Policy Research, Australian National University, Canberra.

Anderson, I., Clarke, A., Renhard, A., Otim, M. and Andrews, S. (2002c) Aboriginal acute care and national strategy. Linking acute care to a strategy for improving Aboriginal health. *Australian Health Review.*

Anderson, I. and Sanders, W. (1996) *Aboriginal health and institutional reform within Australian Federalism.* Centre for Aboriginal Economic Policy research, ANU, Discussion Paper No 117/1996. Canberra.

Attwood and Markus (1998) Representation Matters: the 1967 referendum and citizenship. In N. Peterson and W. Sanders (eds) *Citizenship and indigenous Australians: changing conceptions and possibilities*, pp. 118–40. Cambridge University Press, Cambridge.

Australian Bureau of Statistics (1997) *The health and welfare of Australia's Aboriginal and Torres Strait Islander peoples.* Commonwealth of Australia, Canberra.

Australian Bureau of Statistics (1999) *The health and welfare of Australia's Aboriginal and Torres Strait Islanders.* Australian Bureau of Statistics and Australian Institute of Health and Welfare, Canberra.

Australian Bureau of Statistics (2001) *The health and welfare of Australia's Aboriginal and Torres Strait Islander people.* Commonwealth of Australia, Canberra.

Australian Institute of Health and Welfare (2001) *Expenditures on health services for Aboriginal and Torres Strait Islander people 1998–1999.* Commonwealth of Australia, Canberra.

Burgman, V. (1993) *Power and protest, movements for social change in Australian society.* Allen and Unwin, St Leonards, NSW.

Chesterman, J. and Galligan, B. (1997) *Citizens without rights, Aborigines and Australian citizenship.* Cambridge University Press, Cambridge.

Codd, M. (1993) *Developing a partnership: A review of the Council of Aboriginal health.* Council of Aboriginal Health Review Team, Canberra.

Commonwealth Department of Health and Aged Care (1989) *Expenditures on health services for Aboriginal and Torres Strait Islander people.* Commonwealth of Australia, Canberra.

Commonwealth Department of Health and Human Services (1994) *The National Aboriginal Health Strategy: an evaluation.* Commonwealth of Australia, Canberra.

Commonwealth Grants Commission (2001) *Report on Indigenous Funding.* Commonwealth Department of Health and Aged Care, Canberra.

Cunningham, J. (2002) Diagnostic and therapeutic procedures among Australian hospital patients identified as indigenous. *Medical Journal of Australia,* **176**, 58–62.

Department of Health and Ageing (2002) Available at http://www.health.gov.au/hsdd/gp/branch/ds.htm.

House of Representatives Standing Committee on Community Affairs (2000) *Health is life: Report on the Inquiry into Indigenous Health.* Commonwealth of Australia, Canberra.

Human Rights and Equal Opportunity Commission (1997) *Bringing them home. National inquiry into the separation of Aboriginal and Torres Strait Islander children from their families.* Commonwealth of Australia, Canberra.

Johnston, E. (1991) *Royal Commission into Aboriginal deaths in custody.* Australian Government Publishing Service, Canberra.

Kunitz, S. (1994) *Disease and social diversity: the European impact on the health of non-Europeans.* Oxford University Press, New York.

Mackay, D. (1989) The politics of reaction: the AMA as a pressure group. In H. Gardner (ed.) *The politics of health: the Australian experience.* Longman, London.

National Aboriginal and Torres Strait Islander Working Party (1989) *A national Aboriginal health strategy.* Commonwealth of Australia, Canberra.

National Aboriginal Community Controlled Health Organisation (2000) *Report to the United Nations Committee on social cultural and economic rights.*

Office of Aboriginal and Torres Strait Islander Health (2001) *Better health care. Studies in the successful delivery of primary health care services for Aboriginal and Torres Strait Islander Australians.* Available at http://www.health.gov.au/oatsih/pubs/bhcs.htm.

Office of Aboriginal and Torres Strait Islander Health (2000) *Consultation draft.* National ATSI Strategic Workforce Framework Canberra.

Sabatier, P. and Jenkins-Smith, H. (1993) *Policy change and learning – an advocacy coalition approach.* Westview Press, San Francisco, CA.

Saggers, S. and Gray, D. (1991) *Aboriginal health and society.* Allen and Unwin, Sydney.

Schwab, R. and Anderson, I. (1998) *Trends in indigenous participation in health sciences education: the vocational education and training sector.* Discussion Paper 171. Centre for Aboriginal Economic Policy research, Australian National University, Canberra.

Treasurer (2002) *Portfolio Budget Statements 2001–02.* Commonwealth of Australia, Canberra.

World Health Organization (1978) Declaration of Alma-Ata. Available at http://www.who.int/home-page.

World Health Organization (2001) *Jakarta Declaration on leading health promotion into the twenty-first century.* Available at http://www.who.int/home-page/.

World Health Organization (1986) *Ottawa charter for health promotion.* Available at http://www.who.int/home-page/.

Chapter 15

Māori in Aotearoa/New Zealand

Sue Crengle, Peter Crampton and
Alistair Woodward

Indigenous peoples are defined in terms of collective
aboriginal occupation prior to colonial settlement.
They are not to be confused with minorities or ethnic
groups within states. Thus 'indigenous rights' are
strictly distinguished from 'minority rights'.
Trask 1999 p. 33

Introduction

Māori are the indigenous people of Aotearoa (New Zealand) and indigeneity
should form the basis of the Māori claim on the state. In practice this claim is
operationalized through the 1840 Treaty of Waitangi.

This chapter focuses on the provision of health services to Māori in
Aotearoa. It includes a brief discussion of the Treaty of Waitangi and its relevance to health followed by general information about the health sector.
Māori demographic and health information, including a discussion of the
factors that contribute to and maintain disparities in contemporary times,
also is presented. The provision of health services to Māori by the so-called
'mainstream' services is described. Finally the development and activities of
Māori health services are described.

Historical overview

After the Treaty of Waitangi (the Treaty) was signed in 1840 the rate of
European settlement accelerated, as did an active process of colonization. This
was followed in the first half of the twentieth century by Government policies
and actions that were characterized by ongoing oppression and attempts to
assimilate Māori into the colonial society (Walker 1990). Post World War Two

government policies resulted in the urbanization of the majority of the Māori population (Metge 1995).

The processes of colonization, assimilation and urbanization resulted in the loss of Māori land, loss of the Māori economic base, poverty and the imposition of non-Māori institutions and laws that were associated with the destruction of Māori cultural practices, language and institutions. As a consequence, Māori experienced increased socio-economic deprivation, poorer health, poorer education, fewer employment opportunities and many other disadvantages. A government programme of structural reform based on 'New Right' economic and social philosophies commenced in 1984, and Māori bore the brunt of the losses in the labour market, as shown by rising unemployment, increasing bene-fit dependency and falling incomes (Kelsey 1995). Māori living today in Aotearoa continue to experience the effects of these processes through inequitable access to society's goods and resources.

Despite the assaults on Māori society, culture and language during the last half of the nineteenth century and the early and middle parts of the twentieth century, Māori *iwi* (tribes), *hapu* (subtribes), *whānau* (families), individuals and institutions have continued to assert their belief in, and right to, cultural identity and self-determination (Durie 1998; Walker 1990). Although Māori have asserted this right since the 1840s it was not until the 1970s that protest action reaffirmed the Treaty as the founding document of Aotearoa, highlighted the government's failure to honour the Treaty, sought restoration of justice according to the Treaty and, in a broad sense, expressed Māori desire for self-determination. Since then Māori language and cultural practices have been revitalized and Māori development has progressed, particularly in the education and health sectors, which have seen the development of Māori education institutions and an increase in the number of Māori health care providers.

The Treaty of Waitangi

Representatives of Queen Victoria and Māori signed the Treaty of Waitangi (the Treaty) in 1840. Two versions of the Treaty were written: one in Māori, the other in English. There are substantial differences in meaning between the two versions. For example, article one of the English version confers on the Queen of England sovereignty over Aotearoa; in the Māori version she has the right to govern. Article two (Māori version) conferred on Māori chiefs *tino rangatiratanga* (absolute chieftainship, sovereignty) over 'their lands, homes and all their treasured possessions', whereas the English version guaranteed 'full, exclusive and undisturbed possession of their lands and estates, forests, fisheries, and other properties'. The differing uses of sovereignty and governance, as well as the use of 'all their treasured possessions', has resulted in different understandings of the extent of the government's obligations and Māori rights arising from the Treaty of Waitangi. From the time of its signing, the letter and the spirit of the Treaty were not honoured by representatives of Queen Victoria, and successive governments continued to breach the Treaty. Māori, recognizing that their Treaty partner was not behaving honourably, began protesting, and petitioned the Queen and her representatives in Aotearoa, the government and various commissions of inquiry from the 1840s onwards.

In 1975 the Treaty of Waitangi Act, which established the Waitangi tribunal and empowered it to hear claims and make findings relating to potential breaches of the Treaty, was passed through Parliament. The Tribunal was not able to hear claims about historical breaches of the Treaty until the Act was amended in 1984. Throughout the late 1970s and the 1980s government policy with respect to Māori continued to evolve and increasingly recognized Māori rights, acknowledged Māori grievances, and encouraged Māori participation in government policies and programmes.

Despite this progress, the Treaty, while being recognized by government as the founding document of Aotearoa, is not used as the basis of government policy. A recent analysis of Māori health policy asserts that the failure of successive governments to meaningfully implement the Treaty of Waitangi in health policy is a key factor that has limited Māori health outcomes (National Health Committee 2002). Three principles that are derived from the Treaty appear to have guided government responses to Māori health over the last decade. These principles, which were developed by the Royal Commission on Social Policy (Royal Commission on Social Policy 1988), are partnership (between Māori and government), participation (by Māori) and protection of Māori interests (equity between Māori and non-Māori). The extent to which these principles have been implemented has varied over time. Throughout the 1990s, successive governments focused on participation; resource allocation that took into account Māori health needs; and culturally appropriate practices and procedures in purchasing and providing health services (Department of Health 1992). Consequently throughout the decade there was more consultation with Māori, strategies to develop the Māori health workforce were implemented, and the number of Māori health service providers increased significantly. Current Māori health policy has been extended to include objectives relating to ensuring access to and the effectiveness of the 'mainstream'[1] (non-Māori) health service providers; working across sectors; and fostering *whánau* (family) development (Ministry of Health 2001a). However, current government policy is not formulated on a Treaty rights basis, but is based on a social justice approach that focuses on reducing disparities for Māori, low

[1] We use quotes around 'mainstream' and 'race' as we believe the use of these words is odd in relation to Māori and Aotearoa.

income and other population groups, rather than using the Treaty as the basis for determining its relationship with Māori and developing programmes to improve the status of Māori within Aotearoa.

The health sector

Since the early 1980s, the New Zealand health care system has undergone four major episodes of restructuring, including the introduction of a quasi/internal-market based system during the 1990s (Gauld 2001). As part of the changes during the early 1990s, the government introduced contracting into the health sector, which brought with it for the first time an opportunity for the state to exert centralized planning approaches to issues such as the distribution of general practitioners and control over demand-driven expenditure. Previous attempts at central planning control had been piecemeal and only partially successful. Overall, New Zealand spends about 8 per cent of its gross domestic product on health care, which is very close to the OECD average (Ministry of Health 2000).

The majority of health care services in Aotearoa are publicly funded. About 77 per cent of total health care expenditure is from public sources, and about 23 per cent from private sources, such as out-of-pocket payments for general practitioners and health insurance premiums (Ministry of Health 2000). Since 2001, twenty-one District Health Boards are responsible both for purchasing health services and providing secondary health services to the whole population within their district. Most hospital and related services, laboratory and radiology services, are funded entirely by the government (although around 40–50 per cent of elective surgery operations are privately funded and are carried out in private hospitals). Government subsidies for pharmaceuticals vary, depending on the cost of the drug to the government, and patient co-payments are determined by the level of government subsidy of the prescribed drug and the individual patient's eligibility for a targeted benefit.

Public health programmes (e.g. public health nurses, mammography screening and health promotion programmes) are also funded in full by the government.

Aotearoa does not have a universal primary care system that is free at the point of use. Independent general practitioners, who traditionally have adopted a self-employed, for-profit small business model, deliver most primary health care. General practice services are funded in part by the government but out-of-pocket charges levied on people using primary care services contribute a significant amount to the funding received in primary care. About 40 per cent of total primary care expenditure is from private sources, and about 60 per cent from public sources (Ministry of Health 2000). Reforms during the 1990s promoted a range of developments, including the grouping of general practitioners into well organized negotiating bodies for contracting purposes (independent practitioner associations), the introduction of population-based management approaches within primary care organizations, the development of new services for Māori, and also have enabled midwives and nurses to gain access to resources and expand their professional roles (Crampton 2000; Crampton and Brown 1998). Over 70 per cent of general practitioners belong to independent practitioner associations (IPAs) or similar groups. These groups undertake contracting and reporting to funding agencies and provide quality assurance programmes and continuing education programmes (Malcolm and Wright 2000).

Aotearoa is currently reorienting its health services with an increasing focus on primary care. Accompanying this reorientation is the increasing use of capitation funding for primary care services and the formation of new, non-profit primary health organizations that have responsibility for enrolled populations. Furthermore, primary care providers are being encouraged to increase the health promotion, prevention, screening and early detection programmes within their organizations (Ministry of Health 2001b).

A single health system provides services to both Māori and non-Māori through the so-called 'mainstream' (non-Māori health service providers) services and Māori health service providers. That is, there are not parallel health systems for Māori and non-Māori. Funding for Māori health providers is sourced through the government budget, Vote: Health. The proportion of total health expenditure that goes to Māori health providers is very small: approximately NZD$180 million from a total health expenditure of approximately NZD$8000 million (French *et al.* 2001). Māori providers have similar contracts to non-Māori services. Māori are able to make use of both 'mainstream' and Māori health services and people of any ethnic group are able to attend Māori providers' services.

Demography, Māori health status and Māori experience of health services

Demographic information

The 2001 census enumerated 526,281 Māori, representing 14.7 per cent of the total population normally resident in Aotearoa (Statistics New Zealand 2002a). The total resident population in New Zealand is nearly 3.8 million with 85 per cent residing in urban areas, and roughly three-quarters living in the North Island (Statistics New Zealand 2002b). The main ethnic groups are European/other (80.8 per cent), Māori (14.7 per cent), Pacific Island people

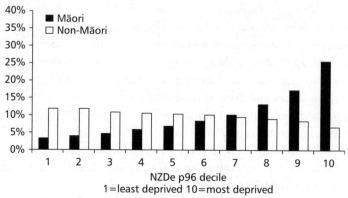

Figure 15.1 Distribution of Māori and non-Māori populations by deprivation decile, 1996 (From Reid *et al* (2000) Disparities in health: common myths and uncommon truths. With permission from *Pacific Health Dialogue* **7**, 38–47)

(6.5 per cent) and Asian (6.6 per cent) (Statistics New Zealand 2002c). (Note that these figures add up to more than 100 per cent due to self-identification with more than one ethnic group.) The Māori population is younger than the non-Māori: children aged less than 15 years make up 37.3 per cent of the Māori population and 20 per cent of the non-Māori population (Statistics New Zealand 2002d). Social and economic policies have resulted in a very uneven distribution of social and material resources across different ethnic groups. Māori are over-represented in areas of high socio-economic deprivation. The New Zealand Deprivation Index (NZDep96) is a measure of small area deprivation based on nine variables from the 1996 census (Crampton *et al.* 2000) and 25.8 per cent of Māori reside in the most deprived 10 per cent of areas (compared with 4.9 per cent of non-Māori). Conversely only 3.2 per cent of Māori reside in the least deprived 10 per cent of areas (compared with 12.6 per cent of non-Māori) (Salmond and Crampton 2000). The distribution of Māori and non-Māori across the deprivation deciles is shown in Figure 15.1.

Other consequences for Māori of the uneven distribution of social and material resources include poorer performance by the education system (for Māori children), limited employment opportunities, lower income levels and lower levels of home ownership (Te Puni Kokiri 2000).

Māori health status

Although Māori life expectancy has improved over the last few decades, on almost every health status indicator, Māori still have poorer health status than the non-Māori population. Current estimates of morbidity and mortality are likely to underestimate Māori rates because the collection of ethnicity

Table 15.1 Leading causes of death for Māori and non-Māori

Māori	Non-Māori
Total cancer	Total cancer
Ischaemic heart disease	Ischaemic heart disease
Diabetes	Cerebrovascular disease
Other heart disease	Other heart disease
Cerebrovascular disease	Chronic obstructive respiratory disease

Source: adapted from New Zealand Health Information Service 2001.

information in the databases used for the numerators in these statistics is incomplete and inconsistent through time and across datasets (Robson and Reid 2001). A recent study linking mortality information and the census databases estimated that routine mortality statistics underestimated Māori deaths by 29 per cent (Blakely *et al.* 2002a). Even so, reported Māori life expectancy at birth is currently 8.6 years lower than that of the non-Māori/non-Pacific population (Ministry of Health 1999a).

For all age groups combined the leading causes of death are similar in the Māori and non-Māori populations, with the exception of diabetes, which is the third leading cause of death in the Māori population. Non-communicable diseases are the most common cause of death for both groups (see Table 15.1).

Māori experience of health services

Health promotion, prevention and screening

National cervical and mammography programmes have been less successful for the Māori population. Coverage (adjusted for hysterectomy prevalence) in the cervical screening programme is 50.9 per cent for Māori and 77.7 per cent for non-Māori/non-Pacific women (University of Otago 2001a). Coverage of Māori women in the mammography screening programme is also low. During its first two years of operation the national programme engaged 41.7 per cent of eligible Māori women compared with 60.2 per cent of non-Māori/ non-Pacific women (University of Otago 2001b).

Other preventive programmes also fail to provide services as effectively to the Māori population. Childhood immunization coverage rates for Māori children are lower than those of non-Māori. A coverage survey undertaken in the northern part of the North Island in 1996 reported that 44.6 per cent of Māori and 72.3 per cent of non-Māori/non-Pacific children aged two years had received the full childhood immunization schedule (North Health 1997).

Similarly, public health programmes have been less effective for Māori. Public health information and education regarding the health risks associated with tobacco use have resulted in a significant reduction in the number of non-Māori who continue to use tobacco products, but less dramatic reductions among Māori. The impact of recent health promotion and nicotine cessation programmes that target Māori has yet to be determined.

Utilization of primary medical care services

The 1996/97 New Zealand Health Survey found that a higher proportion of Māori (19 per cent) were high users of services (over six visits to a general practitioner in the preceding twelve months) than European/Pakeha (15 per cent) people. However, Māori also reported much higher levels of unmet need (not visiting a general practitioner when the person felt that they needed to) with 19 per cent of Māori reporting unmet need compared to 12 per cent of European/Pakeha (Ministry of Health 1999b).

Hospitalization

The causes and rates of hospitalization vary across age groups and gender, and the patterns of hospitalization are complex. Age adjusted total hospitalization relative risks for Māori (compared to the non-Māori/non-Pacific ethnic group) are 1.2 (females) and 1.1 (males) (Ministry of Health 1999a). But, after controlling for deprivation, total hospitalization rates for Māori men and women are similar to, or lower than, those of non-Māori/non-Pacific people across all age groups, except the 45–64 year group for which Māori rates are similar to or slightly higher than non-Māori/non-Pacific people (Salmond and Crampton 2000).

For some conditions, for example congestive heart failure, Māori have higher rates of hospitalization than non-Māori (Westbrooke and Baxter 2001). However, congestive heart failure mortality rate differences are even greater than those for hospitalization and the increased hospitalization rates may, in fact, represent relative under-utilization taking into account need for services. For other conditions, hospitalization rates, when controlled for gender, age and deprivation are lower for Māori than other ethnic groups. For example, hospitalization rates for cardiac interventions are lower for Māori than non-Māori (Westbrooke and Baxter 2001). Further research is required to elucidate these issues more clearly.

Finally, in Aotearoa there is some evidence of ethnicity-related differences in the management of some conditions, including access to 'best practice' treatments. This has been documented for cardiac interventions, since after controlling for age, gender and deprivation, Māori have lower hospitalization rates for cardiac procedures (Westbrooke and Baxter 2001) despite an ischaemic heart disease mortality rate ratio (Māori:non-Māori) of 1.8. Several studies have demonstrated that people of Māori and Pacific ethnicity are less likely to receive asthma preventive medication and asthma action plans (Garrett *et al.* 1989; Mitchell 1991). The causes for these disparities are likely to be multifactorial; however, consideration must be given to whether the quality of care received by Māori differs from that received by non-Māori and the role that health services play in causing and maintaining disparities. Further work is required to elucidate these issues.

Understanding these differences

This brief overview of Māori health status has illustrated the poorer health status, relative under-utilization of primary and secondary services, and possible differences in quality of care. Furthermore, as noted earlier, Māori living in contemporary Aotearoa continue to be over-represented in areas of high socio-economic deprivation; experience disparities in almost every health and social indicator; and experience poorer outcomes from health, education and other public services. These findings are consistent with the experiences of colonized indigenous peoples around the world and originate within the processes of colonization. Several factors are often identified as important when attempting to understand the basis of these differences in contemporary societies. These factors include colonization, low socio-economic status, accelerated ageing and the inability of health services to adequately meet the needs of Māori.

Colonization results in the destruction of indigenous societies, cultural practices, values and beliefs and imposes the laws, institutions, values and beliefs of the colonizing society on indigenous peoples. As the colonizing society became dominant, Māori were (and continue to be) denied equal access to the resources, goods and services provided within New Zealand society.

Low socio-economic status is associated with poorer health status. However, not all of the disparities in health status between Māori and non-Māori can be explained by differences in socio-economic status. Analysis of health outcomes by ethnicity and deprivation show that Māori have worse outcomes than non-Māori within the same deprivation decile (Reid *et al.* 2000).

Premature morbidity and mortality, and accelerated ageing are evident among Māori who, in general, have more numerous and complex health problems at younger ages than their non-Māori peers. For example, the relative risk for mortality amongst Māori adults aged 25–44 years compared with non-Māori is 2.68 for men and 2.87 for women (Blakely *et al.* 2002b). Jones's (Jones 1999) work in the United States and Aotearoa suggests an accelerated ageing process may in part explain the observed premature morbidity and mortality.

Health services have not adequately met the needs of Māori. The international literature has documented a number of barriers that 'disadvantaged' people face when accessing health services. Broadly speaking these barriers can be divided into three categories: financial, organizational and personal (Adler *et al.* 1993; Ginzberg 1994; Margolis *et al.* 1995; Riportella-Muller *et al.* 1996; Schorr 1989). Financial barriers result in an inability or reluctance to use health care because of the cost of these services; organizational barriers are health care system or service related factors that reduce access to care; and personal barriers are the difficulties people face in mobilizing resources to obtain health care. Many Māori are exposed to such barriers. The effect of these barriers is to reduce access to health services and adversely impact on health outcomes.

In addition, Māori, like other colonized indigenous groups, face cultural barriers that operate in a variety of ways and result in reduced access to and utilization of health care services. Health care services, which are grounded within non-Māori culture, are generally unable to provide services that incorporate or value Māori cultural practices, values and beliefs. Health-related information is not provided in a way that is likely to reach and impact on the intended recipients. Health professionals may be unable to develop effective relationships and communicate well with Māori service users. Furthermore, as described above, there is evidence that points to different quality of care for Māori and non-Māori.

Although some of these factors may be interlinked, others seemingly are independent of one another. Internationally, researchers are exploring overall mechanisms that may account for the observed experiences and disparities. Jones (2001) argues that although 'race' is often thought to capture a combination of social class, culture, or genes, it is in fact an inadequate proxy for these factors. She goes on to argue that 'race' as a variable 'is a social classification in our race-conscious society that conditions most aspects of our daily life experiences and results in profound differences in life chances' (Jones 2001 p. 300), and asserts that the variable 'race' is a strong measure of exposure to racism. Three levels of racism can be identified: institutionalized; personally-mediated and internalized (Jones 2000, 2001). All three levels of racism can impact on health outcomes. Institutionalized racism affects socio-economic status and access to health care; personally-mediated racism results in differences in treatments and causes increased stress in recipients of racist behaviour; and internalized racism impacts on the health behaviours of an individual (Jones 2001). The racial climate, consisting of all three levels of racism, can account for many of the seemingly independent or loosely related factors associated with differences in health outcomes. In Aotearoa the role that the racial climate may play in determining health outcomes is coming under increasing scrutiny.

How are health services delivered to Māori?

As previously stated, Māori access both 'mainstream' and Māori provider services. This section first describes the delivery of services to Māori by 'mainstream' services, followed by a description of Māori health service providers.

'Mainstream services'

Public health programmes

Public health programmes such as health promotion and population-based screening programmes are, in general, universally delivered. Recent years have seen the introduction of health promotion targeted to Māori, for example, the *Auahi Kore* (Smokefree) programme. Mammography and cervical screening programmes are universal but have Māori providers who deliver some of the health promotion and education components of these programmes. Māori units or staff within health promotion organizations and programmes are utilized to increase the effectiveness of these programmes in delivering their service to the Māori community. This is achieved through ensuring that programme content, resources and methods of delivery are appropriate for use with Māori.

Hospital and related services

Hospitals and their related services (for example, outpatient clinics, district nurses), in general, deliver services in the same way to patients regardless of their ethnicity. Many hospitals contain Māori health units whose primary role is to provide support and advocacy for Māori patients and their families while they are in hospital. Some hospitals have become more responsive to the cultural needs of Māori, for example, by allowing family members to stay with their sick relative and by allowing new parents to take the placenta with them to be buried (as is traditional custom). Others have instituted more detailed programmes, for example, the Auckland District Health Board has recently proposed a set of standards for hospital staff response to many important Māori cultural values and practices. A few institutions, particularly within mental health services, have units that cater specifically to Māori patients and their families.

Primary care

Most general practitioner groups are, at the present time, largely unresponsive to Māori health needs. That is, they do not provide specific services or programmes that target Māori and employ few Māori staff. The current government policy objective to improve the health of Māori, in combination with the implementation of the primary health care strategy (which emphasizes primary care organizations taking responsibility for the total population in their area) may see increasing responsiveness to Māori health needs in the future.

Māori health service providers

Māori have been involved in the delivery of health care since 1899 – the year that Maui Pomare (the first Māori medical practitioner) graduated. However, the involvement of Māori as health professionals was very limited until the late 1980s when hospitals began to institute 'bicultural services' (Māori health units within hospital settings), and a small number of *marae* (meeting places for a Māori community) based health programmes were established (Durie 1998). For a number of reasons, the Māori community had, for a considerable time, wanted to realign 'mainstream' health services and to become more involved with the provision of health services. These reasons included the Treaty based right to self-determination including the right of Māori to deliver health services to Māori; awareness of the disparities in health status and the many barriers to accessing care; and belief that services provided by Māori would better meet the needs of Māori, be more appropriate, acceptable and accessible to the Māori community, and would result in the reduction/elimination of disparities and Māori health gains.

The alignment of government policy and Māori desire for participation resulted in the growth of Māori health service providers throughout the 1990s. At the time, it was commonly stated that Māori health organizations would provide services that were more appropriate for use by Māori, more acceptable to the Māori community, more accountable to the community and more affordable.

Māori responded to this opportunity and there are now around 240 Māori health provider organizations. Māori health provider organizations (Māori providers) are only available in some parts of the country. Māori health providers mainly deliver primary care services, health promotion and education services, and mental health and disability support services, but do not own hospitals that provide secondary and tertiary care.[2] Māori providers are of variable size ranging from providers that deliver a single health promotion programme to those that deliver a wide range of primary care services (Crengle 1999). However Māori providers are small in comparison to

---

[2] However, because of the difficulties that Māori experienced in accessing services during the 1918 influenza epidemic, Te Puea Herangi developed her own services to manage outbreaks of infectious diseases and planned a hospital to cater for Māori with infectious diseases. See M. King (1977) *Te Puea – a biography.* Hodder and Stroughton, Auckland).

Independent Practitioner Associations (IPAs) (Malcolm and Wright 2000). For these reasons, despite the increase in Māori providers over the last decade, most Māori receive care in 'mainstream' services.

Many Māori providers are governed and operated by Māori groups or organizations that often have a wider focus than health alone. The nature of these organizations varies. Some are *iwi* (tribal) organizations i.e. governed and operated by an *iwi* (tribe). Others are governed and operated by urban Māori authorities[3] or by Māori organizations that have evolved independently from an *iwi* or urban authority. In addition to the usual legal and constitutional arrangements necessary for the establishment of a provider organization, Māori providers have mechanisms in place that allow the community to have their say in the development and function of the service and provide a level of accountability by the provider to their local community (Crengle 1999).

Māori providers are scattered around the country in a range of locations, varying from urban locations in the largest city in New Zealand to remote rural locations. Some providers cover geographical areas that include a mixture of towns and rural environments.

Two philosophical approaches are shared by all Māori providers. First, the philosophy of positive Māori development underpins all Māori providers. Positive Māori development refers to Māori social, cultural and economic advancement within a framework of Māori self-sufficiency and control (Durie 1992). Second, Māori providers are based within *kaupapa* (philosophy, purpose) Māori; developing and delivering services within a Māori paradigm of health and well-being rather than the Western, illness-focused paradigm. These two philosophies form the basis of the approach used by Māori providers. Māori working within the health sector believe that the economic, cultural, education and employment factors that impact on the health of an individual and their family must be addressed when considering their health and well-being. The differing philosophical approaches used by the Māori providers and the funding agencies they contract with can cause tension. Māori providers are reluctant to ignore issues that are, in the Western definition, non-health-service related. Funding agencies are reluctant to fund activities that are not traditionally paid for by health sector funding. As a consequence many Māori providers find themselves undertaking work that is not funded within their contracts (Bevin 2002; Crengle 1997).

----

[3] Organizations established within urban areas, particularly the larger cities, to cater to the needs of Māori living in urban areas away from their tribal areas.

Services are delivered using *tikanga* Māori (Māori customs, practices, protocol or lore) and, where appropriate, *te reo* (Māori language). For example, when visiting homes, Māori health workers will greet all people within the home in a culturally appropriate manner and will ensure that their behaviour and actions when delivering the service do not contravene Māori protocols (Crengle 1997, 1999). Where available, providers use resources e.g. reading material, posters and videos, which are based within Māori culture, use Māori design and are appealing to Māori.

Many of the staff employed by Māori providers are Māori. The employment of Māori staff ensures that staff are aware of and comfortable with working within Māori *kaupapa* and *tikanga* (customs). This results in greater rapport between health workers and service users (Crengle 1997). The Māori health workforce is extremely small, particularly in health professions such as medicine and nursing. Only 2.3 per cent of the medical workforce were Māori in 2000 (Medical Council of New Zealand 2000). Māori are similarly under-represented in the other health professions. Māori providers also employ non-Māori health professionals, particularly doctors. Community health workers are the largest group in the Māori health workforce. Until recently there was no formal training programme available for this group, despite the fact that they are essential components of the Māori health workforce. The community health worker provides information and education for the community, is a health advocate within the community, works alongside health professionals with families, provides advocacy and support for families during their interactions with services in the health sector, is essential for outreach and follow-up activities and is a link between Māori services and the communities they serve.

What programmes are delivered?

Māori providers deliver a range of preventive, primary care, mental health and disability programmes including:

(1) intervention/clinical services

    (a) general practitioner services

    (b) dental services

    (c) midwifery services

    (d) counselling and intervention programmes for specific issues such as anger management, sexual abuse and substance abuse.

(2) community health programmes (health promotion, education and screening programmes

    (a) targeting specific age groups

        (i) *tamariki ora* (well child) services

    (ii) health checks to *kohanga reo, kura kaupapa, kura tuarua* (Māori immersion pre-schools, primary and secondary schools)

    (iii) *rangatahi* (youth) health programmes

    (iv) *kaumātua* (older persons) service for example screening for specific health issues such as hypertension and diabetes, health education programmes, exercise and healthy eating programmes

  (b) targeting specific health issues

    (i) healthy *kai* (food) and nutrition programmes

    (ii) women's health

    (iii) asthma

    (iv) diabetes

    (v) smoking

    (vi) exercise

    (vii) substance abuse education

(3) health promotion and opportunistic screening at community events and meetings

(4) disability support services

  (a) programmes/services for people with disabilities

(5) mental health services

  (a) residential and respite care people with psychiatric illnesses

(6) community support e.g. home support services, community support workers

(7) Māori traditional healing services.

Unlike most 'mainstream' (non-Māori) providers, Māori providers deliver services at a range of sites. In addition to a base site many Māori providers have clinics in other locations. This increases access to the services for clients who may live some distance from the base site and/or have difficulties with transport. Some providers have mobile clinics that visit a variety of venues on a regular basis or for opportunistic screening, health promotion and health education purposes. Regular venues can include the providers' offices, local pre-schools, schools and *marae* (Māori meeting-places). Opportunistic screening occurs at a variety of forums including *hui* (meetings), cultural events, sports events and other local community events and venues.

    Programmes, apart from general practitioner services, are provided free of charge. General practitioner services within Māori providers are cheaper than their 'mainstream' counterparts and may be free for some population groups, including children under age seventeen.

A number of Māori providers also have a range of social and education/ training programmes (funded from non-health sources) within their organizations or have strategic relationships with local social and education/training organizations (Māori or non-Māori) that provide the services that are not available within their own organizations. In addition to relationships with organizations that provide social, education and training programmes some Māori health providers have strategic relationships with other organizations that provide health services that are not delivered by Māori providers. Both organizations benefit. Clients of the Māori provider are able to access services delivered by the other provider, and patients of the other provider can access the programmes offered by the Māori provider. An example is the relationships between *Tipu Ora* (a Māori well child programme) and the local general practitioners.

In general Māori providers address a number of the reported structural (service related) barriers to accessing care (Crengle 2000). Some of these barriers and the solutions offered by Māori providers are detailed in Table 15.2.

Over the last approximately eight years a number of governance organizations, known as Māori Co-Purchasing Organisations and Māori Development Organisations, have been developed. These have several roles including providing an interface between funding bodies and the group of providers that are engaged with the organization; providing corporate and management support to the providers; and having a corporate governance relationship with funding agencies. The operating principles are based on the Treaty of Waitangi principles, Māori leadership and a geographical location inclusive of all Māori.

How effective are these health services?

Publicly available information on the effectiveness and efficiency of any health service in Aotearoa is very limited. Available data about hospital and public health programmes are limited to population-based data such as mortality rates, hospital discharge rates, smoking rates and population coverage for screening programmes such as cervical and breast screening, while information on primary care, including Māori providers, is even more limited. There are some indications that Māori providers may be more effective; for example, a home visiting programme in West Auckland achieved childhood immunization schedule coverage rates of 90 per cent in 1996 (Crengle 1997). However, as discussed earlier in this chapter, there is a good deal of evidence that the mainstream health system is not effectively addressing Māori health needs. Mortality, morbidity, public health and health service utilization statistics show wide disparities between the Māori and non-Māori populations.

Table 15.2 Barriers to care and solutions used by Māori providers

Barrier	Solution
Financial barriers:	
Unable to afford payment for general practitioner (GP)	Cheaper GP fees
Unable to afford prescription payment	Agreement with pharmacist to discount or abolish drugs charges for low income patients
Geographic and transport barriers:	
	Use mobile and satellite clinics to improve service access
	Transport patients to clinic/service
Lack of knowledge:	
Of health issues, health services and how to access health information	Provide these services at a wide variety of locations and venues and community activities
	Provide information in ways understood and appreciated by Māori
Barriers within the health system:	
Inability to receive care at the needed time	Flexible appointment systems; ability to walk in and be seen
Failure to identify and reach those at risk	Provide services in satellite or mobile clinics
Lack of confidence/inability to negotiate health care system	Assist with appointments including attending clinic with the person
Limited follow-up	Proactive outreach using various locations and methods
	Proactive follow-up using health service staff and community networks
	Integrate community health and general practice with a focus on health promotion
Cultural barriers:	
Failure to provide health information in ways that are appropriate for use in Māori communities	Deliver services using Māori cultural practices and beliefs
	Employ Māori staff
Failure to provide services that are appropriate and acceptable to the clients	Present information in ways that are appropriate and acceptable for use with Māori community
	Use resources appropriate and acceptable to the Māori community

Source: Crengle, S. (2000) The development of Māori primary care services, with permission from Pacific Health Dialogue 7, 48–53.

What are the advantages and disadvantages of different service delivery models?

The development of Māori providers has gone some way towards meeting Māori desires for self-determination in the delivery of health services and towards fulfilling government obligations under the Treaty of Waitangi. Furthermore, this process has afforded Māori the opportunity to address perceived deficiencies in the delivery of health services to Māori by 'mainstream' health services.

The development of Māori providers has afforded Māori in some parts of the country the choice between 'mainstream' services and Māori providers. Comparative data are scarce, but there are signs that Māori providers deliver services that are more accessible, appropriate, affordable and acceptable to the Māori community and that Māori take advantage of Māori providers when there is one available in their area.

Māori providers attempt to provide health services within an holistic model incorporating Māori models of health as well as working intersectorally with services/agencies addressing other social, educational and training needs. Furthermore, health promotion, education and screening activities are significant components of services delivered by Māori providers.

The Māori providers' approaches to service development and provision take forward current government policies for primary care and Māori health, including involvement of the community, better provider accountability mechanisms and the provision of a range of health promotion, education and screening activities within primary care services (Ministry of Health 2001b).

Māori providers also play a critical role in meeting government policy objectives for Māori provider development and Māori health workforce development. Māori providers also lead the way in attempts to address several other Māori health policy objectives, particularly whānau health and development and working across sectors (Ministry of Health 2001a). The meaningful incorporation of Māori models of health (as the basis for a health service), family health and development objectives and intersectoral initiatives into contractual arrangements with health funding agencies is a challenge for policy makers, funding agencies and providers.

A number of other challenges face Māori providers. The small Māori health workforce, and limited opportunities for workforce and capacity development are major challenges, although recent governments have provided additional funding (the Māori Provider Development Scheme) to enhance capacity in Māori providers. Areas that need strengthening in the future include information management, quality assurance programmes, integration with secondary and tertiary services, and strengthening the foci on family health/development and intersectoral programmes. Needless to say, these areas are also challenges for 'mainstream' providers. Additional challenges for 'mainstream' providers are ensuring the development of and maintenance of culturally competent services and workforce, addressing issues of quality of care across ethnic groups and improving ethnicity data collection. Finally, mainstream providers must recognize that the presence of Māori providers within the sector does not absolve them of the responsibility to provide high quality, culturally competent services to Māori.

Conclusion

Māori, the indigenous people of Aotearoa, account for about 15 per cent of the population. The experience of colonization and the ongoing contemporary expression of colonial power have resulted in remarkable similarities in the health and social status of Māori and other indigenous peoples who have been colonized and become minorities in their own lands. The basis of indigenous peoples' claims upon the state lies within their indigeneity. In Aotearoa, Māori claims on the state are operationalized through the Treaty of Waitangi, and Aotearoa is unique amongst colonized nations in the manner and extent to which Māori and the government have worked to implement a treaty-based relationship. Current government approaches to implementing the Treaty are centred on equity rather than a full expression of the Treaty, and while this is less than ideal, it has facilitated Māori development within the health sector, including the institution of Māori health service providers. The role of Māori providers is supported by many elements of the health sector and current indications suggest that the development of Māori providers has, to date, been a successful process. Further development of Māori services will require successful management of a variety of challenges. Information on the effectiveness and efficiency of different ways of providing services to Māori is sparse, but in general, it appears that mainstream services have not met Māori health needs. In order to reduce and ultimately eliminate Māori health disparities, mainstream health services must increase their responsiveness to Māori health. To achieve these goals the wider society within Aotearoa must implement the Treaty of Waitangi in a meaningful manner, including recognizing Māori right to self-determination, and work towards eradicating the contemporary expressions of colonial power that impact on the lives and well-being of Māori today.

Acknowledgements

The authors would like to thank Papaarangi Reid, Gwen Tepania-Palmer and Rob Cooper who provided comments on earlier drafts of this paper.

References

Adler, N., Boyce, W., Chesney, M., Folkman, S. and Syme, L. (1993) Socio-economic inequalities in health: no easy solution. *Journal of the American Medical Association*, **269**, 3140–5.

Bevin, N. (2002) *An evaluation of the impact and effectiveness of diabetes care as administered by a Māori community based health initiative.* Unpublished research report. Wellington School of Medicine, Wellington.

Blakely, T. and Woodward, A. (2002b) Unlocking the numerator–denominator bias. II: adjustments to mortality rates by ethnicity and deprivation during 1991–94. The New Zealand Census-Mortality Study. *New Zealand Medical Journal*, **115**, 43–8.

Blakely, T., Robson, B., Atkinson, J., Sporle, A. and Kiro, C. (2002a) Unlocking the numerator–denominator bias. 1: adjustments ratios by ethnicity for 1991–94 mortality data. The New Zealand Census Mortality Study. *New Zealand Medical Journal*, **115**, 39–43.

Crampton, P. (2000) Policies for general practice. In P. Davis and T. Ashton (eds) *Health and public policy in New Zealand.* Oxford University Press, Auckland.

Crampton, P. and Brown, M. (1998) General practitioner funding policy: from where to whither? *New Zealand Medical Journal*, **111**, 302–4.

Crampton, P., Salmond, C., Kirkpatrick, R., Scarborough, R. and Skelly, C. (2000) *Degrees of deprivation in New Zealand: an atlas of socioeconomic difference.* David Bateman Ltd, Auckland.

Crengle, S. (1997) *Ma papatuanuku, ka tipu nga rakau: A case study of the well child health programme provided by Te Whanau o Waipareira Trust.* Unpublished Masters of Public Health thesis, University of Auckland.

Crengle, S. (1999) *Māori primary care services: a paper prepared for the National Health Committee.* Available at http://www.nhc.govt.nz/pub/phc/phcMāori.html.

Crengle, S. (2000) The development of Māori primary care services. *Pacific Health Dialogue*, **7**, 48–53.

Department of Health (1992) *Whaia te ora mo te Iwi: strive for the good health of the people.* Department of Health, Wellington.

Durie, M. (1992) *Māori development, Māori health and the health reforms.* Paper presented at Hui Hauora a Iwi, 11 April 1992. New Zealand, Takapuwahia Marae, Porirua, Aotearoa.

Durie, M. (1998) *Whaiora: Māori health development*, second edition. Oxford University Press, Oxford.

French, S., Old, A. and Healy, J. (2001) *Health care systems in transition: New Zealand.* World Health Organization Regional office for Europe, Copenhagen.

Garrett, J., Mulder, J. and Wong-Toi, H. (1989) Reasons for racial differences in A & E attendance rates. *New Zealand Medical Journal*, **102**, 121–4.

Gauld, R. (2001) *Revolving doors: New Zealand's health reforms.* Institute of Policy Studies and Health Services Research Centre, Wellington.

Ginzberg, E. (1994) Improving health care for the poor: lessons from the 1980s. *Journal of the American Medical Association*, **271**, 464–7.

Jones, C. P. (1999) *Māori-Pakeha health disparities: can treaty settlements reverse the effects of racism?* Ian Axford Fellowship report. Ian Axford Fellowships Office, Wellington.

Jones, C. P. (2000) Levels of racism: a theoretic framework and a gardeners tale. *American Journal of Public Health*, **90**, 1212–15.

Jones, C. P. (2001) Invited commentary: 'Race', racism and the practice of epidemiology. *American Journal of Epidemiology*, **154**, 299–304.

Kelsey, J. (1995) *The New Zealand experiment: a world model for structural adjustment?* Auckland University Press with Bridget Williams Books.

Malcolm, L. and Wright, L. (2000) Emerging clinical governance: developments in idependent practitioner associations in New Zealand. *New Zealand Medical Journal*, **113**, 33–6.

Margolis, P., Carey, T., Lannon, C., Earp, J. and Leininger, L. (1995) The rest of the access-to-care puzzle: addressing structural and personal barriers to health care for socially disadvantaged children. *Archives of Pediatric and Adolescent Medicine*, **149**, 541–5.

Medical Council of New Zealand (2000) *The New Zealand medical workforce in 2000.* Medical Council of New Zealand, Wellington.

Metge, J. (1995) *New growth from old: the Whanau in the modern world.* G.P. Print, Wellington.

Ministry of Health (1999a) *Our health, our future, Hauora Pakari, Koiora Roa.* Ministry of Health, Wellington.

Ministry of Health (1999b) *Taking the pulse: the 1996/97 New Zealand health survey.* Ministry of Health, Wellington.

Ministry of Health (2000) *Health expenditure trends in New Zealand 1980–1999.* Ministry of Health, Wellington.

Ministry of Health (2001a) *He korowai oranga: Māori health strategy: A discussion document.* Ministry of Health, Wellington.

Ministry of Health (2001b) *The primary health care strategy.* Ministry of Health, Wellington.

Mitchell, E. (1991) Racial inequalities in childhood asthma. *Social Science and Medicine*, **32**, 831–6.

National Health Committee (2002) *Tena te ngaru whati, tena te ngaru puku. There is a wave that breaks, there is a wave that swells.* Ministry of Health, Wellington.

New Zealand Health Information Service (2001) *Mortality and demographic data 1998.* Ministry of Health, Wellington.

North Health (1997) *1996 regional immunisation coverage report.* North Health, Auckland.

Reid, P., Robson, B. and Jones, C. (2000) Disparities in health: common myths and uncommon truths. *Pacific Health Dialogue*, **7**, 38–47.

Riportella-Muller, R., Selby-Harrington, M., Richardson, L., Donat, P., Luchok, K. and Quade, D. (1996) Barriers to the use of preventive health care services for children. *Public Health Reports*, **111**, 71–7.

Robson, B. and Reid, P. (2001) *Ethnicity matters: review of the measurement of ethnicity in official statistics, Māori perspective.* Statistics New Zealand. Available at http://www.stats.govt.nz

Royal Commission on Social Policy (1988) *The April report: report of the Royal Commission on social policy.* Wellington.

Salmond, C. and Crampton, P. (2000) Deprivation and health. In P. Howden-Chapman and M. Tobias (eds) *Social inequalities in health: New Zealand 1999.* Ministry of Health, Wellington.

Schorr, L. (1989) *Within our reach: breaking the cycle of disadvantage.* Anchor Press/Doubleday.

Statistics New Zealand (2002a) *Population summary for the Māori ethnic group census usually resident population counts, 1991, 1996, 2001.* Available at http://www.stats.govt.nz.

Statistics New Zealand (2002b) *2001 Census of population and dwellings: population and dwelling statistics.* Statistics New Zealand, Wellington.

Statistics New Zealand (2002c) *2001 Census of populations and dwellings: regional summary Volume 1.* Statistics New Zealand, Wellington.

Statistics New Zealand (2002d) *Age group by sex for the Māori ethnic group census usually resident population count, 1991, 1996, 2001.* Available at http://www.stats.govt.nz.

Te Puni Kokiri (2000) *Progress towards closing the social and economic gaps between Māori and non-Māori.* Te Puni Kokiri, Wellington.

Trask, H. (1999) *From a native daughter,* revised edition. University of Hawaii Press, Honolulu.

University of Otago (2001a) *Independent monitoring group of the national cervical screening programme quarterly report 2 National Cervical Screening Programme January–March 2001.* Hugh Adam Cancer Epidemiology Unit, Department of Preventive and Social Medicine, University of Otago, Otago.

University of Otago (2001b) *BreastScreen Aotearoa independent monitoring group breastScreen Aotearoa monitoring report No. 7.* Hugh Adam Cancer Epidemiology Unit, Department of Preventive and Social Medicine, University of Otago, Otago.

Walker, R. (1990) *Ka whawhai tonu matou: struggle without end.* Penguin Books.

Westbrooke, I. and Baxter, J. (2001) Are Māori under-served for cardiac interventions? *New Zealand Medical Journal,* 114, 484–7.

Chapter 16

The History and Politics of Health Care for Native Americans

Stephen J. Kunitz

Provision of care by the federal government

Since the early nineteenth century, the federal government has provided health care to American Indian people, both as a treaty obligation and as a consequence of its role as trustee (Office of Technology Assessment 1986). Care was first provided by military doctors until 1849, when the Bureau of Indian Affairs (BIA) was transferred from the War Department to the newly created Department of the Interior.

The Department of the Interior has always been in a difficult position with regard to Native Americans. On one hand, it is charged with acting as trustee for Indian rights and resources. On the other hand, federal legislators, primarily those from western states whose constituents covet those same resources, often subject it to intense pressure not to be too zealous in its defense of Indian rights and resources. Moreover, presidential administrations that were unsympathetic to Indians have often appointed as Secretaries of the Interior and Commissioners of Indian Affairs, people who themselves had interests other than the Indians' at heart. It is a fair generalization to say that non-Indians in states with substantial Indian populations often resent the presence of Indians and the role of the federal government in awarding them what are perceived to be special privileges and services.

Thus the Department of the Interior has often been less than zealous in protecting Indian rights and resources. During the 1930s, however, under Secretary Harold Ickes and his Commissioner of Indian Affairs, John Collier, the department was unusually protective of Indian rights – so much so, indeed, that a number of western legislators attempted to have the Bureau of Indian Affairs abolished and its responsibilities moved to other federal agencies or levels of government. But Collier was adamant that all responsibility should remain within the bureau; in 1936 for example, he resisted an attempt to move the health care function to the US Public Health Service (Kelly 1983;

Philp 1977). The bureau remained intact as long as the Democrats were in the White House, but major changes began to occur in the 1950s.

The First Hoover Commission

When Harry Truman became president upon the death of Franklin Roosevelt, one of his major concerns was to reorganize the government. He believed that his predecessor had not been a good manager and that the executive branch required rationalization. At the same time, the Republican-dominated Congress, which was elected in 1946, wanted to trim the executive branch for the purposes of 'economy and efficiency' and, many Democrats feared, to undo the reforms of the New Deal (Moe 1982 p. 23–4).

The result was legislation that empanelled a bipartisan Commission on Reorganization of the Executive Branch of the government under the chairmanship of former president Herbert Hoover. One observer wrote:

> There is no doubt that the Commission's ultimate plan was to have been keyed to a Republican Administration which everyone, except Truman and some 23,000,000 Americans who voted for him, anticipated in November, 1948. The Commission's findings and recommendations for changes in executive organizational structure were to have been the grand overture of a new Republican era.
>
> Moe 1982 p. 24

Despite the fact that the Republicans did not win the presidential election of 1948, the commission's recommendations were of enormous significance and had not been forgotten when the Republicans did win four years later.

The Hoover Commission's Task Force on Indian Policy had advocated the integration of Indians into the larger US population, a policy completely antithetical to the one pursued by the Bureau of Indian Affairs under John Collier in the 1930s and early 1940s. The members recommended that, '[P]ending achievement of the goal of complete integration, the administration of social programs for the Indians should be progressively transferred to State governments' (U.S. Commission on Organization of the Executive Branch of the Government 1949; U.S. Public Health Service 1957). This was to include, of course, all health services. The policy of assimilation and the steps to achieve it became federal Indian policy during the Eisenhower years. This involved terminating the federal recognition of Indian tribes, encouraging the relocation of Indian people from reservations to cities, and weakening and ultimately dismantling the Bureau of Indian Affairs.

It was recognized, however, that termination of federal oversight could not occur overnight. The economic, educational, and health status of many Indians was so inadequate compared with that of the rest of the US population that in many instances services would have to be improved before the government could withdraw entirely. Moreover, state and county governments were simply unwilling to shoulder the responsibilities recommended for them by the task force. Thus to both weaken the Bureau of Indian Affairs and improve Indian health, transfer of health service to another federal agency, the U.S. Public Health Service, part of what was then the Department of Health, Education and Welfare, was recommended. However, when legislation was introduced in both houses of the 82nd Congress in 1952 authorizing the transfer, it was defeated. It was passed in 1954 by the 83rd Congress as PL568.

Testimony in the hearing before the bill was passed revealed several important differences of opinion about the desirability of transfer. Indian tribes were themselves divided on the issue. Some expressed fear that the result would be hospital closures, decreasing access to health care, and discrimination in non-Indian facilities. Others believed that the level and quality of health care provided by the Bureau of Indian Affairs were simply inadequate and that a professional corps of commissioned officers would be more numerous and better trained, would have access to more resources, and would provide better care. Professional opinion was decidedly in favor of the transfer for the same reasons. Indeed, the sponsor of the House bill, Rep Walter Judd from Minnesota (himself a physician), claimed that the original idea had come to him from the American Public Health Association after its annual meeting in 1951. And of course there were the assimilationists, many of whom wished to weaken the Bureau of Indian Affairs, the primary guardian of Indian rights and resources.

The Department of the Interior, under a Republican administration, now favored the transfer of responsibility. Assistant Secretary Orme Lewis wrote to Senator Hugh Butler, chairman of the Senate Committee on Interior and Insular Affairs:

> For over 100 years the Indian has had a relationship to the Bureau which has resulted in dependency for certain services. The Department believes that a new relationship with the need to work out problems and services through normal community and agency facilities will be worth any administrative difficulties which may be encountered.
>
> Lewis 1954 p. 2927–30

Oveta Culp Hobby, Secretary of Health, Education, and Welfare, had what were perceived to be primarily administrative objections and resisted transfer to her department. Her concerns were largely dismissed.

Thus the bill passed both houses of Congress. Senator Edward Thye of Minnesota, who introduced the bill into the Senate, had said that the purpose was several fold: '1. To improve health services to our Indian people; 2. To coordinate our public health program; and 3. To further our long-range objective integration of our Indian people in our common life' (Thye 1954 p. 12). The authors of the legislative history of the bill were equally clear as to its purpose.

> The proposed legislation is in line with the policy of the Congress and Department of the Interior to terminate duplicating and overlapping functions provided by the Indian Bureau for Indians by transferring responsibility for such functions to other governmental agencies wherever feasible, and [to enact] legislation having as its purpose to repeal laws which set Indians apart from other citizens.[1]

The result of the transfer was to create the only truly national health service for civilians in the United States, one that provided nearly the full range of public and personal services to a defined population. In the more than 40 years that have passed since the transfer was made, many Indian and non-Indian people have come to see the provision of these services by the Indian Health Service (HIS) as an entitlement, something owed to Indians as a result of treaty rights and trust obligations. That is not how the government regarded its obligation at the time of the creation of the IHS. And indeed it is not an entitlement, for the services provided are dependent upon annual congressional approval of the budget for the IHS, and the benefits are not portable when people leave reservations for urban areas.

The Indian Health Service

The system of care that was developed by the Public Health Service may be characterized as hierarchical regionalism, a term one writer used to describe the series of attempts by reformers to reorganize the American health care system in the 1920s and 1930s (Fox 1986). The Indian Health Service (or Division of Indian Health, as it was then known) was highly integrated in terms of both services and administration, with field stations linked to general hospitals and referral centers. Administration followed the same chain of command, with service units (catchment areas) reporting to area offices, which in turn reported to headquarters in Washington. A Public Health Service document that was published at the time the Division of Indian Health was created stated that 'Indian health services on the reservation

---

[1] They listed three, all enacted August 15, 1953: P.L. 83–277, repealing federal statutes prohibiting the use or possession by or the sale and disposition of intoxicants to Indians; P.L. 83–280, conferring civil and criminal jurisdiction over Indians upon certain states; and P.L. 83–281, repealing statutes applicable only to Indians having to do with personal property, the sale of firearms, and the disposition of livestock. Senate Report 1530 to accompany H.R. 303, 83rd Congress, second session, June 8, 1954, 2919.

should be tied in more closely to a regional pattern so that services of larger medical facilities would be available for diagnostic, consultative and treatment services for complicated cases' (U.S. Public Health Service 1957).

This highly integrated regionalized system dominated by white professionals (some Public Health Service career officers, some individuals serving two-year military obligations, some civil servants) began to change significantly within two decades of its establishment. The demand for community control, which originated in the civil rights movement of the 1960s, enshrined 'maximum feasible participation' of the poor in the Economic Opportunity Act. The result was the increased hiring of Indian paraprofessionals, the creation of community health boards, and the beginnings of decentralization of what had begun as a highly centralized system.

Decentralization and community control accelerated throughout the 1970s after President Nixon specifically rejected the policy of 'forced termination' which had been instituted when he was vice president during the Eisenhower administration. In a message to Congress he wrote, 'The policy of forced termination is wrong, in my judgment, for a number of reasons. First, the premises on which it rests are wrong.' He said that federal responsibility was not simply an act of generosity toward a 'disadvantaged people' that could therefore be discontinued 'on a unilateral basis whenever [the federal government] sees fit.' The relationship rests on 'solemn obligations' – that is to say, on 'written treaties and through formal and informal agreements'. Second, 'the practical results [of forced termination] have been clearly harmful in the few instances in which [it] has actually been tried.' And third, forced termination has made Indians suspicious:

> The very threat that this relationship may someday be ended has created a great deal of apprehension among Indian groups and this apprehension, in turn, has had a blighting effect on tribal progress ... In short, the fear of one extreme policy, forced termination, has often worked to produce the opposite extreme: excessive dependence on the Federal government.
>
> Nixon 1979 pp. 2–3

The policy his administration was to pursue was to steer a middle course. Nixon went on to say:

> I believe that both of these policy extremes are wrong. Federal termination errs in one direction. Federal paternalism errs in the other. Only by clearly rejecting both of these extremes can we achieve a policy which truly serves the best interests of the Indian people. Self-determination among the Indian people can and must be encouraged without the threat of eventual termination. In my view, in fact, that is the only way that self-determination can effectively be fostered.

> This, then, must be the goal of any new national policy toward the Indian people: to strengthen the Indian's sense of autonomy without threatening his sense of community. We must assure the Indian that he can assume control of his own life without being separated involuntarily from the tribal group. And we must make it clear that Indians can become independent of Federal control without being cut off from Federal concern and Federal support.
>
> Nixon 1979 p. 3

The Nixon administration's Indian policy was embodied in two central pieces of legislation: the Indian Self-Determination and Education Assistance Act (PL 93–638), passed in 1975, and the Indian Health Care Improvement Act (PL 94–437), passed a year later. Title I of PL 93–638 created mechanisms whereby tribes could, if they wished, contract with the Secretaries of Interior and of Health, Education, and Welfare (now Health and Human Services) to develop new services or assume control over services previously provided by the federal government (Kunitz 1983; Urban Associates 1974). Contracting was limited to health and social service programs; it did not extend to natural resource management.

There does not appear to be any reason to believe that the Nixon administration was insincere in advocating the policy of self-determination without termination, although clearly there were important political calculations involved as well.[2] One of President Nixon's staff, John Erlichmann, explained the President's interest in Native Americans as follows:

> Nixon did have a personal interest in Indian issues. There were three reasons. First, he was a 'strict constructionist' who believed that treaties were meant to be observed. Second, he believed that because they were relatively few in number, Indians were a manageable minority and that their problems *could* be addressed by the government. Finally, he was favorably disposed towards Indians because of his high regard for his football coach at Whittier, 'Chief' Newman.
>
> Bergman *et al.* 1999

....

[2] In his testimony on behalf of the self-determination bill, Frank Carlucci, Undersecretary of Health, Education, and Welfare, echoed the president's message to Congress: 'As we advance the propriety of self-determination . . . we must also be sensitive to the need for maintaining Federal support and concern for the Indian people. As we strengthen the Indian's sense of autonomy, we must be sure not to threaten his sense of community and tribal life. That means making it clear to Indians that they can become independent without losing their unique relationship with the Federal Government and that self-determination and the assumption of control of H.E.W. programs and services by Indian tribes represents a reinforcement rather than a termination of this unique relationship.' Statement of Frank Carlucci before the Senate Committee on Interior and Insular Affairs, Subcommittee on Indian Affairs, on S. 1017, Indian Self-Determination and Education Reform Act, 93rd Congress first session 62–63, Washington, DC, June 1 and 4, 1973.

Whatever the reasons, the consequences of the policy change were far-reaching. First, there was an increase of federal funds for health and social services. And second, tribal termination was replaced by self-determination. I shall address each briefly in turn.

Federal spending

Figure 16.1 displays the total federal appropriations in current dollars since 1956, when the responsibility for health care was shifted from the Bureau of Indian Affairs to the IHS. There has been a slow increase in the amount available for services each year, with a discernible upward deflection in the 1970s. These increases have not been as rapid as increases in the costs of health care, however.

To account for the increases in the costs of health care, Figure 16.2 displays the amounts available each year from 1990 through 1999, in both current and constant dollars (adjusted for health care costs). It is clear that in constant dollars there has been no increase. Indeed, because the Indian population is growing, the amount available per capita is actually declining.

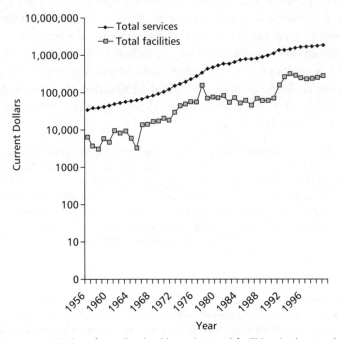

Figure 16.1 Appropriations for Indian health services and facilities, in thousands of current dollars, 1956–1999, semilog scale.

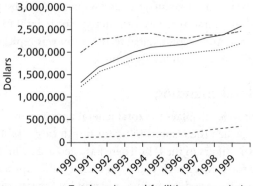

Figure 16. 2 Indian health service budget, 1990–99, in current and constant dollars.

······ Total service and facilities appropriations
--- Third party payments
—— Total budget, current dollars
---- Total budget in constant dollars

Moreover, the amount spent per capita on health services is substantially less than that spent on health for the entire US population. Excluding construction and research costs, the per capita expenditure on health for the entire US population in 1990 was $2,629 (National Center for Health Statistics 1993) whereas the IHS appropriation for American Indians, excluding facilities, was $976 per capita ($1,052 if Medicare/Medicaid and private insurance reimbursements received by the IHS are included). If one adds about another $600 per capita for out-of-pocket expenditures by Indians, the average increases to about $1,600 ($1,700 including Medicaid, Medicare, and private insurance), or between 60 per cent and 65 per cent of the national figure.[3]

A study by the (IHS) in 1999

> used actuarial methods to compare Indian health funding with costs of a mainstream personal medical services plan, the Federal Employees Health Benefits Plan (FEHBP). The FEHBP Disparity Index (FDI) study did not address public health deficiencies and needs for safe water and waste disposal. After discounting for Medicare, Medicaid, and private insurance coverage, the FDI study found that IHS funding fell $1.3 billion short of parity with the benchmark health plan in 1999.
>
> Dixon and Roubideaux 2001; Indian Health Service 2002

[3] I am grateful to Peter Cunningham for providing me with an estimate of out-of-pocket expenses of $504 based on the 1987 National Health Expenditure Survey. I have rounded this amount up by about $100 for the 1990 estimate. Medicare, Medicaid, private insurance reimbursement, and 1990 service population data are from IHS 1994: 20 and 28. According to the U.S. Census, the service population in 1990 was 1.2 million people.

Table 16.1 Indian health service allocations by area, 1993

Indian Health Service area	Allocation per user	Allocation per person enumerated
Aberdeen	976	1223
Alaska	1908	1906
Albuquerque	867	915
Bemidji	888	838
Billings	922	1091
California	1000	562
Nashville	1322	831
Navajo	608	717
Oklahoma	575	534
Phoenix	1002	886
Portland	946	525
Tucson	1051	799

Source: Indian Health Service (1994) *Regional Differences in Indian Health, 1994*. Rockville, MD: U.S. Department of Health and Human Services.

Average figures blur very considerable variations in allocations among the 12 IHS area offices (see Table 16.1). In 1993 these allocations ranged from $1,908 in Alaska to $575 in Oklahoma per IHS user (defined as anyone who has used program services in the three previous years), and from $1,906 in Alaska to $525 in Portland, Oregon, if the program (census-defined) population issued. There is a high correlation between the two measures ($r = 0.77$), but the differences are important. There have been complaints about the inequitable allocations, some of the reasons for which are based on historical precedent, regional differences in cost and accessibility to care, the different ways that services are provided (e.g., whether in IHS or contract facilities), and the relative influence that Indian tribes and Alaskan Native corporations have with their states' congressional delegations. Indeed, the IHS sites were 'funded at less than 60 per cent of comparable mainstream plans'. Whatever the reason for the disparities among regions and regardless of whether the method of allocation is equitable, the fact is that even those areas with the highest allocations per person get considerably less than does the average US citizen.

One consequence of this low level of expenditure has been that IHS hospitals provide a more limited range of services, both diagnostic and therapeutic, than community hospitals in general. Thus, they have shorter average lengths of stay and lower occupancy rates. Because a full range of services is not provided in IHS facilities or even the major referral centers, an increasing proportion of services must be provided by non-Health Service personnel, paid for with contract funds and costing more than such services would if they were provided internally. The reason for high costs is twofold: the IHS has failed to negotiate aggressively with private providers; and in some areas where private providers are scarce, there is not sufficient competition to force them to lower their prices (Office of Technology Assessment 1986).

Self-determination

Increasingly throughout the 1980s and 1990s responsibility for care has devolved to tribal organizations. There were several reasons for devolution. One has to do with a widespread rejection of governmental responsibility for many different types of services, and growing suspicion of governments' ability to operate as efficiently as non-governmental organizations. Devolution should thus be seen in part as a manifestation of a larger trend toward outsourcing and, in the government sphere, privatization. For instance, Senator John McCain (Republican, Arizona), chairman of the Senate Committee on Indian Affairs, said in 1994:

> [T]his administration like its predecessor is committed to reducing federal regulatory burdens. I can think of no better place to start to reduce the crippling effect of regulations than in the area of Indian self-determination. It is time that the BIA and the IHS get the message. Self-determination is not simply another federal program and it is not an excuse for federal officials to continue seeking domination over the affairs of tribal governments. In this instance, the BIA and the IHS suffer from the delusion that tribal programs can only be operated in the way that the BIA or IHS have operated them. To the contrary, self-determination requires a diminishment of the federal presence in tribal affairs. This includes reducing the federal work force and minimizing regulatory interference. Since the BIA and IHS seem unable or unwilling to accomplish these goals, I believe it has become necessary to repeal their authority to promulgate regulations under the Self-Determination Act.
>
> McCain 1994.[4]

A corollary is the assumption by tribal governments of responsibility for programs previously provided by the IHS and the Bureau of Indian Affairs (BIA). This exercise of tribal sovereignty is thought by many to be good in itself but also to lead to better services more responsive to local conditions than were those provided by a centralized organization such as the IHS.

---

[4] Indeed, a continuing theme of those critical of the BIA and the IHS has been the corruption and incompetence of federal employees. See, for example, *A Report of the Special Committee on Investigation of the Select Committee on Indian Affairs. A New Federalism for American Indians*, 101st Congress, first session, 1989.

There are two ways in which tribes can assume responsibility for health services, contracting and compacting. Contracts require that tribes provide the same level and types of services as were provided by the BIA and IHS programs they replace. 'Compacting,' which is a looser arrangement than contracting, gives tribes more flexibility in their use of government funds (Dixon *et al.* 2001; Hagstrom 1994 p. 90–1). Both the IHS and the BIA have been criticized by federal legislators and tribal leaders for exercising excessively microscopic oversight of contracts and thus stifling tribal initiative, as Senator McCain's comments quoted above suggest. Compacting is a mechanism to reduce just such allegedly excessive regulation, although in the future it may also raise serious questions about accountability for the use of federal funds, which is at least as great a cause of regulatory proliferation as the bureaucratic hunger for control.

Indian and Alaska Native corporations and tribes differ widely in their willingness to sign contracts and compacts with the IHS. Some have done a great deal in this regard; others, very little. A study of 107 federally recognized tribes sought to discover some of the reasons underlying the decision to assume responsibility for health services 'Tribes residing in California, Alaska, and the Northeast were excluded from the analysis because these tribes had never served under the traditional IHS structure' (Adams 2000). The single most important variable was a measure that seemed to reflect inadequate responsiveness to tribal concerns by the local IHS. Among other significant predictors was tribal poverty rate: the higher the level of poverty, the lower the probability that a tribe would make the decision to manage its own services.

There are other reasons for assuming or rejecting control of health services, of course. One is the concern by non-contracting/compacting tribes that IHS resources will be inequitably consumed by the tribes that already have contracts and compacts. This is an issue that has led to conflict between various tribes and the IHS as Congress has not appropriated sufficient funds to pay for 100 per cent of contracts but only for 90 per cent.

> Most tribes have historically taken the position that the law requires the Federal Government to pay 100 per cent of tribal CSC [Contract Support Costs] and, if necessary, the Indian Health Service should use other parts of its appropriation to fund CSC as the 100 per cent level. The Indian Health Service position is that the funds for CSC are subject to the availability of funding appropriated for CSC, and that to take funds from other programs would have an adverse impact on administration and health services provided to non-compacting/contracting tribes. This difference in interpretation has led to congressional oversight hearings and litigation. The U.S. Court of Appeals (Federal Circuit) has affirmed the Indian Health Service position in their 1999 ruling.
>
> Indian Health Service 2002

The Navajo Tribe is one that has been reluctant to engage in contracting:

> The Navajo Nation is aware of its option to request that an entire program like the dental department become a '638' contract. However, the Navajo Nation views contracting as a problematic option because there is no available 'pool' of contractors in the area. Contracting for clinical services or medical professionals can cost 2 to 3 times as much as an Indian Health Service employee. The problem of inadequate resources to meet growing needs will not be solved by transferring the operating responsibility while continuing to fund the program at 1/8 the national rate of expenditure.
>
> Navajo Nation 1994

The Navajo statement points out an important problem for tribal organizations, which is that, in remote areas especially, it is likely to cost tribes more than it would cost the IHS to provide services, an issue to which I return below. It also illustrates some of the conflicts around the assumption of responsibility for health care. The executive branch of the Navajo Nation government began to plan for and advocate assumption of responsibility, thinking that they could do as good a job as the IHS. The matter came to a vote in January 2002, when the Navajo Nation Council (the legislative branch of the tribal government) voted against assuming responsibility for the provision of services. Navajo employees of the IHS were very much opposed to the assumption of responsibility by the tribe and lobbied for defeat of the measure. One of the issues was allegedly concern over job security and benefits, although opposition was voiced in terms of the tribal government's inability to manage other large undertakings successfully.

The problem for the Navajo Nation and others like it is that they feel forced by events to undertake contracting and compacting. If they do not, they fear that the limited money available in the IHS budget will be absorbed at an increasingly disproportionate rate by those that do contract and compact, and that they will be left with very little. One study suggests that this is not a real problem (Dixon and Roubideaux 2001). Nonetheless, while contracting is supposed to be a matter of choice for tribal governments, many fear losing what services they have (Johnson 1994). The litigation described above, in which contracting/compacting tribes attempted to extract more money from the IHS budget, would appear to confirm the validity of those fears, even though the attempt was defeated. Indeed, there is a significant correlation ($r = 0.58$, $p < 0.05$) between the amount allocated per user of services (see Table 16.1) and the proportion of service units in an area that are under tribal management.

Finally, as tribes have been given increasing responsibility for managing their own health and other services and as the costs of those services rise, the inadequacy of government appropriations has become increasingly evident.

Tribes are thus being encouraged to provide resources to supplement the government appropriations, which accounts in part for the epidemic of casino gambling that has swept through Indian country in recent years.

Changes in Indian health

Despite difficulties enumerating Indian people and tabulating vital rates, there is little doubt that, since 1955, Indian mortality has declined and life expectancy has improved substantially – from about 60 years at birth in the 1950s to 73.2 years at birth in 1989/91. The most recent figures are two years less than those for all US races and three years less than those for US Whites in 1990 (Indian Health Service 1994) p. 75.

Not unexpectedly, the major improvements have been in infant and child mortality, and the major declines have been in infectious diseases. Among Indian people, deaths from tuberculosis, gastroenteritis, and pneumonia-influenza have dropped significantly. In addition homicide, other deaths due to violence, and alcohol-related deaths have also declined. On the other hand, deaths due to non-insulin-dependent diabetes are unusually high and rising, compared with those among non-Indians. Neoplasms, which are less common among Indian than among non-Indian people, are also rising (Indian Health Service 1994 p. 75).

This data suggests that the IHS has been effective in reducing preventable and treatable conditions such as infectious diseases but that it has not yet had an impact on certain chronic conditions such as diabetes and some cancers, most notably, perhaps, cervical cancer. Evidence from New Mexico, however, indicates that the IHS has been effective in providing early detection and intervention services for both infectious and non-infectious disease equivalent to those provided to, and utilized by, other Americans, at least in one state (Gilliland *et al.* 1999). Furthermore, alcohol abuse has been the focus of much tribal and IHS attention, which may have contributed to the decline in alcohol-related deaths (Kunitz and Levy 1994 Chapter 9). While some very important preventable problems remain, it is clear that, overall, the IHS has contributed significantly to the improvement of Indian health.

Thus the organizational changes I have described have occurred as the health conditions of greatest concern have shifted from acute infectious to chronic non-infectious in nature. The argument that some advocates of devolution make is that such conditions are best addressed by health care programs that are locally based and managed by people who know the community, its culture, and its people well. This is a reasonable hypothesis, but whether it is the case or not is far from clear.

Some consequences of devolution

It is difficult to assess the impact of devolution of services on the meaningful exercise of tribal sovereignty, and I shall not attempt to do so here. I shall simply note that contracts and compacts with the IHS account for a very large proportion of some tribal budgets, and that jobs in health care and other service occupations are among the most common in many of these populations with high unemployment. Thus control of health programs represents a substantial source of political and economic influence and even patronage in some tribes.[5]

It is almost as difficult to assess the impact of devolution on the quality and consequences of public and personal health services, but some weak tests are possible. A significant body of work over the past 20–30 years has been devoted to the assessment of the medical contribution to the improvement of the health of contemporary populations (Rutstein *et al.* 1976). Most of the studies in this tradition classify causes of death as either amenable or not amenable to medical care.

> Here medical care is defined in its broadest sense, that is prevention, cure and care, including the application of all relevant medical knowledge, the services of all medical and allied personnel, the resources of governmental, voluntary, and social agencies, and the co-operation of the individual himself. An excessive number of such unnecessary events serves as a warning signal of possible shortcomings in the health care system, and should be investigated further.
>
> Holland 1993 p. 1

Avoidable deaths may thus arise for a variety of reasons, including inadequate funding, inaccessible services and/or populations, incompetent staff, or non-compliant patients. Though all of these factors may be contributory, the fact that some populations have higher rates than others is an indication that adequate health services responsive to the unique needs of particular populations may not be available.

I have correlated death rates from a variety of causes thought to be more or less amenable to medical intervention with the median household income and with the proportion of tribally managed service units in each of the IHS areas. Because the number of service units in each area differs, I have weighted the

---

[5] It is thus understandable why IHS employees who are protected by civil service regulations might be resistant to changes that would ultimately make them tribal employees and leave them less protected from what they perceive to be political pressures. Civil service protection, like academic tenure, is of course a double-edged sword, for it can be used to protect the inept, the lazy, and the unaccountable as well as political dissidents.

analysis by number of service units. This is a weak test because the duration of time service units have been managed (either under contract or compact) by tribal organizations is not taken into account, because areas are more or less diverse, and because there are too few areas for multiple regression analysis. Nonetheless, it is worth pursuing, for if the results indicate that mortality rates are lower in areas in which tribally managed programs predominate, it would support the hypothesis that tribally managed programs are more responsive to the unique health needs of the populations they serve. On the other hand, if the results do not show lower mortality rates in areas in which tribally managed programs predominate, that is not a truly convincing argument that they are not effective for the reasons noted above. I have included median household income in the analyses as well because so many health conditions are associated with economic status.

First, there is a strong and positive correlation between median household income and proportion of service units in an area that are under tribal management ($r = 0.83$, $p < 0.0008$). This strong association is consistent with the results reported above on the predictors of tribal decisions to assume control of services; that is, tribes in which the poverty level was low were more likely than others to make the decision to undertake contracting and compacting. I can only speculate about the reasons for the association. It may mean that more affluent areas have a higher proportion of people with private insurance that can supplement IHS funds. Thus a tribal health program could bill the private insurance carrier for services provided to a tribal member. Or it may indicate proximity to urban areas where more providers are available, competition among them greater, and thus the costs of contracting lower. There is no association with educational attainment. The association also suggests that median income is likely to confound attempts to detect a relationship between the management of services and health outcomes.

Table 16.2 displays the results of the correlations between median household income and proportion of service units under tribal management on the one hand, and various causes of death and one measure of preventive health care utilization on the other. To the list of causes of death widely considered to be amenable to medical interventions I have added motor vehicle accidents, diabetes, and alcoholism because these are among the conditions that are especially significant in many Native American and Alaskan Native communities.

The results indicate that median household income is inversely and significantly associated with age adjusted death rates from diabetes, tuberculosis, alcoholism, and motor vehicle accidents. That is to say, the higher the median income in an IHS area, the lower are the death rates from these conditions.

Table 16.2 Correlations (Pearson's *r*) between median household income, proportion of service units under tribal management in an IHS Area, and age adjusted death rates from various causes

Cause of death	Median household income	Proportion of tribal service units
Lung Cancer	−0.11	0.13
Heart disease	−0.31	0.12
Diabetes	−0.71*	−0.37
Tuberculosis	−0.79*	−0.72*
Cerebrovascular disease	0.003	0.12
Breast cancer	−0.19	−0.15
Cervical cancer	−0.23	−0.05
Infant mortality rate	−0.46	0.02
Alcoholism	−0.71*	−0.54
Motor vehicle accidents	−0.86*	−0.64†
Prenatal care in the first trimester	0.42	0.67*

* $p > 0.01$.

† $p > 0.05$.

Source: All the data are from *Regional Differences in Indian Health 1998–99*. U.S. Department of Health and Human Services, Indian Health Service, Office of Public Health, Division of Community and Environmental Health, Program Statistics Team, Rockville, MD. No date.

The results also indicate that the proportion of service units under tribal management is inversely and significantly correlated with death rates from tuberculosis and motor vehicle accidents (that is, death rates are lower where health services are tribally managed), and positively correlated with the proportion of women who receive prenatal care during the first trimester of pregnancy. The correlations with the death rates are weaker than the correlations between median income and those same death rates.

This admittedly weak test therefore indicates that for a few selected conditions there is a significant association in the expected direction with proportion of service units under tribal management but that the relationships are stronger with, and confounded by, median household income. Thus at this very gross level of analysis there is no evidence that tribal management produces better health outcomes than management by the IHS. On the other hand, the results also suggest that preventive services, as measured by early prenatal care, may be better in tribally managed than in IHS managed service units. If this is the case, however, it is not reflected in differences in infant mortality rates. (The number of maternal deaths is very low in all areas and the differences among them are substantively meaningless.)

A much stronger test of the impact of tribally managed services would require a comparison of the morbidity and mortality amenable to medical interventions of compacting/contracting tribes with that of non-contracting/ compacting tribes, while adjusting for such confounding variables as income and isolation. Such data do not exist, nor, given the generally poor quality of data collected at the tribal and service unit level, are they likely to exist in the future. What does exist is a survey of tribal leaders, which indicates that leaders of compacting/contracting tribes

> more commonly perceived that the overall quality of their health care had improved if they were operating their own health care systems as compared to those who received Indian Health Service direct services. Also, a greater proportion of tribal leaders of compacting and contracting tribes perceived improvements in waiting time, types of services, and number of people served, than tribal leaders from tribes with direct Indian Health Service services.
>
> Dixon *et al.* 2001 p. 98

The difficulty with such a survey, of course, is that the very people who are responsible for the management of the system are the ones being asked to opine about the improvements since they assumed responsibility. The unfortunate result is that it is at present impossible to tell whether devolution of services has had a beneficial impact on health status. It will very likely not be possible to make a convincing determination in the future either, for outsourcing has led to a decline in the quality of data collected from different tribes and areas (Roubideaux and Dixon 2001), which has been far from ideal even under the best of circumstances.

Conclusions

This brief history raises a number of issues and questions. It exemplifies the century-long debate in the United States between assimilationism and pluralism (now called multiculturalism). Native Americans are, of course, different from many other racial and ethnic groups inasmuch as they did not ask to be invaded, and many have treaties that give them a unique status in the eyes of the law. This unique status is perhaps why many conservatives have been supportive of Indian self-determination with federal support when they would not support similar claims by other ethnic groups.

Self-determination is more complicated than that, however, for it is also embedded in a much larger ideological movement that minimizes the role government, especially the federal government, has to play in the management of programs and services of all sorts. That is to say, outsourcing, or devolution in the case of Indian health programs and services, is part of the trend away from the centralizing impulse of the New Deal years that has pervaded all aspects of public policy. For entirely understandable reasons, this change in policy has been welcomed by many tribal governments, for it requires recognition of their rights as domestic sovereign nations. But this history also suggests that self-determination is a double-edged sword (Noren 1998).

When funding is sufficient, tribally managed programs may be very innovative and responsive to the special needs of their particular populations, just as their advocates assert. In addition to the arguments in favor of tribal sovereignty, this is of great potential value given the enormous variability in socioeconomic, cultural, and health conditions described previously. As we have seen, however, the data so far available do not offer compelling evidence for this position. When funded insufficiently, however, the results may be worse than those achieved when the federal government was the provider. Because investment in Indian programs has historically been barely adequate, in many instances the programs taken over by tribes may not have been functioning optimally from the start. Moreover, as is the case with outsourcing in general, transaction costs (e.g. the costs of monitoring contracts) may be high. Further, tribes may not benefit from economies of scale (e.g. with regard to the purchase of goods and services) although some assert this has not proven to be a problem (Dixon and Roubideaux 2001 p. 104), recruitment and retention of professional staff may be difficult; and tribal and state regulations (for instance with regard to Medicaid) may conflict with one another.

None of these problems is inevitable or insurmountable. Indeed it appears likely that there is, and will continue to be, great diversity in the funding, functioning and success of tribally run programs. Nonetheless, to the degree that budgetary constraints influence all programs to some degree, serious problems are likely to be more or less widespread and may well have a greater impact on preventive than on clinical programs (Noren *et al.* 1998; Weiner 1999).

Clearly, self-determination is a highly problematic concept. As generally used, it derives from the attempts after the First World War 'to make state frontiers coincide with the frontiers of nationality and language' (Hobsbawm 1992 p. 132–3). For the most part, this has turned out to be impossible to accomplish in more than a handful of nations. Indian reservations are among the few places where boundaries often do encompass one self-identified ethnic or linguistic group, although such groups are not sovereign nations as the term is usually understood. It is important to recognize that the concept is most readily applied to a territorially bounded group, not to individuals.

Thus, it makes some sense to talk about self-determination of reservation populations. The issue becomes more problematic when applied, for instance, to people from many tribes who live scattered throughout Los Angeles County, people who may be as different from one another as any of them is from non-Indian people.

It can be argued, of course, that it is 'Indianness' rather than tribal identity that is important. This raises issues that go well beyond the scope of this paper but are nevertheless important because, with growing intermarriage and mobility, it becomes increasingly difficult to determine who is an Indian and is entitled to federal and tribal benefits, and who is not. Recall that the transfer of responsibility for Indian health services was part of a larger policy that also included relocation of many Indians to urban places. The migration of the past 40 years means that, at present, about 50 per cent of Indians live in metropolitan areas. There has been an ongoing debate between Indian urban and reservation leaders about support for health services to urban residents. Urban leaders understandably consider health benefits to be an entitlement that ought to be portable; reservations leaders just as understandably fear the loss of support for reservations health programs. In fact, urban programs receive only a small fraction of the IHS budget: $22.8 million out of a total appropriation of $1.94 billion in 1994 (Indian Health Service 1994 p. 20). This simply shows that health services for Indians are not an entitlement, that is, a package of fixed and portable benefits for each individual simply by virtue of membership in a federally recognized tribe. The level and distribution of services are shaped by annual appropriations.

Policy and demographic changes have thus worked to alter profoundly both the IHS and the care available to Indian people. Self-determination is forcing Indians into the expensive private market for health care without increasing appropriations to cover the costs equitably across Indian country. And the massive movement from reservations to cities will require urban residents to depend increasingly on the same sources of health care as the rest of the population. The policy of integration that gave birth to the Indian Health Service almost 50 years ago seems to be coming to fruition.

Acknowledgments

The present chapter is a much revised version of an article titled 'The history and politics of US health care policy for American Indians and Alaskan Natives,' originally published in the *American Journal of Public Health*, **86**, 1464–73, 1996. It is published here in revised form with the permission of the editor of the journal.

References

Adams, A. (2000) The road not taken: how tribes choose between tribal and Indian Health Service management of health care resources. *American Indian Culture and Research Journal*, **24**, 21–38.

Bergman, A. B., Grossman, D. C., Erdrich, A. M., Todd, J. G. and Forquera, J. A. (1999) A political history of the Indian health service. *The Milbank Quarterly*, **77**, 571–604.

Dixon, M., Mather, D. T., Shelton, B. L. and Roubideaux, Y. (2001) Organizational and economic changes in Indian health care systems. In M. Dixon and Y. Roubideaux (eds) *Promises to keep: public health policy for American Indians and Alaska Natives in the 21st century*, pp. 89–118. American Public Health Association, Washington DC.

Dixon, M. and Roubideaux, Y. (2001) *Promises to keep: public health policy for American Indians and Alaska Natives in the 21st century*. American Public Health Association, Washington DC.

Fox, D. M. (1986) *Health policies, health politics: the British and American experience, 1911–1965*. Princeton University Press, Princeton, NJ.

Gilliland, F. D., Mahler, R., Hunt, W. C. and Davis, S. M. (1999) Preventive health care among rural American Indians in New Mexico. *Preventive Medicine*, **28**, 194–202.

Hagstrom, J. (1994) Treaties treatment. *Government Executive*, **26**, 34–39.

Hobsbawm, E. (1992) *Nations and nationalism since 1780: programme, myth, reality*, second edition. Cambridge University Press, Cambridge.

Holland, W. W. (1993) *European community atlas of 'avoidable death'*, vol. 2. Oxford University Press, Oxford.

Indian Health Service (2002) Available at http://info.ihs.gov/Resources/Resources4.pdf.

Indian Health Service (1994) *Regional differences in Indian health*. Department of Health and Human Services, Rockville, MD.

Indian Health Service (1994) *Trends in Indian health*. U.S. Public Health Service, Rockville, MD.

Johnson, E. (1994) *Statement of Emery Johnson, M.D., M.P.H., assistant surgeon general, retired, U.S. Public Health Service, before the Committee on Indian Affairs of the U.S. Senate, Hearings on S. 2067, 8 June, 1994*. From the Indian Health Service Internet address available in 1995.

Kelly, L. C. (1983) *The assault on assimilation: John Collier and the origins of Indian policy reform*. University of New Mexico Press, Albuquerque, NM.

Kunitz, S. J. (1983) *Disease change and the role of medicine*. University of California Press, Berkeley, CA.

Kunitz, S. J. and Levy, J. E. (1994) *Drinking careers: a twenty-five year follow-up of three Navajo populations*. Yale University Press, New Haven, CT.

Lewis, O. (1954) C. Letter to Sen. Hugh Butler, Senate Committee on Interior and Insular Affairs,U.S. Code Congressional and Administrative News, 83rd Congress, 2nd session. Washington, DC, U.S. Government Printing Office.

McCain, J. (1994) Statement before the Senate Committee on Indian Affairs, Hearings to accompany S. 2036, the Indian Self-Determination Contract Reform Act, June 15, 1994. Washington, DC, U.S. Government Printing Office.

Moe, R. C. (1982) *The Hoover Commission revisited*. Westview Press, Boulder, CO.

National Center for Health Statistics (1993) *Health United States 1992*. U.S. Public Health. Service, Hyattsville, MD.

Navajo Nation (1994) *Statement of the Navajo Nation before the Senate Committee on Indian Affairs on S. 2067, A Bill to Establish an Assistant Secretary for Indian Health, June 8, 1994*. From the Indian Health Service Internet address available in 1995.

Nixon, R. M. (1979) Message from the President of the United States transmitting recommendations for Indian Policy. 91st Congress, second session, July 8, 1979. H. Doc. 91–363. Government Printing Office, Washington, DC.

Noren, J., Kindig, D. and Sprenger, A. (1998) Challenges to Native American health care. *Public Health Reporter*, **113** (1), 22–33.

Office of Technology Assessment (1986) *Indian Health Care*. U.S. Congress, OTA-H-290. U.S. Government Printing Office, Washington, DC.

Philp, K. (1977) *John Collier's crusade for Indian reform, 1920–1954*. University of Arizona Press, Tucson, AZ.

Roubideaux, Y. and Dixon, M. (2001) *Health surveillance, research, and information. Promises to keep: public health policy for American Indians and Alaska Natives in the twenty-first century*, pp. 253–73. American Public Health Association, Washington DC.

Rutstein, D. D., Berenberg, W., Chalmers, T. C., Child, C. G., Fishman, A. P. and Perrin, E. B. (1976) Measuring the quality of medical care: a clinical method. *New England Journal of Medicine*, **294**, 582–8.

Thye, E. J. (1954) *Comments, U.S. Senate, Hearings of the Subcommittee of the Committee on Interior and Insular Affairs, on H.R. 303, 83rd Congress, second session, An Act to Transfer the Maintenance and Operation of Hospital and Health Facilities for Indians to the Public Health Service*. U.S. Government Printing Office, Washington, DC.

U.S. Commission on Organization of the Executive Branch of the Government (1949) *The Hoover Commission Report*. McGraw-Hill Book Company, New York.

U.S. Public Health Service (1957) *Health Services for American Indians*. PHS publication 531, U.S. Government Printing Office, Washington, DC.

Urban Associates (1974) *A study of the Indian Health Service and Indian tribal involvement in health*, published as an Appendix to the Hearing on Indian Health Care before the Permanent Subcommittee on Investigations of the Committee on Government Operations. 93rd Congress, second session, September 16, 1974. U.S. Government Printing Office, Washington, DC.

Weiner, D. (1999) Ethnogenetics: interpreting ideas about diabetes and inheritance. *American Indian Culture and Research Journal*, **23**, 155–84.

Chapter 17

The Value and Challenges of Separate Services

First Nation in Canada

Josée G. Lavoie

Introduction

The colonization of what is now known as Canada, first by France in the early 1500, and then by Britain in 1759, impacted on hundreds of culturally distinct indigenous groups. Armitage (1995) suggests that the relationship between the Crown and indigenous groups can be divided into five periods: domination, at the time of contact until 1860; paternalistic forms of protection, from 1860 until the 1920s; assimilationist policies, from the 1920s until the 1960s; integration through the 1960s and 1970s; and lately, pluralism and self-government. Since 1982, the Constitution of Canada recognizes Aboriginal peoples' inherent right to self-government, affirms Aboriginal and Treaty Rights, and promotes Aboriginal people (including First Nations formerly known as Indians, Inuit, formerly known as Eskimos and Métis) participation in decision-making over issues that directly affect them.

The Health Transfer Policy is an outgrowth of this recent shift. It was announced in 1986, aiming to provide First Nations with the opportunity to take over the administration and delivery of health services existing on their reserve. It was a natural progression from the 1979 Indian Health Policy, which claimed to address

> [T]he intolerably low level of health of many Indian people, who exist under conditions rooted on poverty and community decline. The Federal Government realizes that only Indian communities themselves can change these root causes and that to do so will require the wholehearted support of the larger Canadian community.
>
> Health Canada 2000b

Ever since their emergence in the early 1920s, primary health care services for First Nations have been the jurisdiction of the federal government, whereas all secondary and tertiary, as well as primary health care services for other Canadians have been the domain of provincial governments. With the Health Transfer Policy, Canada has gone one step further by not only maintaining the historical separation in matters of health care, but also supporting culturally distinct, community-based services in the pursuit of better health.

As of December 2001, Health Canada reports that nearly 70 per cent of eligible communities have taken over their health services, and that another 12 per cent are engaged in pre-transfer discussions (Health Canada 2002). Fifteen years after it was first announced, it is obvious that the policy has had some relevance in meeting First Nation's aspirations. But it has not been without criticism. Touted as a measure of community control, it defines very neatly the space over which First Nations may exercise this control. And while promoted as a mechanism to improve Aboriginal health, it has yet to be evaluated to assess whether it meets this stated goal.

Health care services to marginalized populations can be provided in various ways. Separate services are one option. In the Canadian context, separate health services emerged primarily for historical, legal and Constitutional reasons. Although it may be important to ask whether separate services are better, it is equally important to investigate how separate services are financed and structured, and how these administrative choices affect their potential effectiveness. This chapter provides a case study of the Health Transfer Policy, including both the opportunities and challenges it offers to participating First Nation communities. The chapter begins by reviewing the historical and Constitutional basis for separate health services for First Nations; the second section explains the context in which the Health Transfer Policy emerged; the third section explores how complexities in the areas of governance and financing impact First Nations; and the fourth section reviews some of the benefits reported to date. The final section summarizes conclusions.

The historical and constitutional basis for separate services

The Health Transfer Policy relates to primary health care services provided by First Nations themselves with funding from the federal government, for 'status Indians' living on-reserve. The expression 'status Indians' refers to those First Nations who are recognized by the federal government as Indians according to the definition provided in the Indian Act (explored below). The expression on-reserve refers to Indian reserve land held in trust by the Minister of Indian Affairs for First Nations who were signatories of Treaties at the beginning of the twentieth century, in exchange for a surrender of their ancestral territory.

Simply put, the British Crown issued the Royal Proclamation in 1763, following the 1759 conquest of what was known as New France. The Royal Proclamation was an attempt to contain a westward expansion from the American colonies and to create an alliance between the Crown and the indigenous population to ensure the sovereignty of the British Crown (Coates 1999). It essentially stated that the indigenous peoples of Canada were not conquered and retained title to their ancestral territory. Any encroachment on the part of settlers was to be approved by the Crown, negotiated through the Treaty process and duly compensated (King George 1763).

The Constitutional Act of 1867 defined health care as a provincial jurisdiction, and Indian affairs as a federal jurisdiction, thereby beginning a jurisdictional debate over Indian health that remains current one 135 years later. The federal responsibility for Indian Affairs changed hands a number of times, each move reflecting the ideological and political place of First Nations within the Canadian context. Jurisdiction was first vested with the Department of Secretary of State (1867), and moved to the Department of Indian Affairs (1880) during the negotiation of Treaties. It was moved to the Department of Mines and Resources in 1936 after the dissolution of the Department of Indian Affairs, and then to the Department of Citizenship and Immigration in 1950. The Department of Indian Affairs and Northern Development (now named Indian and Northern Affairs Canada) was revamped in 1966 (Indian and Northern Affairs Canada 1999). Indian health was initially included under Indian Affairs. It was moved to the Department of National Health and Welfare upon its creation in 1944 (now known as Health Canada), where it has remained ever since.

Following Confederation and the push to create a sustainable agrarian economy, the Crown engaged in Treaty negotiations with First Nations throughout the Prairie Provinces. The 11 numbered Treaties, as they are known, are land surrenders agreed to in exchange for reserve land, calculated at 128 acres per family of four at the time of signature, as well as other provisions, such as rations in time of famine, medicines, and agricultural implements. The signature of the Treaties must be understood as an exercise in self-preservation for First Nations, in light of the American Indian Wars, the demise of the buffalo, and the devastating impact of epidemics (Coates 1999).

The Royal Proclamation still has currency today. Modern Treaties, such as the James Bay and Northern Quebec Agreement (1975), the Inuvialuit Land Claim Agreement (1984), the Nunavut Land Claim Agreement (1995) and the Nisga'a Agreement (1997) (among others), were motivated by the need to clarify (and/or legalize) the Crown's access to land and resources.

Since Confederation, the federal government has worked to limit the sphere of influence of the Royal Proclamation and the Treaties, by carefully defining who can and cannot be included under the legal category 'Indian', to which is attached eligibility to live on a reserve, and certain individual-based benefits. Thus the term 'Indian' has become a bureaucratic construct first defined in the 1876 Indian Act. It is a questionable proxy for cultural affiliation. The Treaties were signed with 'full blood Indians' and those of mixed ancestry who were deemed to live as Indians. From then on until 1985, a First Nation woman who married a man who was not First Nation lost her Indian status. The same applied to children from this marriage. In contrast, a non-First Nation woman (of European or other origin) who married a First Nation man gained First Nation status. This discriminatory provision was repealed from the Indian Act with the adoption of the 1985 Bill C-31, and replaced by an equally problematic concept. As the legislation stands now, members of First Nations who never lost their Indian status (through marriage, and by opting out of status in order to get employment, drink alcohol prior to 1962, access medical care when denied by the Indian Agent, etc.), are registered as an 'Indian' under the Indian Act article 6(1). Those who lost status by marriage or other means prior to 1985 are eligible for registration under the Indian Act article 6(2). Both 6(1) and 6(2) classification categories imply full status and Aboriginal Rights. Children of parents classified as 6(1) are classified as 6(1). Children of a 6(1) parent and 6(2) parent are classified 6(1). Children of a 6(1) parent and a non-status are considered 6(2). Finally, children of a 6(2) parent and non-status parent are considered non-status, and therefore the responsibility of the provinces. In human terms, it means that status can be lost within two generations of mixed relationships; and First Nation governments are funded for 6(1) and 6(2) members only. When non-status children are born on-reserve, First Nation governments are placed in the position of either denying services to them, or of spreading the funding thinner to satisfy a moral obligation towards these children.

The collective term 'First Nations' hides a multiplicity of distinct Indian nations, including Nisg'aa, Cree, Ojibway, Salish, Mohawk, Micm'ac, and Innu, to name a few. In administrative terms, there are currently 625 First Nations recognized by the federal government (Canada Department of Indian Affairs and Northern Development 2002a). These are political and administrative organizations that emerged to satisfy the requirements of the Indian Act. They may or may not be members of one of the 79 regional Tribal Councils. These numbers do not represent the whole of indigenous organizations, nor the number of indigenous cultures: Inuit and Métis are excluded. Further, it was the practice of the federal government at the turn of the century to divide large cultural groups into more 'manageable' administrative subgroups, thus there are in fact considerably less cultural groups than there are First Nations.

The original impetus for the development of health services to First Nations came from the settlers who arrived at the turn of the twentieth century to farm the land. They found themselves living close to Indian reserves where appalling health conditions prevailed. It was the fear of epidemics, mostly tuberculosis, which led the federal government to begin to invest funding in health services, with the hiring of a General Medical Superintendent in 1904 and a mobile nurse visitor program in 1922 (Waldram *et al.* 1995). The first federally funded on-reserve nursing station was set up at Fisher River, Manitoba in 1930. The Indian Health Branch was incorporated into the Department of National Health after its formation in 1944. This was followed by a sustained expansion of health services to First Nations. Currently, nearly all First Nation reserves (with the possible exclusion of a few located at proximity to urban centres) have access to services delivered by a health centre located on-reserve. These health centres offer primary health care services delivered by nurses and local Community Health Representatives (see below). Other services include addiction counselling, and medical transportation. Physicians funded by the province visit these communities on a regular basis. Patients requiring secondary, tertiary or emergency care are transported to the nearest provincial referral centre (Waldram *et al.* 1995). In some respects, the transition between the federal and provincial systems is relatively smooth. The Canadian health care system is a publicly financed, publicly administered, and partially privately delivered national health care system.

As shown in Figure 17.1 (Health Canada 1999a) primary, secondary and tertiary care is entirely funded through progressive income tax garnered at the provincial and federal levels. Individual Canadians, including First Nations, access these services through the Medicare, the national health insurance plan. Private insurance does play a role, but only as a top-up to Medicare. For example, private insurance may be used for medication, dental and eye health coverage, and to pay for the added cost associated with a single, as opposed to a free double room in a hospital. Physicians are remunerated on a fee-for-service basis. Unlike other OECD countries, Canada has resisted pressures to further privatize health care (Deber and Baranek 1998). The Canada Health Act 1984 defines the five principles the provinces must respect to secure their full federal transfer payment, namely:

♦ Public administration: The health insurance plan of a province must be administered and operated on a non-profit basis by a public authority accountable to the provincial government.

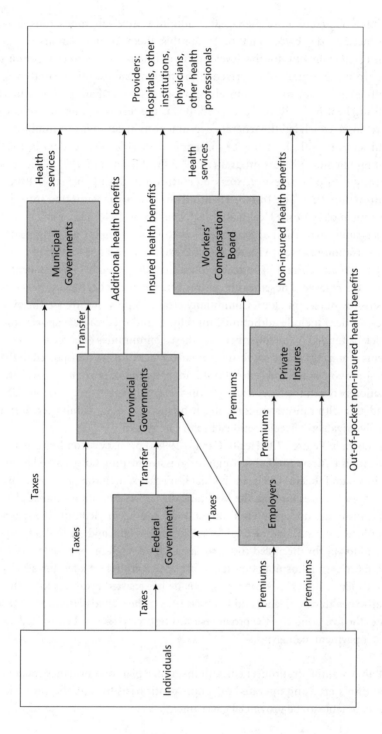

Figure 17.1 The Canadian health financing system (Health Canada 1999a).

- Comprehensiveness: The plan must insure all medically necessary services provided by hospitals and physicians. Insured hospital services include inpatient care at the ward level and all necessary drugs, supplies and diagnostic tests, as well as a broad range of outpatient services. Chronic care and public health services are also insured.

- Universality: The plan must entitle 100 per cent of the insured population, i.e. the Canadian population and all landed immigrants, to insured health services on uniform terms and conditions.

- Accessibility: The plan must provide, on uniform terms and conditions, reasonable access to insured hospital and physician services without barriers. Additional charges to insured patients for insured services are not allowed. No one may be discriminated against on the basis of income, age, health status, etc.

- Portability: Residents are entitled to coverage when they move or travel to another province within Canada or, to a more limited extent, abroad (Health Canada 1999a).

Currently, most on-reserve health funding comes from federal public funding. Some First Nations may secure funding through agreements with their respective provincial or regional health authority (for examples, diabetes or urban services), but this is still public funding, and minor in terms of total revenue.

The Health Transfer Policy is neither a national strategy to create a separate First Nations' health care system, nor conceived by the federal government as a response to Aboriginal rights or Treaty obligations. Only Treaty 6 (1876) makes a provision for health care. It is known as the Medicine chest clause, and reads:

> That a medicine chest shall be kept at the house of each Indian Agent for the use and benefit of the Indians at the direction of such agent …
>
> That in the event of the Indians comprised within this treaty being overtaken by any pestilence, or by a general famine, the Queen, on being satisfied and certified thereof by Her Indian Agent or Agents, will grant to the Indians assistance of such character and to such extent as Her Chief Superintendent of Indian Affairs shall deem necessary and sufficient to relieve the Indians for the calamity that shall have befallen them.

> Morris 1880

First Nations have argued that this is the basis for a Treaty right to free health care that encompasses all contemporary aspects of health care delivery in Canada. Their position was supported by a court ruling in the 1965 Johnston case, but the Saskatchewan Supreme Court overturned the lenient ruling for a much more literal interpretation. According to this ruling, the provision of health services is at the discretion of the federal government, and therefore a matter of policy (Backwell 1981). Consequently, the Health Transfer Policy is simply an initiative aimed at transferring the administration of existing federally-funded on-reserve services to First Nation governance. Its area of influence does not extend to the provincial health care system: it rather remains at the periphery, yet closely tied to that system.

The emergence of the Health Transfer Policy

The emergence of the Health Transfer Policy is linked to a series of events that reshaped relations between First Nations and the nation-state. I can only present a synopsis that cannot possibly do justice to the complexity of the process. One of the events that acted as a catalyst was the Hawthorn Report (Hawthorn 1966), the first comprehensive survey of on-reserve social and economic conditions, which brought considerable embarrassment to Canada. The report emphasized the dismal living conditions on Indian reserves, and recommended a shift from caretaking to economic development. The Trudeau liberal government was elected in 1968, having fought a campaign couched in liberal ideology under the slogan '*The Just Society*', advocating for equality and human rights on an individual basis. Its answer to the Hawthorn report, articulated in what became known as the 1969 White Paper, called for:

- The repeal of the Indian Act;
- The dismantling of the Department of Indian Affairs; and
- The transfer of reserve land to First Nations, subject to provincial legislation.

Trudeau's vision was to put an end to the differentiated citizenship of First Nations, thereby welcoming them into the fabric of Canadian society on an 'equal basis'. First Nations rejected the assumptions on which this vision was based, as illustrated by Indian leader Harold Cardinal's landmark book *The unjust society* (Cardinal 1969). The rationale behind the liberal government's position lay in the post Second World War rise of welfarism, the realm of the provinces, which had pushed First Nations into administrative ambiguity. Provincial authorities have historically been opposed to a reserve system that placed land and resources outside of their control. Consequently, they were reluctant to consider First Nations full provincial citizens, and unwilling to extend the same services as other provincial residents, unless they gave up their Treaty and Aboriginal Rights (Hawthorn 1966). The gap was widening under the federal government's caretaking policies.

The White Paper was met with a political mobilization of First Nations, for a number of reasons. While the historically oppressive Indian Act maintained First Nations in a continued state of underdevelopment, nevertheless, along with the Treaties and the Royal Proclamation, it reaffirmed First Nations' status as nations within a nation, and the fiduciary obligation of the Crown towards them. At less than 3 per cent of the Canadian population, First Nations preferred to continue to negotiate with the federal government, and to have the federal government deal with the provinces, rather than having their collective voice fragmented between ten governments, each with different and at times less than favourable priorities (Long and Boldt 1988). Unrest over the White Paper led to the formation of the National Indian Brotherhood (now the Assembly of First Nations), the tabling of grievances in the 'Red Paper' (1970) and finally, the withdrawal of the White Paper. This marked a change in federal policy, and the integration of Aboriginal political organisations into a formal, on-going process of consultation on matters of policy (Weaver 1981). The Assembly of First Nations is now part of a complex First Nation governance structure, as represented in Figure 17.2. As it stands today, First Nation local government is termed Chief and Council (really an invention of the 1876 Indian Act that displaced traditional forms of governance). Some, not all, First Nations are united under regional cross-sectorial umbrella organizations called Tribal Councils. Tribal Councils provide expertise in a wide range of areas under First Nation control, including governance, education, economic development, health, child and family services, addiction services, etc. These organizations allow small First Nations to pool resources in order to improve their access to expertise.

Each province has a cross-sectorial political organization that is independent from but advises and monitors provincial developments relevant to First Nations. The Assembly of First Nations is the national cross-sectorial political organization. The leaders of provincial and national organizations are elected by the Chiefs of individual First Nations. Each layer retains the autonomy to speak directly with the federal departments, and to bypass layers within the First Nation governance as they see appropriate.

The mobilization of the 1960s acted as a catalyst and led to numerous debates over 'the Indian problem' between the federal government and First Nations. This eventually resulted in the formulation of the 1979 Indian Health Policy that recognized three pillars: community development, the traditional relationship of the Indian people to the Federal Government, and the Canadian health system (Health Canada 2000b). By 1982, the Community Health Demonstration Program was in place to allow First Nations to

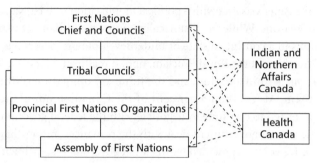

Figure 17.2 First Nations political structure.

experiment with different models of community-based service delivery. Thirty-one such projects were funded for two years, although only seven dealt with transfer issues (Garro *et al.* 1986). The Health Transfer Policy was developed on the strength of this limited experience and announced in 1986. The first transfer was implemented in 1988 (Bird and Moore 1991).

The transfer process was and remains presented as entirely voluntary and progressive. First Nations are encouraged to first apply for funding for a Pre-transfer study, where communities are expected to engage in a community based needs assessment, leading to a community health plan. The second phase is that of negotiations with Health Canada. The third phase is implementation, with contracts signed for three or five years depending on the First Nation's previous experience with program administration. Each phase has clearly defined deliverables, shown in Table 17.1 (Health Canada 1999c; Health Canada 2001c; Health Canada 2001d).

The services targeted for transfer are defined by the federal government, and include mandatory services such as communicable disease control, environmental/occupational health and safety, and treatment services (available in health centres located either off the road system and/or at least 60 km from the nearest referral centre) (Health Canada 1999c). Public health and addiction counselling are optional programs. Medical and Hospital Insurance Services are excluded (under provincial jurisdiction), as well as what is commonly known as Non-Insured Health Benefits (NIHB) which include medication, medical transportation, eye and dental care. These are services that Health Canada offers outside the umbrella of Medicare (insured services) and have been made available free of charge to Indians and Inuit. Indigenous people argue that these services are an Aboriginal Right entrenched in the Medicine Chest Clause of Treaty 6, whereas the federal government argues that these services are offered on humanitarian grounds.

Table 17.1 Phases of health services transfer with components of the community health plan to be completed

Phase 1: Pre-transfer planning (1 year)	Community health priorities and needs (as identified in the Community Needs assessment) Proposed health management structure Management and delivery of mandatory programs Management and Delivery of Community Health Programs

Phase 2:
Bridging
(9 months)
	Items for negotiation:
	  Medical officer of health services
	  Liability and malpractice insurance
	  Drugs and medical supplies
	  Moveable assets reserve
	  Confidentiality procedures
	  Accountability and reporting mechanisms
	  Professional supervision
	  Comprehensive budget

Phase 3: Implementation (3 or 5 year contracts)	Training plan Emergency preparedness plan Evaluation plan

Source: adapted from Health Canada (1999c, 2001b).

More recently, the federal government introduced two alternatives to the original transfer model: the Integrated Community-based Health Services (1994) and Self-Government (1995). Details are shown in Table 17.2. Under the Integrated Community-based Health Services model, First Nations can opt to sign one Contribution Agreement to administer selected community health services, in partnership with Health Canada. Alternatively, the Self-Government option provides an opportunity for First Nations to reconcile all federal and provincial government funding agreements (including education, health, economic development, governance, etc.) under one framework agreement.

The self-government model has successfully been implemented in the Yukon Territory and some parts of British Columbia, but attempts at broad implementation everywhere else appear to have failed. One issue may be related to the complexity of bringing two federal government departments and a multitude of provincial governmental departments to the table to nego-tiate 'a fair deal'. But it may also have to do with the Government of Canada's claim that the signing of such an agreement will lead to a 'corresponding diminution of Crown fiduciary obligations' (Health Canada 1999c). Jurisprudence on the issue, namely from the *Kruger et al.* v. *The Queen* [1985], clearly establishes that the fiduciary responsibility of the Crown cannot be

Table 17.2 Health Canada's three models of transfer

	% of First Nations in each model	Features
Integrated Community-based Health Services Approach (1994)	21%	Funded 1 year planning phase; One master agreement for all Health Canada health programs operating in the community; Additional health management funding (50% of what is allocated under the Health Transfer Policy) to enable to development of community health management capacity; Programs funded at historical levels; Health Canada retains 100% of the risks; Limited budgetary line flexibility
Health Services Transfer Approach (1986)	Pre-transfer 14% Transferred 45%	Funded 1 year training and planning process, plus 9 months negotiation process; Agreements for 3 to 5 years; Greater budgetary line flexibility, one master reporting system, limited ability to negotiate for program enhancement, greater flexibility in program planning and delivery; Community take over of moveable assets; Community assumes a much greater part of the risks.
Self-government approach (1995)	1%	Brings together all funding by Health Canada, Indian and Northern Affairs Canada and provincial funding under one master agreement, including Indian and Northern Affairs: funding for First Nation governance, infrastructure, economic development, welfare, primary and secondary education, on reserve housing; Health Canada: funding for health services; and Provincial government: child protection, as well as other more minor programs. Health remains funded at the same level as that of the Health Transfer Policy.

Sources: Adapted from Health Canada (1999c, 2001b), Health Canada First Nations and Inuit Health Branch Health Funding Arrangements (2000).

reduced or overridden (O'Neil *et al.* 1999). Another issue may be linked to this model's stated goal 'to achieve economies in administration' (Lemchuk-Favel 1999).

Of these models, the Health Transfer Policy remains the most prevalent.

The administrative maze

The Health Transfer Policy aims at increasing First Nation control over their lives and services, and improving Chief and Council's accountability to community members (Health Canada 2001a). However, the policy was designed to transfer pre-existing services, and to be revenue neutral to Health Canada. Over time, Health Canada has responded to additional demands and documented needs by funding Aboriginal and other vertical strategies for which First Nations can compete. Other funding was tagged on to the transfer agreement, following different distribution formulae and processes. The result has been the creation and maintenance of an administrative maze that is inefficient, and impedes the policy's stated goals. The following discussion is but a snapshot of this maze.

Resource allocation issues

A number of issues have been raised with regards to the funding allocated to First Nations who have pursued a transfer. First, it is based on historical expenditures plus 15 per cent for administration, and does not provide for population increases as a result of natural growth or a return to the reserve associated with improved infrastructure. Health Canada had implemented in the Community Workload Increase System (CWIS), which accounted for population figures in the allocation of resources prior to transfer, as well as a nursing reporting system to monitor workload. Thus, the resources allocated to each clinic prior to the transfer were to some extent formulae-based, with a strong emphasis on clinical activities by nurses. It did not necessarily match existing needs. The reporting system also failed to document health activities performed by other members of the health care team, namely the Community Health Representatives (CHRs) and the Alcohol and Drug Abuse Counsellors (known as NNADAP Workers). These resources were transferred based on historical funding. The NNADAP program was initially transferred to Chief and Councils in 1975. While usually located at the Health Centre, these staff were considered employees and supervized by Chief and Council (O'Neil *et al.* 1999).

First Nations on-reserve continue to grow at an annual rate of 3 per cent (Indian and Northern Affairs Canada 2000). Much more significantly, the funding formulae accounts for First Nations living on-reserve at the time of the signing. In the prairie provinces, the signature of transfer agreements coincided with another process, called the Treaty Land Entitlement (TLE). A detailed discussion of the TLE lies beyond the scope of this chapter. Suffice to say that First Nations in the prairies were recently compensated for a short-fall of reserve land that had been promised at the signature of Treaties, but never provided. As a result, First Nations have been successful in securing additional land, either in their traditional territory or in the urban centres where many now reside (Lavoie 1999). Some First Nations thus expect their on-reserve numbers to expand as a result. This issue was brought up to Health Canada's attention as early as 1995. Health Canada's latest Annual Report mentions that a process has been set up to deal with TLE issues if new communities are formed (Health Canada 2002). The non-enrichment clause however remains, so increased population as a result of natural growth or TLE related movement back to existing reserves associated with improved infra-structure remains outstanding.

Third, there is a concern about equity between First Nation and provincial services, and between First Nations themselves. Much has been made in the Canadian popular discourse and in official literature of the overall amount of funding dedicated to First Nation health services. The popular opinion is that 'money is just being thrown at the problem'. The article 'Canada's Bottomless Medicine Chest' (S.C. 1994) is a typical example. Citing the Medicine Chest as the cause of the problem (see earlier discussion), the article goes on to cite First Nations' high utilization rate of hospital services (allegedly twice that of the Canadian population, a figure I do not contest). The argument is con-structed as if the Treaty Clause was the cause of utilization and therefore high health care cost for First Nations, rather than needs. However, the literature suggests that this is not quite the case. The following examples illustrate the complexity of the issue:

◆ The 1993 Royal Commission on Aboriginal Peoples (Canada Royal Commission on Aboriginal Peoples 1996) showed that the 1992–93 com-bined per capita expenditures from federal and provincial governments for Aboriginal health is $2,282 compared to $1,652 for Canadians, a 38 per cent difference. These figures are provincial and territorial aggregates and should be interpreted in the knowledge that service delivery in the far north is expected to be much more expensive than the rest of the country. It is not clear whether the figures include Métis and off reserve First Nations.

◆ Looking at 1991/92 federal and provincial expenditures net of transporta-tion, Manga and Lemchuk-Favel (1993) documented that the combined funding for a comparable set of services for Ontario First Nations was only 8.6 per cent higher than that of other Ontarians.

♦ A similar analysis for Manitoba documented that the combined expenditure for First Nations was only 0.8 per cent higher (Manga and Lemchuk-Favel 1993).

The above analyses look at actual expenditures, reflecting utilization rather than needs. If First Nation's health status has improved considerably over the past thirty years, it nevertheless continues to compare poorly to that of other Canadians. A recent Health Canada report (Health Canada 1999b) shows that the life expectancy of First Nations rose by about ten years between 1975 and 1995. The difference between First Nations and other Canadians remains around six years, reflecting a neonatal death rate that is two times higher, a postnatal death rate that is almost five times higher than in the general Canadian population (Health Canada 1999b) and a higher incidence of heart diseases, hypertension, diabetes, and tuberculosis. These are based on 1995 figures for all provinces except the Maritimes. The self-reported prevalence of diabetes (type II) on reserves is 2.5 times that of the general population, a figure that is believed to under-represent the problem because of delays in diagnosis (Health Canada 2000a). The age standardized tuberculosis incidence rate among on-reserve First Nations has dropped from 58.1 in 1991 to 35.8 in 1996, still nearly six times the national rate (Health Canada 1999b). Social pathologies such as violence and addictions remain a major source of morbidity and mortality. The incidence of suicide in 1997 was three times the national average (Health Canada 1999b). This suggests that First Nation health care needs are much higher than that of other Canadians. In fact, two separate analyses show that First Nation services are indeed inequitably financed when compared to provincial services. Manga and Lemchuk-Favel (1993) suggested that the optimal level of per capita expenditure on health services is actually 6.8 per cent lower for Ontario First Nations than for other Ontarians, despite documented higher needs. Assessing what may be a fair allocation, Eyles et al. (1994) show an actual shortfall of over $700 per capita for First Nations living in the remote Sioux Lookout area of Ontario. They calculate what a fair allocation would be using with the Ontario per capita expenditures, adjusted (1) for demographic differences (age and gender) and (2) for health risks that cannot be explained by age or gender alone. More work is required in this area, as inequities are likely to vary across the country, and across an urban to remote gradient.

Fourth, a majority of transferred First Nations funding comes from the transfer agreement, but many initiatives (the day care program, Aboriginal

Healing Foundation, Aboriginal Headstart, for example) may be introduced on a competitive basis outside the transfer framework. This means that the allocation is proposal driven, thus favouring larger First Nations with better access to professional services, as opposed to need based. These initiatives are theoretically designed to address pressing needs identified within the on-reserve or the larger Aboriginal community, but may not be available to small First Nations, no matter how pressing their needs actually are.

Fifth, the funding is calculated on the basis of the First Nation population living on reserves. But others also live on reserves: non-Aboriginal spouses, nurses and teachers; or children of First Nations who 'fell out of status' under Article 6 of the Indian Act. Also, many reserves serve an adjacent non-reserve based population, and offer the only health service available regionally. But they are not funded for providing services for these people, since they fall under provincial jurisdiction. In such cases, First Nations may find themselves morally obligated to provide services at a loss.

Sixth, Lemchuk-Favel (1999) has documented a number of cases where the federal and provincial dual jurisdiction in health leads to cost shifting. The position of the federal government is that it complements services offered by the provinces. During the 1990s, however, the list of services provided by the provinces has shifted or simply shrunk. In some cases, the federal government's response has lagged, simply leaving First Nations without. For example, the recent shift from institution to community care, in the areas of mental health and home care, has occurred in many provinces without any consideration for its impact on First Nation communities, who are not resourced to provide care to these patients. The federal response in the area of home care lagged by two to three years, leaving First Nation patients in need of care in a very difficult situation. The de-institutionalization of severely dis-abled mental health patients to under-resourced First Nation communities has yet to be addressed.

First Nation governance

As a result of Health Canada's interpretation of the Constitutional framework and Indian Act, First Nations remain precluded from providing services to the whole of their constituency. The Health Transfer Policy is designed to serve the First Nation population living on-reserve only. Although a few provin-cially funded facilities have emerged over the years to serve urban First Nation needs, the off-reserve population is expected to use mainstream services. These people are effectively caught in a federal-provincial cost shifting exercise, where the federal government argues that off-reserve health care is a provincial jurisdiction and the provincial government argues that First Nations are a federal jurisdiction (Canada Royal Commission on Aboriginal Peoples 1993).

The 2001 census results show that there are now 690,101 First Nations people in Canada, of which 43 per cent live off reserve (Canada Department of Indian Affairs and Northern Development 2002b). The Health Transfer Policy thus theoretically applies to less than 400,000 First Nations. But the First Nation population remains mobile, a percentage moving between urban centres and the reserve following educational, housing, medical or employment needs. This issue continues to pose an enumeration challenge and affects funding for on-reserve services. It also poses governance problems, as Chief and Council are elected by the whole membership, but can only offer services to the on-reserve population. Until recently, the Indian Act allowed First Nations to restrict voting rights to those First Nations living on reserve only. However, a 1999 Supreme Court decision (*John Corbiere et al.* v. *the Batchewana Indian Band and Her Majesty the Queen*) ruled that section 77 of the Indian Act violated the Canadian Charter of Rights. First Nations now find themselves culturally, politically and legally obligated to First Nation members living off-reserve, while at the same time receiving virtually no funding to provide services to them.

Impact on First Nations

The Assembly of First Nations summarizes the situation as follows:

> First Nations have less money, a larger services population and fewer options with each passing fiscal year. By attempting to offer the same services for the same money and to avoid default on their agreements, First Nations can incur enormous debt for which they will be stigmatized for being fiscally irresponsible.
>
> Assembly of First Nations 2002

It is hardly surprising to find that almost 60 per cent of respondents to the First Nations and Inuit Regional Health Study 2001 believe that their health services are substandard. It is however important to note that First Nations who have transferred are less likely to identify a disparity in the quality of their services, as compared to Canadians (Canada First Nations and Inuit Regional Health Survey National Steering Committee 2001).

Health Canada has yet to address the concerns explored above. Outwardly, the only tangible step forward has been the production of a three-page document that failed to mention some of the issues raised above (Health Canada 2001b). This may go a long way to validate previous fears that the Health Transfer Policy may be a 'dump and run process' (Auditor General of Canada 1997) adopted by the federal government to offload a politically costly and embarrassing problem onto First Nation shoulders (Culhane Speck 1989). However, discussions are moving along at another level. In a report commissioned by both the Assembly of First Nations and Health Canada, Lemchuk-Favel (1999) proposes that integrated health care funding – the pooling of both federal and provincial funding – may be the solution. An integrated funding strategy would allow First Nations to control all primary health care funding, thus allowing a more flexible approach to planning and delivery. The Lemchuk-Favel proposal is a good start. However, it falls short on two main points. First, it does not resolve the issue of historical and inequitable funding by proposing an alternative, although capitation is mentioned briefly. In fact, a capitation model adjusted for demography, remoteness and needs could resolve some of the concerns expressed above. Second, the proposal fails to address the on-off-reserve debate. But this could be resolved by implementing a registration process allowing on-reserve non-First Nation residents, and off-reserve people wishing to receive services on-reserve, to register for a First Nation health service, thereby redirecting a capitation-based funding allocation to that service. The Lemchuk-Favel report was based on an Ontario case study. Case studies in other provinces have also been conducted. This would suggest that Health Canada is considering alternatives to this administrative maze. Any proposal to pool federal and provincial funding is likely to require a great deal of political goodwill.

The benefits of separate services

In federally-controlled services, nurses are the primary health care service providers and managers, benefiting from a direct line of authority with federally employed supervisors living in urban centres. This is the situation today in services that have not been transferred, and was the situation in services prior to transfer. Although consultations occur, the Health Centre entirely bypasses the authority of the local Chief and Council. This administrative structure evolved out of the bureaucratic culture of Health Canada. The nursing-focused model of care evolved out of necessity: many communities are too small to make the presence of a physician economical; and recruitment and retention issues are compounded for physicians. Finding physicians to work in remote communities was a challenge in earlier days, but it turned to a crisis at the end of the 1960s. Canadian medical schools stepped in to palliate to this situation, each 'adopting' a region, and providing services both on-reserve and in hospital, thereby improving the continuity of care. Residencies and rotations in northern communities are promoted (Waldram *et al.* 1995).

Historically, nurses provided the best care they could, at times going beyond their level of comfort and skills to save lives and limbs. The rise in the nursing profession, better transportation, the northern expansion of expectations and legalities in quality of care, led to a tightening of the nursing scope of practice. Nurses working on reserves now benefit from a legally defined extended scope of practice.

Although the number of Aboriginal nurses is increasing, the majority of nurses remain non-Aboriginal. Their average stay has been said to be between three to six months, making continuity of care a real challenge. Health Canada began a Community Health Representative program in the early 1960s to support the nurses working on reserve. The role of the Community Health Representative is crucial. These workers were to assure a linguistic and cultural liaison with the community, thus supporting the nurses in the delivery of clinical and public health services. They were not and still are not considered professionals. In the early years, the role of the Community Health Representative expanded and contracted at the whims of the nurse in charge, spanning the direct delivery of midwifery services to a strictly clerical and translation role. They received little formal training, other than what nurses were prepared or able to deliver on the job. In informal discussions, senior Community Health Representatives have pointed out that in the early years of the program, these workers often performed tasks that are no longer allowed under the current legislative framework. The current role is more likely to be that of translation, health promotion, tracing infectious diseases contacts and collaborating with nurses in immunization or prenatal clinics. Although the Community Health Representative program was initially seen as a step towards training Aboriginal nurses, this has proven difficult to implement.

First Nations who have opted to take over health services have generally revised the hierarchy in the Health Centre. The organizations I am aware of have opted to hire a community member as Health Director. Some are former Community Health Representatives. Although there were discussions on expanding the role of the Community Health Representatives, aspirations were generally thwarted by their lack of formal training. The Saskatchewan Indian Institute of Technology has developed a two years certificate qualification to address this issue. Clinical service delivery has remained focused on nurses, an increasing number being of Aboriginal ancestry. Under the transfer framework, physicians continue to be paid by the province, and make weekly or so visits. Transferred First Nations may be in a better situation to negotiate for an expansion of those services, but do not have the funding to hire physicians.

Advocates of community control have often pointed out that responsiveness to local needs, local employment and the use of local language and vernacular, are likely to make services more relevant to First Nations and to improve outcomes. This reasoning has obvious intuitive value. The literature on potential health benefits is rather slim and epidemiological investigations nearly non-existent. Transferred health services are required to conduct a thorough evaluation of their services every five years. These reports generally do not provide strong epidemiological evidence because the population they report on is rather small, the five year time span too short, and because Health Canada has not been able to provide baseline data (Angees *et al.* 1999). Anecdotal reports of positive results in the areas of access, use and outcome have been noted. For example, The Montreal Lake Band, who implemented transfer in 1988, has reported a number of such improvements:

- Increased on-reserve health services, making services more accessible;
- Increased access as a result of community ownership and use of local language;
- More extensive and effective health promotion and prevention activities; and
- Lower hospitalization rate (Bird and Moore 1991).

Warry (1998) relates the experience of the North Shore Tribal Council, pointing out that the planning phase of the transfer provided an opportunity to engage the community in a process of reflection leading to the revitalization of traditional medical practices. Further, a study by Chandler and Lalonde (1998) on cultural continuity and suicide among First Nation youth in British Columbia is now attracting considerable attention. The authors looked at suicide in First Nation communities, and were able to show that the prevalence of suicide is significantly lower in communities where the police and fire services, education, health, and local facilities for cultural activities are under local government control, and where land claims have been pursued. Thus they conclude that communities that have pursued measures to rehabilitate or protect their cultural integrity are less likely to see their youth commit suicide. A recent review by Kirmayer *et al.* (2000) of the literature on Canadian Aboriginal people's mental health supports this conclusion. Community control may also help alleviate the feelings of invalidation and racism reported by some First Nations relying on provincial services (Browne and Fiske 2001).

Conclusion

Today, both the federal government and First Nations seem to agree that 'only Indian communities themselves can change [the] root causes [of ill health in their communities]' to paraphrase the 1979 Indian Health Policy (Health Canada 2000b). Once implemented in the microcosm of First Nation communities, the jurisdictional divide and piecemeal approach to transfer create an unmanageable administrative maze. To date, First Nations remain limited in their ability to address the needs of their constituency for a number of reasons.

- The services are not funded on an equitable basis when compared to provincial services.
- The funding allocation does not reflect the actual population being served.
- Access to funding is fragmented, and at times competitive, rather than needs-based and administratively efficient.
- Federal and provincial cost shifting at times leaves First Nations in a substandard or no care situation.
- The current system perpetuates the on-off-reserve debate that fragments Aboriginal people into different administrative categories based on jurisdiction rather than identity or needs.
- The resulting structure limits First Nation's ability to offer services that are holistic and responsive to their own priorities.

Most of the issues listed above are not new (Assembly of First Nations 2002; Canada Royal Commission on Aboriginal Peoples 1996). Given this situation, how does one explain that a large majority of First Nations nevertheless continue to engage in this process? Quiet acceptance is not the answer. At less than 3 per cent of the overall population, First Nations are not likely to find and maintain their place in Canadian society through the democratic process alone. The transfer process appears to offer First Nations a far from perfect yet helpful step forward in the pursuit of self-government. Active participation in health service planning and delivery is not only likely to improve responsiveness, but also provide opportunities for First Nations to access high level decision-making tables previously not accessible to them, and improve their ability to shape the policies and programs that affect them. The recent Assembly of First Nation submission to the Commission on the Future of Health Care in Canada, and the Aboriginal consultative forum that followed on 25 June 2002, are cases in point. Commissioner Romanow has made a commitment to recommend a solution to Parliament (Romanow 2002). It however appears that any solutions will have to fit within rather than benefit from a change in the current Constitutional division of power (Leeson 2002), hence, First Nations will continue to deal with both federal and provincial governments in health care. Further, it is unlikely First Nations will agree to turn on-reserve health to the provinces (Assembly of First Nations 2002), for a number of reasons ranging from the historical relationship between First Nations and provincial governments, to negative experiences in provincial health services (Browne and Fiske 2001; Farkas and Shah 1986). Separate services are here to stay.

And the process continues. The Northern Intertribal Health Authority, a consortium organization uniting two very large First Nations and two Tribal Councils representing 25,000 First Nations altogether signed its first three-year agreement in 2001. This is a first in Canada, and takes over yet another level of services previously provided by Health Canada. The authority is funded to deliver the following services: a Community Health Status and Surveillance Unit, a tuberculosis screening and treatment program, nursing program support, program planning in the areas of mental health, addictions and environmental health, research capacity building, and health information capacity building and training (Merasty 2001). This new venture will go a long way to address issues of access to capacity and infrastructure building experienced by First Nations in the areas. Administratively, however, this is yet another piecemeal transfer, a reflection of the climate explored above.

It is hoped that the Commission on the Future of Health Care in Canada will find solutions, and convince the Canadian parliament to adopt them. Considerable provincial and federal political goodwill will be required to reshape the current system. This may very well require 'the wholehearted support of the larger Canadian community' as predicted by the 1979 Indian Health Policy (Health Canada 2000b).

Acknowledgements

This paper is part of a larger research project on indigenous health providers in Canada, Australia and New Zealand, undertaken as part of a Ph.D. with the Health Policy Unit of the London School of Hygiene and Tropical Medicine. I would like to thank my supervisors Dr Lucy Gilson and Stephen Jan for the insightful comments on an earlier draft, and their ongoing support. Funding for this research is provided by the Fondation Ricard of Canada, a charitable foundation that supports French-Canadians by providing graduate and post-graduate scholarships. Madame Ricard, avec toute ma gratitude.

References

Angees, E., Anderson, C., Young, T. K., O'Neil, J. D. and Hiebert, S. (1999) *Evaluation of transferred health services in the Shibogama First Nations council communities of Kingfisher Lake, Wapekeka, and Wunnumin Lake.* University of Manitoba, Center for Aboriginal Health Research, Winnipeg.

Armitage, A. (1995) *Comparing the policy of Aboriginal assimilation: Australia, Canada and New Zealand.* UBC Press, Vancouver.

Assembly of First Nations (2001) *Assembly of First Nations – the story (Internet).* Assembly of First Nations, Ottawa.

Assembly of First Nations (2002) *Presentation notes to the commission on the future of healthcare in Canada.* Assembly of First Nations, Ottawa.

Auditor General of Canada (1997) *Health Canada – First Nations health,* chapter 13. Auditor General of Canada, Ottawa.

Backwell, P. (1981) The medicine chest clause in treaty No. 6. *Canadian Native Law Reporter,* 4, 1–23.

Bird, L. and Moore, M. (1991) The William Charles Health Centre of Montreal lake band: a case study of transfer. *Arctic Medical Research,* 50 (1–4), Suppl. 47–49.

Browne, A. J. and Fiske, J. A. (2001) First Nations women's encounters with mainstream health care services. *Western Journal of Nursing Research,* 23 (2), 126–47.

Canada Department of Indian Affairs and Northern Development (2002a.) *First nation profiles.* Canada department of Indian Affairs and Northern development. Available at http://esd.inac.gc.ca/fnprofiles/, accessed 9 February 2002.

Canada Department of Indian Affairs and Northern Development (2002b) *Registered Indian population by sex and residence 2001* (QS-3620–010-EE-A1, Catalogue No. R31–3/2001E) Minister of Public Works and Government Services Canada, Ottawa.

Canada First Nations and Inuit Regional Health Survey National Steering Committee (2001) *First Nations and Inuit regional health survey.* Health Canada and the Assembly of First Nations, Ottawa.

Canada Royal Commission on Aboriginal Peoples (1993) *Aboriginal Peoples in urban centres.* Ministry of Supplies and Services, Ottawa.

Canada Royal Commission on Aboriginal Peoples (1996) *Gathering strength (Royal Commission on Aboriginal Peoples – final report)* volume 3. Royal Commission on Aboriginal Peoples, Ottawa.

Cardinal, H. (1969) *The unjust society: the tragedy of Canada's Indians.* Hurtig Publishers, Edmonton.

Chandler, M. J. and Lalonde, C. (1998) Cultural continuity as a hedge against suicide in Canada's First Nations. *Transcultural Psychiatry,* 35 (2), 191–219.

Coates, K. (1999) The 'gentle occupation', the settlement of Canada and the dispossession of the First Nations. In P. Havemann (ed.) *Indigenous peoples' rights in Australia, Canada and New Zealand,* pp. 141–61. Oxford University Press, Oxford.

Culhane Speck, D. (1989) The Indian health transfer policy: a step in the right direction, or revenge of the hidden agenda? *Native Studies Review,* 5 (1), 187–213.

Deber, R. and Baranek, P. (1998) Canada: markets at the margin. In W. Ranade (ed.) *Markets and health care: a comparative analysis,* pp. 73–100. Longman, London.

Eyles, J., Birch, S. and Chambers, S. (1994) Fair shares for the zone: allocating health-care resources for the native populations of the Sioux Lookout zone, Northern Ontario. *Canadian Geographer,* 38 (2), 134–50.

Farkas, C. S. and Shah, C. P. (1986) Public health departments and native health care in urban centres. *Canadian Journal of Public Health,* 77 (44), 274–8.

Garro, L. C., Roulette, J. and Whitmore, R. G. (1986) Community control of health care delivery: The Sandy Bay experience. *Canadian Journal of Public Health,* 77, 281–4.

Hawthorn, H. B. (1966) *A survey of the contemporary Indians of Canada economic, political, educational needs and policies part 1 (The Hawthorn Report)*. Indian Affairs Branch, Ottawa.

Health Canada (1999a) *Canada's health care system*. Health system and policy division, Policy and Consultation Branch, Health Canada, Ottawa.

Health Canada (1999b) *A second diagnostic on the health of First Nations and Inuit people in Canada*. Ottawa, Health Canada.

Health Canada (1999c) *Transferring control of health programs to First Nations and Inuit communities, handbook 1: an introduction to all three approaches*. Health Canada, Program Policy Transfer Secretariat and Planning Health Funding Arrangements, Ottawa.

Health Canada (2000a) *Diabetes among Aboriginal (First Nations, Inuit and Métis) people in Canada: the evidence*. Health Canada, Ottawa.

Health Canada (2000b) *Indian health policy 1979*. Canada, Health Canada Medical Services Branch. Available at www.hsc.gc.ca/msb/pptsp/hfa/publications/poli79_e.htm, accessed 19 March 2001.

Health Canada (2001a) *Ten years of health transfer First Nation and Inuit Control*. Health Canada 23 July 2001. Available at www.hc-sc.gc.ca/fnihb/pptsp/hfa/ten_years_health_transfer/index.htm, accessed 14 April 2002.

Health Canada (2001b) *Transfer issues, health Canada, program policy transfer Secretariat and Planning Health Funding Arrangements*. Ottawa, Health Canada.

Health Canada (2001c) *Transferring control of health programs to First Nations and Inuit communities, Handbook 2: The health services transfer*. Health Canada, Ottawa.

Health Canada (2001d) *Transferring control of health programs to First Nations and Inuit Communities, Handbook 3: After the Transfer – The New Environment*. Health Canada, Ottawa.

Health Canada (2002) *Annual report first nations and Inuit control: program policy transfer secretariat and planning directorate, health funding arrangements*. Minister of Public Works and Government Services Canada, Ottawa.

Health Canada First Nations and Inuit Health Branch Health Funding Arrangements (2000) *Reporting and auditing guidelines for health services transfer agreements*. Health Canada, Program Policy Transfer Secretariat and Planning Health Funding Arrangements, Ottawa.

Indian and Northern Affairs Canada (1999) *Individuals responsible for Aboriginal and Northern affairs in Canada 1755 to 1999*. Indian and Northern Affairs Canada. Available at http://www.ainc-inac.gc.ca/pr/info/info38_e.html, accessed October 1999.

Indian and Northern Affairs Canada (2000) *Registered Indian population projections for Canada and regions 1998–2008*. Minister of Public Works and Government Services Canada, Ottawa.

King George (1763) (December 10, 1998) The Royal Proclamation, bloorstreet-com web services. Available at www.miredespa.com/wmaton/Other/L...a/English/PreConfederation/rp_1763.html, accessed 16 February 2002.

Kirmayer, L. J., Brass, G. M. and Tait, C. L. (2000) The mental health of Aboriginal peoples: transformations of identity and community. *Canadian Journal of Psychiatry*, **45** September, 607–17.

Lavoie, J. G. (1999) The Governance and management of the Peter Ballantyne Cree Nation Urban Reserves in Prince Albert. In L. Barron and J. Garcia (eds) *Indian urban reserves in Saskatchewan*. Purich Publishing, Saskatoon.

Leeson, H. (2002) *Constitutional jurisdiction over health and health care services in Canada*. Discussion Paper no. 12, Commission on the Future of Health Care in Canada. University of Regina, Regina.

Lemchuk-Favel, L. (1999) *Financing a First Nations and Inuit integrated health system: a discussion document*, pp. 78. Health Canada, Ottawa.

Long, J. A. and Boldt, M. (1988) *Governments in conflicts? Provinces and Indian Nations in Canada*. University of Toronto Press, Toronto.

Manga, P. and Lemchuk-Favel, L. (1993) *Health care financing and health status of registered Indians*, pp. 200. Health Canada, Ottawa.

Merasty, R. (2001) NITHA, Health Canada Sign Demonstration Project for third level health services, the project is the first of its kind in Canada. PAGC Tribune. (October)

Morris, A. (1880) *The treaties of Canada with the Indians of Manitoba and the North-West Territories including the negotiations on which they were based*, 1991 edition. Belfords, Clarke & Co., Publishers, Toronto.

O'Neil, J. D., Lemchuk-Favel, L., Allard, Y. and Postl, B. D. (1999) Community healing and Aboriginal self-government. In J. H. Hylton (ed.) *Aboriginal self-government in Canada: current trends and issues*, second edition, pp. 130–56. Purish Publishing, Saskatoon.

Romanow, C. R. (2002). *"Building on values: The future of health care in Canada"*. Commission on the future of health care in Canada. Ottawa.

S.C (1994) Canada's bottomless medicine chest. *Newsmagazine, Alberta Report*, **21**, 1–2.

Waldram, J. B., Herring, D. A. and Young, T. K. (1995) *Aboriginal health in Canada: historical, cultural and epidemiological perspectives*. University of Toronto Press, Toronto.

Warry, W. (1998) *Unfinished dreams: community healing and the reality of Aboriginal self-government*. University of Toronto Press Incorporated, Toronto.

Weaver, S. M. (1981) *Making the Canadian Indian policy: The hidden agenda, 1968–1970*. University of Toronto Press, Toronto.

Young, T. K. (1994) *The health of Native Americans: towards a biocultural epidemiology*. Oxford University Press, New York.

Chapter 18

Delivering Health Services in Diverse Societies

Judith Healy and Martin McKee

Diversity and the challenge to collective care

In concluding this book, we return to the two themes of our first chapter. We argued that health policy makers should be responsive to diverse needs within the population of their country. Even the most homogenous societies contain a diversity of health needs due to, for example, age and sex differences. Health systems also must adapt to demographic change over time, such as population ageing in industrialized countries (Organization for Economic Cooperation and Development 2000). Further, societies are becoming more heterogeneous through population movements between countries; for example, migrants accounted for 70 per cent of the population growth in the European Union during 2001 (Eurostat 2002). Thus countries should consider whether established ways of delivering health care are meeting the needs of their changing populations as well as the needs of newcomers.

Our membership of different groups within society substantially influences our health, through causative factors such as genes and biology, and through our physical and socio-economic environments (Marmot and Wilkinson 1999). Our health behaviours are influenced by whether we are rich or poor, white or black, citizens or asylum-seekers; further, these characteristics also influence the responses of health service providers.

The second principle that we espoused was equity, which means that everyone should have access to, and be able to use, appropriate, good quality and affordable health care. Countries vary according to whether they regard health care as a private commodity or a public good or a mixture of both, but even in countries where health care is a universal right, some population groups fare less well than others in accessing and using health services. The service delivery model that a particular group advocates, whether collective or alternative, may have implications for the adequacy and quality of their health care.

This concluding chapter draws upon preceding chapters in analysing the barriers to access and use of health services, and the advantages and disadvantages of separate as opposed to collective services.

Barriers to accessing and using health services

The claim by a population group for special or extra health resources is in large part based upon the view that the 'mainstream' health care system has failed to meet their needs. The chapters in this book document most convincingly the considerable barriers faced by population groups that seek to use health services designed by and for the dominant population group. Table 18.1 lists health system barriers, problems and solutions. This section goes on to discuss four types of barriers (physical, financial, procedural and social) that are encountered. Some groups, such as the Roma in Europe, may encounter all types of barriers: difficulties in travelling to town-based health services, not having money to pay the doctor, filling out many forms, and being treated with a lack of courtesy or even hostility.

Physical barriers

The physical location and design of buildings make it difficult for some groups to access and use health care services. Disability advocacy groups, for example, have achieved some success in raising awareness and in improving physical access for people with disabilities such as wheelchair users (see Chapter 4 by Basnett). Although one might expect hospitals to be accessible to those with disabilities, with entry not barred by flights of stairs, despite calls to redesign hospitals in order to facilitate patient-focused care, many hospitals remain unresponsive to those who need them most (Healy and McKee 2002).

Geography presents another major barrier. Most countries struggle to extend health resources to rural and remote areas through strategies that either take services to rural people or transport rural people to urban health care. The challenges are illustrated by the case of the vast but mostly arid continent of Australia. It contains a population of only 19.5 million people, of whom the great majority live in capital cities or along the eastern seaboard, so that health care is geared more to urban Australia, despite a history of innovative outreach programmes, such as the Flying Doctor Service. In Chapter 5 Humphreys and Dixon discuss the socio-economic, geographic and physical factors that all impact adversely upon the health of Australians in rural and remote regions. Rural Australia is not well served by private health care, since the mainly private general practitioners and specialists are not enthusiastic about living in country towns, given small numbers of patients and hence

Table 18.1 Types of health systems barriers, problems and solutions

Type of barrier	Health system problems	Health service solutions
Physical	Geographic inequities	Improve rural/urban distribution
	Inaccessible location	Re-locate, improve transport
	Poor design	Improve design and ambience
	Inaccessible disabled	Adapt buildings and equipment
	Not advertised	Publicise
Financial	Too costly	Reduce fees, subsidise
	Cost ceilings	Increase expenditure
Procedural	Restrictive eligibility	Lift restrictions, affirmative action
	Rationing health care	Ration by need or expected outcomes
	Restricted hours	Extend hours
	Excessive formality	Allow 'walk-in' appointments
	Complex procedures	Simplify procedures, employ access workers
	Arbitrary decisions	Set criteria agree protocols
	Lack of system knowledge	Set guidelines, train staff
Social	Monocultural	Employ a multicultural staff
	Monolingual	Employ bilingual staff, interpreters
	Social/cultural ignorance	Training on social/cultural factors
	Medical/psychiatric ignorance	Training on specific conditions
	Discrimination	Pass legislation, develop guidelines, change attitudes
	Patriarchal attitudes	Train staff, employ more women
	Psychological	Train and support staff

Source: Healy (1998 p. 110).

limited financial rewards, as well as the limited infrastructure to support medical practice. The dissatisfaction of rural voters since the late 1990s, with the closure of health services, such as hospitals, as well as the rationalization of other services such as banks and post offices, has prompted the national Government to fund a range of strategies intended to improve rural and remote health care. These include training more rural health professionals, offering financial incentives to health professionals to locate in the country, and developing models of rural health service delivery (such as nurse practitioners and multiservice centres), outreach programmes (such as mobile clinics) and technology (such as telemedicine).

Financial barriers

Other than in the United States, industrialized countries have achieved universal or near universal health care coverage, generally funded through mandatory taxation or social insurance, with less than 30 per cent of funds coming from the private sector including out-of-pocket payments by patients (Mossialos and LeGrand 1999). Yet upward pressure on costs, reflecting rising public expectations and the growing scope of health care, means that many countries have put in place policies to contain costs. In reality, these often have the effect of transferring costs from collective to individual funding, such as increased co-payments, with the inevitable consequence that they increase the financial burden on those already disadvantaged.

New Zealand, for example, has undergone four major phases of restructuring since the early 1980s but access to primary health care remained problematic. In the absence of coverage for primary care, low-income people had to apply for a concession card to subsidize their visits to a general practitioner (French *et al.* 2001). Crengle *et al.* (Chapter 15) document the poorer health status of Māori people compared to the rest of the population, with higher proportions (19 per cent compared to 12 per cent) reporting higher levels of unmet need for primary health care. Although many factors are involved, financial barriers are likely to have contributed to poorer health status, prompting the New Zealand government to introduce capitation funding for GP groups.

The health status of Aboriginal people remains abysmal despite a plethora of reports and programs. Aboriginal people live about 20 years less than the rest of the population (Australian Bureau of Statistics 1999) in the midst of a country that enjoys among the best health measures for developed nations. It is clear that the funding for Aboriginal health services is inadequate, although obviously not the only reason for their poor health status, extra funds have been allocated, with 8 per cent per capita higher spending on Aboriginal people in the mid 1990s in addition to mainstream services (Australian Institute of Health and Welfare 2001; Deeble *et al.* 1998), and doubled funding between 1996 and 2001. In Chapter 14 Griew *et al.* argue that the continuing poor health of the Aboriginal population demonstrates that these extra funds are still insufficient, and further, that more control should be devolved to Aboriginal health agenices.

Procedural barriers

Health care services can throw up a myriad of procedural barriers, either through ignorance or in a covert attempt to ration services. People who are not official residents or citizens of a country typically are not regarded as having a legitimate claim upon a country's health care system, and not all countries are prepared to acknowledge their human rights claim.

Refugee policy in Europe, for example, is framed mainly in terms of immigration control and national security, although the European Union demands that member states should comply with basic standards on asylum issues (Kummin 1999). Most European Union governments have introduced restrictions to try and reduce what they perceive as excessive numbers of people seeking protection, including reducing social benefits, detaining asylum seekers and applying a narrow legal interpretation of who can qualify as a refugee. In January 2001, 5.6 million people in Europe were defined as refugees (United Nations High Commission for Refugees 2003). These refugees suffer from a wide spectrum of health problems including communicable disease and mental health problems, which have implications not just for these individuals but also for their host countries (Carballo *et al.* 1998). Their health problems may also reflect, particularly in the case of asylum seekers, the traumas they experienced in their home country, the difficulties of their journey, and the exclusion they experience in the host country. There are good reasons, therefore, for a country to address such special health care needs.

Refugees are regarded as having a limited claim upon the health services even in countries that are widely perceived as having equitable health care policies. Thus, Sweden has a universal health care system, funded mostly through taxes and social insurance, available to all official residents. Sweden applies generally humanitarian policies towards refugees and asylum seekers, with over 30,000 in 2002 applying for residency, a large number for a country with a population under 9 million. Yet Ekblad (Chapter 10) points out that asylum seekers are not eligible for public services until they are registered as official residents and in the meantime county councils have only a limited obligation to assist. Emergency medical and dental care is free but otherwise people must pay 5.4 Euros for a doctor's consultation, perhaps financed through an application to the Migration Board for a daily allowance.

United Kingdom government policy under the Immigration and Asylum Act 1999 is based upon dispersing asylum seekers and refugees out of London, with responsibility decentralized to local government and voluntary agencies (Audit Commission 2000). Coker (Chapter 11) points out that in Britain (with 76,000 applications for asylum in 2001 – the largest proportion of any country), asylum seekers receive restricted housing and cash benefits but are entitled to health care from the National Health Service (NHS). The problem is that in both Sweden and Britain, the lengthy procedures for determining asylum status can undermine the health and well-being of these vulnerable people, as can the barriers thrown up in negotiating access to health care in new and complex health care systems in the context of growing community hostility to asylum seekers. In response to pressure from tabloid newspapers, the British government has substantially hardened its policies on asylum seekers, despite courts subsequently overturning such actions. Further, a Council of Europe report has urged the United Kingdom government to address the hostile climate concerning asylum seekers and refugees (European Commission against Racism and Intolerance 2000).

A more severe regime can be found in Australia, where the current policy, under the catch-cry of 'border protection', established detention centres, both offshore and inside the country, to detain asylum seekers during their often very lengthy application period (Asylum Seekers in Australia 2003). The controversial detention centres in Australia, mostly located in isolated areas, have been the scene of hunger strikes and breakouts by desperate people. Prolonged detention, especially of vulnerable children and adolescents, has resulted in serious mental health problems (Minas and Sawyer 2002).

Social barriers

Social barriers are of many types. Discrimination takes several forms, the root cause being either ignorance or prejudice, and often a mixture of both. Table 18.1 sets out a list of well-known social barriers, but here we focus on age discrimination because this has received relatively little attention until recently in health care systems, and because the share of older people in the population is growing in industrialized countries, making this an increasingly significant issue for the health system.

Older patients may encounter all four types of barriers in accessing and using health care services. Criticisms swelled in Britain during the 1990s that the National Health Service (NHS) was discriminating against older people. These criticisms followed a long period of cost containment, which had involved cost ceilings and the introduction of a quasi-market within the public sector. As a King's Fund review pointed out (Roberts 2000), it was not immediately obvious that age discrimination was occurring, since older people constituted the main consumers of health care, while user surveys generally reported them more satisfied than younger users. Voluntary organisations, such as Age Concern and Help the Aged, however, had publicized many instances of indirect and direct discrimination. Indirect discrimination involved practices that affected older people more adversely than others, such as shorter lengths of stay in hospital, or busy staff having less time for personal care. Active discrimination included staff behaving disrespectfully, denying preventive care, and applying explicit or implicit treatment limits on grounds of age (for example, screening for cervical and breast cancer was restricted to people aged under 65 years). A number of studies throughout the 1990s showed that older people were less likely than younger people to be actively treated, some examples being coronary care (Bowling 1999) and cancer (Turner 1999).

As Victor (Chapter 3) discusses, the National Health Service in the late 1990s acknowledged that age discrimination was occurring, and responded by promulgating a set of eight standards, titled a National Service Framework for Older People, a ten-year program intended to 'root out age discrimination' (Department of Health 2001). This essentially voluntary initiative called for NHS bodies and local authorities to scrutinize their practices, to implement a number of reform measures, and to report on their actions. Critics of such exhortations for voluntary action argue that legislation specific to health and welfare (rather than just conventional and generic anti-discrimination laws) is required to ensure that such agencies do not discriminate, and that staff training and monitoring procedures are required to ensure age equality (Robinson 2002).

The criteria used for prioritizing (or rationing) health care may also disadvantage older people in several ways (Brock 2001). For example, a cost-effectiveness approach means that, other things being equal, life-sustaining treatment for an older person will produce fewer life years than for an older person; since an older person may be assessed as having lower quality of life than a young person, a quality adjusted life years (QALY) approach will produce fewer years; the more complicated medical conditions of the old than the young will make for more costly treatment and less successful outcomes.

Two points of particular relevance to this book emerge from this discussion. First, since it is unlikely that British health services are alone in practicing systematic age discrimination, other countries should also institute similar enquiries. Despite an avalanche of health reforms in industrialized countries that have changed the landscape primarily through restructuring and cost containment (Saltman *et al.* 1998), few countries have looked closely at the impact of these changes upon older people. Second, the British reform proposals call for reforming mainstream services rather than setting up separate and better quality health services for older people. Indeed, some claim that age discrimination has arisen because the NHS fifty years ago set up separate services for frail old people, such as long-term care facilities within hospitals and care homes, which over time became Cinderella services (Robinson 2002). The critique leads to the proposal of various solutions, in essence being a call to reform mainstream services, or else to set up alternative services that eliminate all these barriers.

Service delivery models

The many organizational models for the delivery of health services range from collectivist services for everyone to setting up separate and parallel services for a particular group (Healy 1998). One possible classification of health service delivery models is set out in Table 18.2 and this section goes on to discuss examples under each heading.

Mainstream services

A mainstream model refers to the situation in which health services designed for the majority population are made collectively available to everyone, with minority and indigenous groups expected to use the same health services as everyone else and, arguably, to conform to the dominant conventions. The mainstream model is based on the principle that collective care guarantees a good health care system for everyone, strengthens social solidarity and maintains taxpayer willingness to fund the health care system. The more pejorative view is that such services are assimilationist and ignore cultural differences, as well as, in some countries, the rights of indigenous people.

Perhaps the clearest example of this model, among those considered in this book, is the situation of overseas citizens of France (Halley des Fontaines, Chapter 9). The official view is that people living or born in the overseas

Table 18.2 Service delivery models and population group examples

Service delivery models	Examples
Mainstream (collective)	Women's health care Britain
	Multicultural health care Britain
	Overseas citizens of France
	Refugees in Sweden
	Asylum seekers Britain
	East Germans in the new Germany
	Roma in Europe
	Rural people Australia
Integrationist	The poor in Britain
Participatory	New Zealand Māori
Alternative	Women's health care Australia
	Aboriginal Australians
Parallel services	Military health services
	Prison services
	Native Americans
	Canadian Indians

regions of France are entitled to exactly the same health services as citizens of continental France (the Metropole), and that they should not therefore be treated in any way differently – even though scattered studies suggest that their health status is significantly worse. To ask the question whether overseas citizens experience discrimination is regarded as discriminatory in itself and thus taboo. Further, overseas-born citizens are concerned that making any special claim might undermine their status as full *citoyens de France*. Recent legislation on social exclusion, however, may spark a more open debate.

The situation of east Germans has some similarities. The fall of the Berlin Wall in November 1989 was followed rapidly by formal unification in October 1990, with five East German states (*länder*) created within the German federal system of government. The West German health care system became the dominant model for the unified country, with no debate on whether to retain some good features of the East German model. Busse and Nolte (Chapter 8) point out that although the imposition of the West German health care system must be regarded as a success story in terms of much improved health outcomes, the rapid changes that were implemented, and the lack of consultation with the new citizens, suggests that they may feel little sense of ownership.

In contrast, in other countries a reformist view is now gaining ground, which considers that collective health services should be more culturally responsive and should respect diverse beliefs and needs. Williams and Harding (Chapter 12), in arguing that multicultural Britain is best served by maintaining the National Health Service, cite the policy of mainstreaming that entails 'rethinking mainstream provision to accommodate gender, race, disability and other dimensions of discrimination and disadvantage including sexuality and religion' (Scottish Executive 2000).

Since the 1970s Australia has had explicitly multicultural policies (Borowski 2000; Council for Multicultural Australia), since Australia is an ethnically diverse nation with over 40 per cent of the population either immigrants or the children of immigrants (Australian Bureau of Statistics 2000). Migrants bring to Australia their own unique health profiles, but stringent health requirements in part mean that migrants enjoy good, if not better, health than the Australian-born population, generally known as the 'healthy migrant effect' (Australian Institute of Health and Welfare 2000; Kliewer and Jones 1998). Multicultural health policies in Australia, therefore, are based not upon redressing worse health outcomes, but on addressing differences in specific health conditions and responding to access and equity concerns. Most Commonwealth and State health and social programmes require that specific consideration be given to ethnic groups. For example, culturally appropriate models of preventive health care delivery are being developed in relation to mortality and morbidity for different types of cancer and diabetes (Australian Institute of Health and Welfare 2000).

Access to mainstream services has also been addressed by the disability movement internationally over the last two decades. The context is the history of societal marginalization of people with physical (or intellectual) disabilities so that the push is to 'normalize' service delivery. It is argued that services should be accessible to people with disabilities since separate services in the past, particularly within a medical model, have stigmatized people (Oliver 1990, 1998). 'Access' here is shorthand for a range of barriers that make it difficult for people with disabilities to get to and use the services that are available to the rest of the population. Physical access is just one albeit formidable barrier (Pierce 1998), and there is a growing recognition that it is the environment that is disabling rather than the physical condition of an individual. Greater participation in policy-making is a concern for people with disabilities, as it is increasingly recognized that full access requires the health service delivery system to empower disabled people so as to enable them to participate in decisions on the delivery of care. The quest for improved access must be seen in the context of exclusion from society of people with severe disabilities. Separation is still the norm in many countries where people with severe disabilities attend a separate system of health care services, in the context of their specialized hospital systems, with separate hospitals or dispensaries for the outpatient and inpatient care of those with chronic health problems or disabilities.

Integrationist

Integrationist policies are based on the belief that simply making services available to all does not guarantee that they will be accessed, and that it is necessary to establish a range of activities designed to encourage disadvantaged groups to use collective health services. These activities may include referral services, interpreters and liaison workers, as well as broader policies to direct resources to those who are disadvantaged.

Whitehead and Hanratty (Chapter 5) argue that a variety of social and economic factors are determinants of poor health, through causal pathways such as lack of financial resources, psychosocial stress, and behaviours that increase health risks. A large body of research shows the generally lower use of health services by poor people in industrialized countries, taking into account their greater need for health care, and also identifies the various factors that reduce access. These studies illustrate 'the inverse care law' propounded by Tudor Hart (1971) that the availability of good medical care is in inverse proportion to population need, and the 'inverse equity hypothesis' that new health programmes initially reach people of higher socio-economic status and only later reach the poor (Victora *et al.* 2000). As Whitehead and Hanratty note, the United Kingdom has begun to tackle inequalities that persist despite sixty years of a national health service, for example, by affirmative action to direct extra money to poorer areas through programmes such as the Health Action Zones. However, although barriers to access are well documented, there has been very little research on what strategies work in terms of both better access and better health outcomes.

Participatory services

Participatory services are services within the mainstream health care system that offer avenues for consumer groups to have more say in policy-making and management. Such initiatives may involve setting up area health boards or inviting consumer representatives onto the boards of health agencies. In theory, this makes services more responsive to different groups, such as ethnic minority groups.

Health policies for indigenous populations in each of the four countries considered in this book have seen a shift of responsibility over the years from national departments for indigenous affairs to special sections within national health departments: Canada in 1944, the United States in 1954, New Zealand in 1991, and Australia from a national department for indigenous affairs in 1984 to an indigenous commission in 1989 to an indigenous unit in the health department in 1995. Since then each country, although taking different paths as discussed later, is moving towards greater self-determination by local indigenous communities.

The participatory or partnership model is illustrated by New Zealand where government policy now emphasizes 'partnership' with Māori (French *et al.* 2001). The concept of a 'nation within a nation' (Kymlicka 1995) is apt in that Māori, around 15 per cent of the total population, have six seats in Parliament (with individual Māori voters free to register on either the Māori or General voting register). The 21 district health boards, set up in 2001 to purchase and deliver health care services to their populations, are each required to have at least two Māori members or more where the Māori proportion of the local population is high. In addition, throughout the 1990s, more funds were allocated to community trusts to purchase or provide health services for their local communities, and as part of this thrust and in line with the principles of the Treaty of Waitangi, the number of Māori health care providers doubled to over 240 in 1998, although the bulk of expenditure for Māori health initiatives still went to collective providers. Crengle *et al.* (Chapter 15) argue that the development of Māori health care providers has gone some way towards meeting Māori wishes for self-determination, but that the challenge remains to incorporate Māori models of health into New Zealand health care services.

Alternative services

Alternative services are defined as those that exist in addition to mainstream services, with individuals able to choose between the two. Such services are usually limited in scope and scale (e.g. primary care only) and can be of good quality and designed to meet the needs of particular groups. One example is based on sexual orientation, with some examples in countries, such as the United States, of separate services for gay men and lesbian women (Mayer *et al.* 2001).

The feminist movement in the United States, United Kingdom, Australia and some other industrialized countries, also developed a strong critique from the 1960s onwards that the health care needs of women were not well served by mainstream health care, and indeed that the patriarchal health care system often contributed to the oppression of women. Broom and Doyal (Chapter 2) explain that although the women's health movements in Australia and Britain struggled against similar patterns of discrimination, they chose to go down different paths. Australian feminists campaigned for a range of women's health programs, including the establishment over the next two decades of about 50 community-based feminist women's health centres, which offered an alternative to mainstream primary health care. The key factors were a vigorous women's movement, a progressive reform climate under a national Labour government, the presence of 'femocrats' working for change within the state, and the fact that primary medical care in Australia is delivered mainly by the private sector.

In contrast, the British women's health movement did not develop alternative feminist services but instead concentrated upon reforming the National Health Service. Given the threats to public sector health care under conservative governments throughout the 1980s, the defence of the NHS became the main priority, while the political climate discouraged social reform. Thus while the claims for special attention to women and the barriers to responsive health care services were the same, the political climate and the institutional structure led to different solutions.

Parallel services

By parallel services, we mean a separate but good quality health care system that exists to cater for certain groups and that substitutes for, rather than complements, mainstream services. A common example in many countries is the high quality and comprehensive health care provided for military personnel. Another example, discussed below, is health services designed specifically to cater for indigenous groups. The danger with separate services, especially if they cater for a stigmatized group, is that they may become a second-rate service, as discussed below in relation to prison services.

Indigenous populations in the United States, Canada, New Zealand and Australia all experience worse health than the general population (particularly Australian Aboriginals) and want more responsive health care services. Three factors converge in these countries that allow formal groups to purchase or provide their own health care: their claims for self-determination, the existence of a private market or quasi-market, and a health care system partly funded through a purchaser-provider split. Individuals are not offered extra money (or vouchers) to buy their own services, rather the funds are distributed to formally constituted groups to buy health care for their members through purchase of service contracts or by directly providing their own services.

The federal governments of both the United States and Canada have devolved funds to tribal governments of Native Americans and to First Nation Canada to provide or else to purchase their own health services through compact or contract. Kunitz (Chapter 16) explains that the United States national government has retained responsibility for health care for Native Americans both as a treaty obligation and in its role as trustee of Indian rights and resources, despite proposals over the years to assimilate funding and delivery into mainstream state health services; increasingly since the 1980s, however, funding and responsibility have been devolved to tribal organizations. The transfer was made primarily on grounds of indigenous self-determination, rather than a better health outcome rationale, and also as part of a central government movement towards devolution. As Kunitz explains, the health data so far do not provide compelling evidence that devolution will necessarily produce better health outcomes, particularly if funds are inadequate and transaction costs are high.

Lavoie (Chapter 17) explains that the Constitution of Canada since 1982 has recognized the rights of indigenous people to self-government, affirms treaty rights and promotes the participation of indigenous people in decisions over issues, such as health care, that directly affect them. The national government increasingly is transferring health funds and responsibilities to First Nation Canada.

In Chapter 15 Crengle *et al.* point out that although the New Zealand government bases policy upon social justice rather than treaty rights, the 1840 Treaty of Waitangi has underpinned Māori claims since the 1970s to control their own health services as well as to convince collective health services to incorporate Māori models of health care. Māori are arguing, however, for the right to community self-determination (*tinorangatiratanga*) in managing their own health care.

American and Canadian Indians and Māori in New Zealand, not being nomadic societies and after organized warfare, were able to extract treaties from the colonizing Europeans that have provided a basis for claims to self-determination. In contrast, Aboriginal Australians in the absence so far of a formal treaty or reconciliation agreement, have made strong claims to self-determination on the grounds that they are the indigenous owners of the country (recognized in the Mabo judgement by the High Court of Australia) but also on grounds of social justice, since their health and socio-economic status compare very poorly to other Australians. Griew *et al.* (Chapter 14) argue that the 1989 National Aboriginal Health Strategy has never been implemented fully and that what is required is self-determination by local Aboriginal groups in managing their own primary health care services. One critique of Aboriginal community-controlled organizations is that thus far they have failed to deliver social and health gains (Tsey 1997). Griew *et al.* point out that the criterion for success demanded of Aboriginal primary health care services in terms of improved population health outcomes ignore the many other societal factors that are stacked against such achievement, and further, are not demanded of other primary health care services, such as general practitioners.

Coyle and Stern (Chapter 7) address the long-standing debate over whether health care in prison is better provided by a specialist prison health care service responsible to the prison authorities or by the mainstream health service that looks after all members of the community. The integrationist model stresses a human rights perspective, arguing that independent medical staff are better able to put the interests of their patients first, that their patients would be more likely to trust them, that infections within prisons (such as HIV/AIDS and tuberculosis) spill over into the community, that people moving in and out of prison need continuity of care, and that an integrated service can attract better medical staff. The contrary pragmatic argument for a parallel service is that the health budget can be ring-fenced, that prison health care is a specialism, and that the prison authorities have to be able to control staff working in the prison.

Many countries place prison health care under the control of prison authorities, such as the former Soviet Union where the penitentiary system was a closed world run by the Minister of Interior. Coyle and Stern examine recent changes in three countries that have reduced the isolation of the prison health services although each pursued different structural strategies. France moved prison health care in 1994 from the Ministry of Justice to the health care system; a formal partnership was set up in England and Wales in the late 1990s between the NHS and the prison authorities; and the Australian state of New

South Wales in 1997 set up a new statutory corporation, the Corrections Health Service. The evidence from all three reforms is that forming links between prisons and the health care system has improved the quality of care, although there have been formidable problems in integrating health and prison perspectives.

The case for and against separate services

Which service delivery model is the most appropriate in terms of access, use and outcomes for particular population groups? The examples in this book demonstrate that the answer depends upon context. The models discussed above can be thought of as falling into two broad categories: separate (participatory, alternative and parallel) and combined (mainstream and integrationist). It should, however, be noted that, in most cases, the claim for separate services generally refers to primary health care and to community-based services, as the capital costs and staffing expertise involved in providing more specialized care make it economically problematic to provide separate facilities. The few exceptions are the comprehensive health services, including hospitals, provided in many countries by the military for their armed forces and also veterans, and the comprehensive services once provided by the Indian Health Service in the United States.

Table 18.3 summarizes the advantages claimed for separate services along with the corresponding disadvantages. Thus an advantage on one side of the ledger sheet can sometimes be interpreted as a disadvantage on the other side.

Separate services allow self-determination, an important goal for some indigenous population groups, although this may undermine social solidarity within the nation. More control over their own health services empowers a particular population group, but such a separation may also allow the state to wash its hands of all responsibility for these services and the funds may be vulnerable

Table 18.3 Advantages and disadvantages of separate services

Advantages	Disadvantages
Self-determination	Undermining of social solidarity
More control	Less state responsibility, vulnerability of funding
Greater consumer choice	More limited choice of scope and scale
Better access for some	Limited availability to whole population group
Greater quality in terms of responsiveness	Possibly worse quality in terms of clinical effectiveness
Better targeted services	Higher cost to state
Higher political profile	Greater stigma

to short-term political fluctuations and budgetary pressures. The existence of separate services offers greater consumer choice, since an individual could choose whether to use alternative or mainstream services, such as a women's community health centre, but a completely parallel system usually is unable to offer health services of wide scope and scale. Separate services can improve access for some people but generally a parallel system is not able to extend access across the whole population group.

Separate services may achieve greater responsiveness to cultural and other expectations, but a separate health care system is unlikely to be able to offer comprehensive services. In the case of secondary care, fragmentation and a lower volume of cases for some conditions and procedures may lead to lower clinical quality and make it difficult to recruit and retain health professionals.

Better targeted services may be cost-effective but overall costs may be higher because of duplication of services. For example, special programmes often are established within the framework of the mainstream health care system in order to target particular groups (such as people with a particular conditions such as HIV/AIDS). Funding and/or service delivery are thus separated from mainstream services. The criticism of such separate vertical funding and/or service delivery programs, pejoratively described as 'silo' services, is that the outcome can be a fragmented and inefficient health care system.

A higher political profile may bring more policy attention, but separate services for an already stigmatized group may invite further discrimination and exclusion from mainstream society. For example, Kovats (Chapter 13) argues that although Roma people are discriminated against by mainstream health services, separate services would only further stigmatize and marginalize. Coker (Chapter 11) also argues that while the needs of refugees are not adequately met within the British National Health Service, setting up special services may further stigmatize refugees and thus mark them out for hostile treatment.

Ultimately, arguments often revert to considerations about the nature of citizenship and nationhood. Where there is a consensus about the unitary nature of the state, with members of different groups seeing themselves and being seen by others as part of a common citizenry, then collective health care is often a means of demonstrating commitment to social solidarity, although such collective care may or may not accept the legitimacy of differences in needs and expectations among different groups. Where special needs are accepted then the system may make special provisions for particular population groups via integrationist or participatory programmes, which remain within the mainstream health system.

The main arguments for collective provision are that, first, alternative services would undermine the national health system, and second, collective services strengthen social solidarity within a society. Population groups who have been marginalized and stigmatized may make a second set of arguments for collective provision that also link to social solidarity. These groups include people with disabilities, who are fighting against being marginalized and who favour policies that promote independence and participation in society, and so want better access to mainstream health care. Other groups who wish to overcome social stigma and so prefer to use mainstream services include migrant groups in most countries, poor people in most countries, and perhaps the Roma people in Europe. The third set of arguments in favour of collective health care involve stigmatized people who are the recipients of substandard parallel services, such as those using prison health services, illustrating the potency of the saying that 'a service for the poor is a poor service' (Titmuss 1968).

In contrast, the main argument in favour of special services arises in groups that do not share this sense of shared nationhood, perhaps viewing themselves as a nation within a nation. In these cases the organization of health care is part of a wider quest for self-determination. Groups that advocate alternative or parallel services do so because they want self-determination and more responsive services. These are groups that exert moral and political power within a country and thus have less cause to fear being marginalized. Further, claims for special services are easier to make in countries with a pluralist health care system that offer structural avenues for obtaining special funding and for establishing special services. Women's groups in Australia exerted such power in the 1980s, but in part given some success in reforming mainstream health care, these claims have been overtaken by other groups. The main claim for special services now is made by indigenous people who wish to control their own culturally responsive health services, and who, as conquered and oppressed peoples, have little reason to embrace social solidarity as defined by their colonizers.

References

Asylum Seekers in Australia (2003) www.zip.com.au/~korman/asylum.html. Accessed 9 March 2003.

Audit Commission (2000) *Another country: implementing dispersal under the immigration and asylum act 1999*. Audit Commission, Oxford.

Australian Bureau of Statistics (1999) *The health and welfare of Australia's Aboriginal and Torres Strait Islanders*. ABS and AIHW, Canberra.

Australian Bureau of Statistics (2000) *Yearbook Australia 2000*. Cat. No. 1301.0.0, Canberra, Australian Bureau of Statistics.

Australian Institute of Health and Welfare (2000) *Australia's health 2000*. Australian Institute of Health and Welfare, Canberra.

Australian Institute of Health and Welfare (2001) *Expenditures on health services for Aboriginal and Torres Strait Islander People 1998–1999*. Commonwealth of Australia, Canberra.

Borowski, A. (2000) Creating a virtuous society: immigration and Australia's policies of multiculturalism. *Journal of Social Policy*, **29** (3), 459–75.

Bowling, A. (1999) Ageism in cardiology. *British Medical Journal*, **319**, 1353–5.

Brock, D. (2001) Discrimination against the elderly within a consequentialist approach to health care resource allocation. In D. N. Weisstub, D. C. Thomasma, S. Gauthier and G. F. Tomossy (eds) *Aging: culture, health, and social change*. Kluwer Academic Publishers, Netherlands.

Carballo, M., Divino, J. J. and Zeric, D. (1998) Migration and health in the European Union. *Tropical Medicine and International Health*, **3** (12), 936–44.

Council for Multicultural Australia Available at www.immi.gov.au/multicultural/cma/.

Deeble, J., Mathers, C., Smith, L., Goss, J., Webb, R. and Smith, V. (1998) *Expenditures on Health Services for Aboriginal and Torres Strait Islander people*. AIHW, DHFS and NCEP, Cat. No. HWE 6. Canberra.

Department of Health (2001) *National service framework for older people*. Available at http://www.doh.gov.uk/nsf/olderpeople.htm. The Stationery Office, London.

European Commission against Racism and Intolerance (2000) *Second report on the United Kingdom*. Council of Europe, Strasbourg.

Eurostat (2002) *Migration keeps the EU population growing*. Eurostat, Brussels.

French, S., Old, A. and Healy, J. (2001) *Health care systems in transition: New Zealand*. European Observatory on Health Care Systems, Copenhagen.

Healy, J. (1998) *Welfare options: delivering social services*. Allen and Unwin, Sydney.

Healy, J. and McKee, M. (2002) Improving performance within the hospital. In M. McKee and J. Healy (eds) *Hospitals in a changing Europe*. Open University Press, Buckingham.

Kliewer, E. and Jones, R. (1998) *Changing patterns of immigrant health and use of medical services: results from the longitudinal survey of immigrants to Australia*. Department of Immigration and Multicultural Affairs, Canberra.

Kummin, J. (1999) Europe: the debate over asylum: an uncertain direction. *Refugees Magazine*, (113) Availabe at www.unhcr.ch

Kymlicka, W. (1995) *Multicultural citizenship: a liberal theory of minority rights*. Clarendon Press, Oxford.

Marmot, M. G. and Wilkinson, R. G. (eds) (1999) *Social determinants of health*. Oxford University Press, Oxford.

Mayer, K., Appelbaum, J., Rogers, T., Lo, W., Bradford, J. and Boswell, S. (2001) The evolution of the Fenway Community Health model. *American Journal of Public Health*, **91**, 892–4.

Minas, I. H. and Sawyer, S. M. (2002) The mental health of immigrant and refugee children and adolescents. *Medical Journal of Australia*, **177** (8), 404–5.

Mossialos, E. and LeGrand, J. (1999) *Health care and cost containment in the European Union*. Ashgate Press, Aldershot.

Oliver, M. (1990) *The politics of disablement*. Macmillan, Basingstoke.

Oliver, M. (1998) Theories in health care and research: theories of disability in health practice and research. *British Medical Journal*, **317** (7170), 1446–50.

Organization for Economic Cooperation and Development (2000) *Reforms for an ageing society: social issues.* Organization for Economic Cooperation and Development, Paris.

Pierce, L. L. (1998) Barriers to access: frustrations of people who use a wheelchair for full-time mobility. *Rehabilitation and Nursing,* **23** (3), 120–5.

Roberts, E. (2000) *Discrimination in health and social care: a briefing note.* King's Fund, London.

Robinson, J. (2002) *Age inequality in health and social care.* Paper presented to the IPPR seminar, 28 January. London, King's Fund.

Saltman, R. B., Figueras, J. and Sakellarides, C. (1998) *Critical challenges for health care reform in Europe.* Open University Press, Buckingham.

Scottish Executive (2000) *Towards an equality strategy.* The Stationery Office, Edinburgh.

Titmuss, R. (1968) *Commitment to welfare.* Pantheon, New York.

Tsey, K. (1997) Aboriginal self-determination, education and health: towards a radical change in attitudes to education. *Australian and New Zealand Journal of Public Health,* **21** (1), 77–83.

Tuder Hart, J. (1971) The inverse care law. *Lancet,* **1,** 405–12.

Turner, N. (1999) Cancer in old age: is it adequately investigated and treated? *British Medical Journal,* **319,** 309–12.

United Nations High Commission for Refugees (2003) Available at www.unhcr.ch, accessed 28 February 2003.

Victora, C. G., Vaughan, J. P., Barros, F. C., Silva, A. C. and Tomasi, E. (2000) Explaining trends in inequities: evidence from Brazilian child health studies. *Lancet,* **356,** 1093–8.

Index